LO

Why did she suddenly feel alarmed? Michael just wanted to talk, what was alarming about that? She joined him on the sofa.

'I'm all ears. What do you want to talk about?' she said lightly.

'About us. About our future.'

'Oh!'

His eyes were on her face. 'You must know how I feel about you?'

'Yes, Michael,' she said softly. 'I feel the same way. I love you.'

'I wonder if you really do.'

'What do you mean by that?'

'Is your love strong enough to put me first?'

'I've already said I love you, isn't that enough?'

'It should be, but with you it might not be ...'

About the author

Nora Kay was born in Northumberland but she and her husband lived for many years in Dundee. They now live in Aberdeen, and have one grown-up son.

She wrote more than forty short stories and a newspaper serial before her first novel, *A Woman of Spirit*, was published in 1994.

Lost Dreams

Nora Kay

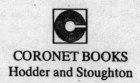

CORONET BOOKS
Hodder and Stoughton

First published in Great Britain in 1996
by Hodder and Stoughton
A division of Hodder Headline PLC
First published in paperback in 1996
by Hodder and Stoughton
A Coronet Paperback

10 9 8 7 6 5

A CIP catalogue record for this title is available from
the British Library.

ISBN 0 340 66999 7

Printed and bound in Great Britain by
Mackays of Chatham plc, Chatham, Kent

Hodder and Stoughton
A division of Hodder Headline PLC
338 Euston Road
London NW1 3BH

For Bill and Raymond

Chapter One

The tea had been served, the best cups and saucers handed round, and hands were eagerly reaching for the sandwiches that seventeen-year-old Laura Morrison had prepared that morning. Some were made with thinly sliced boiled ham from the grocer and some with ox tongue out of a tin she had discovered at the back of a shelf in the cupboard. Her father had used the tin opener to open the tin. After a few false starts when he declared the opener to be useless, it did work and the tongue was eased out and put on a plate. That done, George Morrison removed himself and offered no further assistance.

At the last minute Laura remembered that her aunts liked everything dainty and using a sharp knife she removed the crusts from the bread.

Only when she was in bed did she give way to her tears and then she wept and wept for the loss of her mother. Last night she had tossed and turned with two sodden handkerchiefs under her pillow and sleep seemed just to have claimed her when the alarm went off. Her hand came out of the bedclothes to stifle the sound and with a huge effort Laura forced herself to sit up. A few minutes to come to would have been so very welcome but the risk was too great. She couldn't afford to sleep in, not with all the work she had to get through.

If she had been used to housework it would have been so much easier but her mother had made few demands other than to get her to tidy up her own room, believing as she did that her daughter had quite enough to do with her studies. Now Laura was having to learn and learn fast. Putting on an old overall that had belonged to her mother, she cleaned out the living-room fire and got it going. The fire in the front room was set and just needed a match put to it. She did that right away since the room faced north and took a lot of heating. Laura didn't want any complaints about feeling the cold. With both fires going well she started on the breakfast. The sudden, tragic death of his wife the previous week had left her father shocked, bewildered and grief-stricken but apart from that first awful day when they had all been completely stunned, it hadn't affected his appetite.

Uncle Sam looked at the plate of sandwiches, then raised his eyes to his niece. 'Any with mustard?' he asked.

Laura wondered how anyone could think of mustard at such a time. 'No. Sorry, Uncle Sam, I didn't think, but in any case there is none in the house.'

'That's all right, don't you worry' – as if she was – 'this will do fine, it's just, Laura lass, a wee thing of mustard gives it a bit of taste.' He smiled and she turned away.

Laura, a tall, slim, lovely girl with thick dark blonde hair that fell in soft waves, was paler than usual and there were dark smudges under her blue eyes. Her mother, her darling mother, wouldn't have wanted her to wear black. Her navy blue skirt and jumper would have done. But it didn't do for the aunts who insisted that she must wear black. Too broken-hearted to argue, she had gone to Mathewson's in Cornhill Road and bought a cheap black skirt and black jumper. She wore them with the collar of her white blouse showing at the neck. Her long, shapely legs were in black stockings and her narrow feet in black lacing shoes.

Aunt Peggy took a sandwich, smiled at Laura, then lifted the top to see what was inside. It must have satisfied her and she took a bite.

The house seemed to have taken on the family grief. Without her mother's presence the front room, where they sat, looked dull. As if the life had gone from it just as it had gone from her mother. Laura began to look about her, at the tall oak sideboard with its mirrored back, the long white starched cover that stretched the length and a bit over and in the centre of which was a black marble clock, a wedding gift, that chimed on the half-hour. A Westminster chime, a beautiful sound, but George Morrison had opened the clock, done something to it, and the chime was no more. Laura hadn't seen the sense of it but wisely held her tongue. She rather thought that the suggestion must have come from one of his sisters, she didn't think her father would have troubled otherwise.

The room was very slightly shabby with a comfortable lived-in look though it was seldom used other than on Sundays and when they had visitors. There was a sofa in a tweed mixture of blues and greens and six high-backed chairs in the same material. Over at the window which looked out on the quiet street was a mahogany table with long spindly legs. A plant with a cork mat under it looked dry and in need of watering. The curtains were floral, had plenty of width and brightened the room.

Laura's eyes strayed to her father sitting on the sofa between his sisters, Peggy and Vera. Their husbands, Peggy's Archie and Vera's Sam, sat in armchairs at either side of the fire. The men wore the dark suits and stiff collars they had worn for the funeral and looked as uncomfortable as they felt. Both wondered how soon the real talking would begin and they could get away.

The widower sat with bowed head but raised it to accept a plate on which were two sandwiches, one put there by Peggy and the other by Vera.

George Morrison was good-looking, very tall and in his early forties, and had been served hand and foot all his life. His sisters had been ten and twelve when he was born and just after his sixth birthday their father died. The grandmother immediately gave up her house to go and live with her daughter and the three children and thus it was that George was brought up in a household of women.

In his youth he had gone through a string of girlfriends but only Ellen had captured his heart. Orphaned early in life, Ellen had been brought up by a kindly grandmother. Her only other living relative was a cousin in Canada, and the only contact with her had been a card at Christmas. The romance of George and Ellen was frowned on, George could do better for himself but the truth was that the woman wasn't born who would be good enough for George. But he, despite opposition, had gone ahead and married cheerful, capable Ellen. It was a good, solid marriage, unexciting and without passion, but it suited Ellen and George. He went happily to his job as a minor civil servant, hoping for advancement, and Ellen took charge of everything else including where they would live, and that was at the opposite end of the town to where her in-laws had their homes.

Laura sat down with a cup of tea.

'Laura dear, you haven't taken a sandwich for yourself.'

'I don't want one, Aunt Vera, I don't feel like eating.'

Vera pursed her lips. She was a tall woman, a bit on the hefty side, with a narrow face and a high-coloured complexion. Her sister, Peggy, was smaller and as a girl had been pretty but the prettiness had gone and there was a discontented droop to her mouth. She had, however, kept her figure and dressed well.

'That will not do, Laura, it just won't. You must look after yourself. You owe it to your poor father and young Ronnie, and speaking of the lad, where is he?'

'Next door with Mrs Brand.'

She nodded. 'If I recall correctly she has a lad about the same age?'

'Yes, Ronnie and Alan play together.'

'Poor wee soul, it's going to be hard on Ronnie, he has always been such a mummy's boy. I warned Ellen, warned her often, that he was too timid.' She paused and looked hard at Laura. 'You'll have to be the one to toughen him up, Laura.'

Uncle Archie spluttered over his tea. 'For any favour, Vera, Laura has enough on her plate, she's just a young lass herself.' He beetled his brow, and glowered over at his brother-in-law. 'Time you pulled yourself together, George, and faced up to your responsibilities.'

'I am well aware of my responsibilities, thank you very much,' George said angrily, 'and let me remind you that I have just lost my wife.'

'And Laura has lost her mother.'

Laura got up. Two sandwiches remained on the plate and someone was sure to take them – pity to leave them would be the excuse. Swiftly she picked up the plate and went through to the kitchen. Ronnie might take them with a glass of milk before he went to bed.

All the doors were open and the voices carried clearly.

'College is out of the question but Laura is a sensible lass and she'll realise that.'

'I hope you're right, Vera, but one thing is for sure she is going to be very disappointed.'

'Life is full of disappointments, George,' Vera said briskly, 'Laura has to learn that. None of us has escaped, we've all had our share.' She paused to look at her brother. 'Such a pity we don't live nearer and speaking for myself I would have been only too happy to lend a hand and help Laura but I have my own family to think of.' Her eyebrows shot up as though someone had spoken. 'Yes, I know mine are grown up but with Marie expecting her second and as for Harry, that weak chest of his is a constant worry.' She shook her head as though in despair.

Aunt Peggy nodded gloomily. 'I'm sorry I can't be more supportive but Archie's mother being so poorly I'm having to spend a lot of time with her.' She didn't look at her husband as she said it or she would have seen the sheer disbelief on his face. Only recently his mother had complained to him that she got precious little help from her daughter-in-law. 'And as to college,' Aunt Peggy continued, 'I think we are all agreed that that is a nonsense. A silly idea in the first place and a complete waste, the girl will no doubt be getting married in a year or two. I am not against a good education, far from it, but one should concentrate on the boys. After all they become the breadwinners and the more qualifications they gain the better job they are likely to land.'

'Now you've had your say, do you think I could have mine?' Uncle Archie asked from the depth of the armchair.

'Of course, Archie, don't be silly,' his wife said, shaking her head, 'the whole purpose of this visit is to discuss what is best for George and the family.'

He heaved himself to a more upright position. 'The way I see it, that lass has worked hard to be accepted by the college and the waste would be in not allowing her to take it up.'

Uncle Sam nodded slowly and thoughtfully. 'In happier circumstances I would agree with that, Archie, but these are not happy circumstances.'

'You're making them a deal worse by denying Laura what her mother wanted for her. What's to hinder George getting a woman in for an hour or so each day? I've no doubt Laura would buckle to and do a bit at the weekend and see to what needs to be done in the evening.'

'How like a man to come up with something unworkable,' his wife Peggy said sharply.

'A bit of organising and it could be done.'

'I couldn't afford help in the house,' George said, 'so that is out. You forget, Archie, or perhaps you don't know how expensive it would be to keep Laura at college. There is a lot more than fares to consider.'

Archie's face went a dull red with anger. 'None of it was to come out of your pocket, George, I happen to know that.' He had little time for his brother-in-law but a lot for Laura. 'Ellen, poor lass, had it all worked out. That money she was left was to go on Laura's education, she was adamant about it.'

'What about Ronnie, does he get no consideration?' Vera said in a dangerously quiet voice.

'There would have been no problem about Ronnie. When he was that length, Laura would have finished her studies. In any case the money for the lad's education would have been found somehow.'

'Quite right too,' Peggy came in again, she always had the most to say. 'I'll speak no ill of the dead but to my mind, George, you gave in to Ellen far too much. Too good-natured you are, you should have put your foot down.'

'I would have, but remember it was Ellen's money.'

'Well, it will be yours now and you'll have a better use for it,' she said, sounding smugly satisfied.

'Yes, I've no doubt.'

No one spoke for a little but eyes went to the clock.

'Good! I think that is more or less everything settled,' Peggy said, preparing to get up. 'We should get on our way now but before we do I must draw Laura's attention to that poor plant. Without water she'll lose it.' She shook her head. 'I wonder why young people don't notice these things?'

Chapter Two

Laura stood in the kitchen in rigid silence and listened to her future being discussed. They didn't care that her whole life was in ruins and she was sure that being denied her college place would give her aunts a great deal of satisfaction. Her anger against them and her father was in danger of breaking bounds and Laura had to fight to control herself.

Everything for which she had worked so hard was disappearing, and clutching the back of the chair she closed her eyes and the memories crowded in. So clear was it all that she could recall every word. The present slipped into the past.

Trembling with nervous excitement, she waited for the letter. It must come today, this morning, she was almost sure it would come this morning, and when she heard the rattle of the letterbox Laura dashed to the door. The long brown envelope was on the mat, turned up to show her name. What news was in it? How had she fared? Laura's mouth went dry and her heart began to hammer. Slowly she bent down to pick it up, read her own name and address, checked the postmark and knew she couldn't put it off any longer. Her hand was shaking as she forced herself to open it. The flap came away after a little persuasion and she drew out the single page. The words blurred then cleared and Laura let out a huge sigh, then gave a great whoop of delight.

'Mum! Mum! It's come,' she shouted and ran into the kitchen where her mother was busy at the sink.

'What is it?' Of course she knew and her daughter's face told her the rest.

Laura found she couldn't speak and wordlessly held out the letter.

'Let me get my hands dried before I touch it.' She quickly dried them on a towel, took the letter and began to read it. Her face broke into a broad smile.

13

'Congratulations, Laura, darling. Of course you've got a place, I never doubted but that you would be successful and I'm just so proud of my clever daughter.' She held out her arms and mother and daughter hugged one another. 'A college education is what I dreamed for you and now it is to happen.'

'Thanks to you, Mum,' Laura said quietly, 'you had a fight on your hands, Dad was dead against me staying on at school.'

'That's true, but my dear, you have to make allowances for your father. All his life he has been influenced by those sisters of his. Sour grapes, really, none of theirs had the brains to go on to college.' She smiled and shook her head. 'You owe me nothing,' she said quietly, 'my reward and all I'll ever want is to see you make a success of your life.'

Laura swallowed the lump in her throat. 'Whatever you say I do owe you everything and one day, I promise, I'll make it up to you. No, Mum,' as her mother made to speak, 'let me finish and say what I have to while we are alone!'

Ellen Morrison's brown eyes were soft with love. She was a pleasant-faced woman of medium height with a clear complexion and a smile that lit up her face. She sat down at the kitchen table and poured tea for them both. Laura sat down too and brought the cup in front of her.

'Great-grandma meant that money for you and to be used to make your life easier.'

'I'm perfectly happy with my life.'

Laura ignored the interruption. 'Instead of which it is going towards my education and then, as if you didn't have enough to do, you have been taking in sewing to make extra money.'

'A labour of love.'

'I caused a lot of problems, I do know that. You and Dad were often at loggerheads, he thought that I should have got a job when I was fifteen.'

'That's true enough but your father and your aunts are not alone in their opinion that education, higher education I mean, is wasted on a girl, particularly a lovely girl like you who won't want for admirers.'

'I'm not interested in marriage.'

'Of course you are but you are wise enough not to rush into it. Enjoy your independence, my dear.' She paused to lift her cup and take a drink of tea. 'You are just so lucky that this is nineteen thirty-two and women are not so backward at coming forward.'

Laura giggled. 'Mum, you were never backward.'

'No, and you are a lot like me. As I said, enjoy your time at college and the independence it will give you, then set your sights higher than the young men around here.'

'You do have high hopes for me.'

'I do.'

'What about Ronnie, what are your plans for him?' Ronnie was nine, a quiet, timid boy with no interest in games or sport of any kind but a clever lad who was seldom seen without his nose in a book.

'Ronnie will go on to university.'

'Dad won't object?'

'Oh, no, far from it.'

'Maybe I shouldn't say this, Mum, but Dad doesn't seem to have a lot of time for Ronnie.'

'Only partly true. I didn't give him the son he expected. His son should have loved to kick a ball about, be fond of sport, then they would have had something in common,' She paused. 'Even so, seeing his son top of his class makes him very proud and so it should.'

'I'm glad you fought my corner.'

'I'm a fighter, Laura, and in the end—'

'You usually get your own way,' Laura finished for her.

Her mother went quiet. 'Yes, very often I do get my own way but it isn't an attractive trait in a woman, I have to say that, Laura.' Then she added and sadly, Laura thought, 'In some marriages it is necessary for the woman to lead and take the decisions. The clever wife manages it without it being obvious, I'm not sure if I come into that category.'

'You do, Mum.' They exchanged glances and there was complete understanding.

How long she had been standing there Laura could not have said but at last she opened her eyes and determinedly blotted out the past. She was in no hurry to go back and face them but there was a limit to the time she could remain in the kitchen. Laura took a grip on herself and went through.

'There you are, Laura, I was just about to come through,' Aunt Peggy said with false heartiness. 'Do you want a hand with the dishes before we go?'

'No, thank you, it won't take me long.'

Her thin lips moved into a smile that was meant to be sympathetic and full of understanding. 'Such a sad time and difficult decisions to be made, we have been discussing what would be best—'

'Best for whom, Aunt Peggy?'

Her aunt looked decidedly put out. 'Best for your father, your brother, best for the three of you.'

'Why wait until I was out of the room to discuss my future?'

'You overheard or perhaps you were listening?'

'Since all the doors were open and you weren't exactly whispering I would have had to plug my ears with cotton-wool to keep from hearing.'

Uncle Archie laughed, then smothered it in a cough.

'No call for impertinence, Laura, which is what that is.'

'I'm sure Laura didn't mean it that way,' Uncle Sam said, giving Laura a sharp look. 'Peggy, you should remember that she is just a young lass.'

'Old enough though to take over the running of the house.' Laura sounded bitter and there was an appalled silence.

Aunt Vera broke it. 'That is a terrible attitude to take, Laura, I am deeply disappointed in you and this must be very distressing for your poor father.'

Laura did feel some shame, she shouldn't be so selfish, shouldn't be thinking of herself at a time like this, but they made her so angry and she was almost certain that her mother would have approved of her sticking up for herself and not letting her aunts dictate. What business had they to interfere since they weren't going to put themselves about to help? And as for her dad – she looked over at him with a mixture of affection and exasperation – he was so weak, always taking the easy way out. Without his wife to make the decisions Laura knew that he would once again fall back on his sisters.

There was an uncomfortable silence as they got their coats and prepared to depart but before reaching the door Uncle Archie gripped her arm and said softly and apologetically, 'Sorry, lass, I did my best.'

'I know you did and thanks.'

'Don't give up, maybe there is a way,' he said, but in a voice that gave little hope.

Aunt Peggy, putting up the collar of her coat, turned back to speak to Laura. 'You could give that plant at the window some water, it badly needs it.'

'Yes.'

'Take it to the sink, give it a good soak and be sure there is no water left in the bottom of the pot.' She smiled. 'Plants don't like their feet wet, Mother used to say that.'

'That goes for the rest of us too,' Uncle Sam said as he shrugged himself into his overcoat. He waited for the others to laugh, no one did.

George stood at the front door to see them off.

'George,' his sister gave him a peck on the cheek, 'try and get a good night's sleep and we'll be in touch.'

Vera gave him a hug. 'Always remember, George, you have us.'

Laura stood well back. The door was shut and she breathed a sigh of relief.

'Dad, I'll go round for Ronnie.'

'Yes, you had better, and Laura —'

'What?'

'You'll need to put out my navy suit and a clean shirt, a white one. I could have done with another day or two, so much to see to, but this is all I'm allowed.'

'Better working, Dad, keep your mind off things.'

He sighed and loosened his tie. 'Yes, that's the general idea, isn't it? My black shoes, Laura, put black shoe polish on them before you go to bed then polish them in the morning with a brush and then a polishing cloth. Your mother always did that.'

'I'll get Ronnie,' she mumbled as she went through the kitchen and out the back door.

Mrs Brand opened the door to her knock. She was a good-natured woman in her late thirties with a sweet face and small eyes that disappeared when she laughed which was often.

'Come in, Laura. If your face is anything to go by it was awful,' she said, leading the way into the living-room and all but pushing Laura into a chair. 'The pair of them are in Alan's bedroom playing Snakes and Ladders or Ludo, quite happy anyway, so if you want to talk, then talk. Bert won't be in for an hour yet. I'm not going to ask—'

'Mrs Brand, have you ever felt like murder and that's a terrible thing to say with my mum just—' Her voice broke but she swallowed hard. She'd wept into her pillow every night since her mother died and tonight would be no exception. Until then, however, she would stay dry eyed.

'Often. Some folk should have been drowned at birth and those two aunts of yours among them. Many's the time your mother has come in here after they'd been and not known whether to laugh or cry.'

'Mrs Brand, I'm having to give up my college place,' Laura said quietly.

'No!' She looked shocked.

'Yes, I'm to stay at home and keep house for Dad and Ronnie.'

Mrs Brand had been standing but she sat down abruptly. 'That's a crying shame and the last thing your mother would have wanted.'

'Dad says he can't afford to get anyone in but I know we could manage if he would do his bit.'

'Not often I didn't agree with your mother, Laura, but I have to say she ruined your father. Bert doesn't consider himself hen-pecked but he does see to the fire and getting in the coal and he's not above doing other jobs when it's necessary.' She warmed to her subject. 'Start as you mean to finish. Don't just do things because your mother did. Take my advice and let your father clean his own shoes, Ronnie's too for that matter.'

Laura gave a mirthless laugh. 'Some hope. I've already got my instructions even to how he likes his shoes cleaned and polished.'

'Once you start something it's difficult to stop.'

'Suppose you're right,' Laura said gloomily but seeing no way out of it.

'It shouldn't be impossible for you to go to college, you've worked hard and that should count for something.'

'Not with my father,' Laura said bitterly, 'he couldn't care less about college, as far as he is concerned higher education is for boys but not for their sisters.'

'If it would help Ronnie could stay here until you got home.'

'Thanks, Mrs Brand, you're a gem, Mum always said so, but I'm afraid college is out.' Her voice faltered. 'Uncle Archie did his best for me but his was just a lone voice.'

'Nice to have someone on your side even though it doesn't do any good.'

After seeing Laura and Ronnie out, Mrs Brand was thoughtful. Ellen Morrison's death had greatly upset her, particularly as she believed it could have been prevented. Always so concerned about her family's health but careless about her own. She had got caught in a deluge and been soaked to the skin but instead of immediately changing out of wet clothes she had prepared the meal rather than have it late. A few days in bed and she might have fought off the chill that followed but she wouldn't give in and had paid the price. Now there were two motherless children and their father who wouldn't be much help.

She had to smile remembering her own weakness. George Morrison could make her own heart quicken and her colour would rise when he smiled at her across the hedge that separated the houses. She didn't see Laura's father being alone very long. Selfish and impossible he might be, indeed he was, but few women could resist a handsome face, his brand of charm, and that beautifully modulated voice that made her for one go weak at the knees.

Having these thoughts, Joan Brand occasionally felt guilty and sometimes wondered what plain, ordinary Bert would think if he could read her thoughts and her longings, but then maybe plain, ordinary Bert had his own dreams, his secret desires, and provided they were hidden from each other and kept that way where was the harm?

The marriage of George and Ellen had surprised a great many women. What had he seen in her, they asked each other. She wasn't even pretty, attractive perhaps but no more than that. No one could see it lasting, two maybe three years they gave it but they had been proved wrong. George, as far as anyone knew, had never looked seriously at another woman. Joan Brand was of the opinion that George liked to be mothered and Ellen had excelled in that role.

As to Laura she had come out of it very well. She had her father to thank for her good looks and her mother for her nice nature.

Miltonsands, where the Morrisons lived, was a small, attractive seaside resort on the east coast of Scotland with a good golf course that brought in the visitors. Men in plus-fours were a common sight in Miltonsands and the miles of safe sandy beach made it popular with families. Hotels and boarding-houses were booked up for most of the summer months and those who had a room to spare and the need of a little extra money took in those who couldn't pay the higher prices. Most of the shops were on the High Street which stretched the length of Miltonsands and all made enough in the summer to make up for the dearth of visitors in the winter.

Home for the Morrisons was 9 Fairfield Street which was a street of terraced houses. They had all been built to the same design. Two rooms downstairs with a good-sized kitchen off the living-room which held a table and chairs, and in the Morrison household breakfast was taken there as well as cups of tea. Main meals were served in the living-room. The front room was square-shaped with a double window and used only on Sundays and when there were visitors. Upstairs consisted of three bedrooms and a bathroom. The bathroom had a white bath with clawed feet and linoleum on the floor. The largest bedroom which wasn't large at all held a double bed, a wardrobe, a small dressing-table and one chair – someone had to sit on the bed. The other two had a tight squeeze to fit in a single bed, a single wardrobe and a small chair.

The wind howled, it was bitterly cold, and Laura hurried her young brother from one back door to the other. Before she could turn the knob to get them inside, Ronnie had clutched at her arm and Laura turned in surprise.

'What is it? What's the matter?' She saw his white, strained face.

'You won't go away and leave me, will you?' he whispered fearfully.

'Why would I do that? What made you ask such a thing?' Laura said, shaken at his obvious distress.

'I'm frightened, Laura. Why did Mum have to go and die?' His brown eyes, his mother's eyes, were wide and anxious.

She hugged him, thinking how little and frail he was. 'I don't know, Ronnie,' she said gently.

'She wouldn't have wanted to go away and leave us?'

'I'm sure she wouldn't but God must have decided He wanted her in heaven.'

'He won't want you, will He?'

'Not for a very long time.'

'Promise me,' his fingers dug into her arms with all the desperation of a nine-year-old boy needing reassurance, 'that you won't leave me.

Ever! Ever! Ever!' His voice was rising hysterically.

Laura eased away his fingers. 'You'll have me black and blue.' She bent down. 'Listen, Ronnie, I said I wouldn't leave you and I meant it.' She pushed him in and closed the door behind them.

'You promise? Promise, Laura, and I'll know you'll have to mean it.'

Her words hadn't been enough, she had to use the word promise and perhaps she could understand that. There was something more lasting and binding about it. She would put his mind at ease. 'Ronnie, I give you my solemn promise that I won't leave you and in return I want you to promise me something.'

'What?'

'That you'll do little things to help me.'

He nodded. 'Like carrying the dishes through to the kitchen?'

'Yes, like that.'

'You'll be here when I get home from school? You'll stay in the house like Mum did?'

'Yes,' she said dully, 'that's what I'll be doing, staying in the house like Mum did.'

She saw his relief and he gave her the beginning of a smile.

George Morrison had come into the kitchen then turned back into the living-room and they followed him.

'You've taken your time,' he said irritably, 'surely you could have saved your gossiping for another time.'

'I wouldn't describe it as gossiping.'

'Ronnie, you get to bed, you need your sleep if you are going to school in the morning.'

'Am I, Laura?'

'Yes, but don't go up just yet. It's not that late, Dad, let him stay down for a little while.'

'Do what you like, I'm having an early night. I've had all I can take for one day so I'll say goodnight. Remember to lock up, Laura.'

'Yes.'

He went upstairs and Ronnie followed Laura back into the kitchen.

'Saved you a couple of sandwiches, so go and sit down. I'll pour you a cup of milk.'

'Alan's mum gave me something to eat.'

'Then you won't want—'

'I'm still a little bit hungry, I'll eat them.'

'Good! Then it's off to bed for you. I'll come up later and put out your school clothes.'

'When will you get to bed?'

'I won't be too long, I have some jobs to do.' She looked at the dishes piled up beside the sink. She could have washed and her father dried only it would never have occurred to him. Fleetingly she thought of leaving them until morning, then dismissed that idea, it could be the beginning of a bad habit. She would do them, then see to her father's and Ronnie's shoes. Perhaps she should be taking Mrs Brand's advice but she wouldn't, not this time anyway. She could see herself doing all the jobs her mother had done because if she refused there would be unpleasant scenes and, perish the thought, the aunts might come rushing over.

Laura was tired, desperately tired, but she forced herself to go on. It had been a long, long day but she doubted if she would sleep when she did get to bed. She washed, dried and put away the dishes, put black boot polish on both pairs of shoes – she would have to get another tin, it was almost finished – then set the table for breakfast. The clock showed it to be quarter past eleven, not as late as she'd thought. The tiredness had passed, she'd gone beyond it and now Laura felt fully awake. Sufficiently wide awake to want to be outside in the cold night air, perhaps go for a brisk walk. An absurd notion but then she wasn't herself and nothing was making sense.

Her new duties. Check the doors, back and front, and the windows, she did that and after a last look about her, Laura went upstairs. Opening Ronnie's bedroom door, she tiptoed in. He was out to the world, his breathing regular, and one arm was on top of the quilt. Going to the wardrobe, Laura took out his grey shorts, put them on the chair and his blazer over the back of it. From the drawer she took out clean underwear, a grey shirt, a school tie and a pair of stockings. Then she rescued the elastic bands from his other stockings and gathered up what was meant for the wash. No need to go downstairs, she would leave them outside the door and take them away in the morning. A clean handkerchief, she had forgotten that. She went back and put one in his trouser pocket and one in his blazer pocket. And while she was there she had another look at her sleeping brother. No matter how dreadful it was for her, she had to remember that she had enjoyed her mother's loving care for seventeen years. Poor Ronnie was only nine and desperately afraid and uncertain, it was in his eyes, the way they followed her around. If only there had been a stronger bond between father and son it would have gone a long way to help, to ease the pain of loss, but as her aunt had said and in this case rightly, Ronnie had always been a mummy's boy. It made it all the harder for him and for her too.

As for herself she had to accept the inevitable and for a start she would take a leaf out of her mother's book and get herself organised. Ronnie's welfare would always come first, her mind was made up about that. Her mother would expect it of her and it was what she wanted to do. She hoped it was what she wanted to do.

The alarm wakened her and Laura sat up. No Mum to come up and waken her gently, those days were just a memory. She was in charge and her father and Ronnie were depending on her. After a quick wash, Laura dressed, collected the washing from outside Ronnie's door and hurried downstairs. The fire had been drossed up and there was still a faint glow and a little warmth coming from it. She was saved from going up and wakening her father, she could hear him moving around. Ten minutes later he appeared in his office suit looking smart and every inch the civil servant. He mumbled something and sat down at the table.

'Good morning, Dad, did you sleep?'

'Off and on.'

'Want a boiled egg or I'll scramble one for you if you like?'

'No, toast will do, is that it under the grill?'

'Yes.' She drew out the grill, a minute earlier would have been better but apart from a grimace he made no mention that the toast was overdone. She poured out his tea and went back to the cooker to stir the porridge. Her father didn't like porridge but Ronnie did and she would have a plate herself.

'Time Ronnie was up.'

'Yes, I'll go and waken him.' She lowered the gas under the porridge pot and dashed upstairs. He was still asleep but this was no time for gentle treatment. 'Come on, Ronnie, time to get up.' She shook him and pulled down the bedclothes.

'I'm tired, five more minutes,' he protested and made to haul up the bedclothes.

23

'No you don't, and I'm not leaving here until you have both feet on the floor.'

That struck him as funny and she was glad to see a smile on his face. 'All right, I'm up.'

Laura whipped the clothes right off the bed in case he was tempted to get back. 'A good wash, remember, and don't forget your neck and behind your ears.' She ran downstairs.

Her father had got up from the table and she saw that he had taken only one piece of toast.

'Dad, that'll never see you through the morning,' she said worriedly.

'It'll do, I'll buy something and eat it in the office.'

Laura remembered then that there was a shop nearby where the staff could buy buttered rolls and pastries. She stopped worrying, shouted cheerio when he said he was going and with Ronnie arrived they sat down together to a plate of porridge. Ronnie liked plenty of sugar on his and a liberal amount of milk. Laura, when younger, had liked sugar with hers but not now.

The important thing, she decided, was to keep as near as possible to what had been her mother's routine. Tea with a cookie or biscuit had always been ready for them when they got home from school. When Ronnie came in she saw by his face that he was pleased and just as he always had done he put his schoolbag on the floor behind the door, his blazer on the back of a chair and went to wash his hands at the kitchen sink. Sitting down at the table, he ate his cookie and jam and began to tell Laura about his day at school.

'Laura, it was strange, everybody was looking at me but it was nice. They were all sad about Mum and Miss Campbell asked me if I was all right and patted me on the shoulder. Can I have another cookie and strawberry jam, please?'

'May I, and it'll put you off your proper tea.'

'No, it won't.'

She smiled. 'This once, and go easy on the jam.'

'When it's finished you'll have to make more.'

'No, we'll have to buy it and that's expensive. I don't know how to make jam.'

'You could learn though, couldn't you?'

'I suppose so.' Laura's first big shopping had surprised her and she was alarmed at how much everything cost. What she hadn't been prepared for were the extras like boot polish, Brasso and soap. It wasn't just food. This was something she could do, she could make a list of household expenses and see where she could make savings.

Thank goodness she didn't have to provide a midday meal for her father, he got his in the canteen or dining-room as some of the civil servants called it. For a modest sum they were served with a good meal which was cooked on the premises. It was far superior to what could be had elsewhere at the price and a whole lot better than taking sandwiches.

The evening meal was over. Mince, potatoes and peas followed by stewed apples with custard. The custard was lumpy even though she was sure she had stirred it non-stop. She waited for the complaints, none came. George Morrison pushed back his chair and went through to the living-room and was soon behind his newspaper with his feet on the leather pouffe.

Ronnie, remembering his promise, began carrying through the dishes, one plate at a time until Laura showed him how to pile them up and put all the cutlery together. That finished, he looked up.

'Will that do or do I have to do something else?'

She smiled. 'No, that was a big help and if you've homework to do go and get it done.'

'Not much and it's easy. I got a comic to read from Charlie Adams and he wants it back in the morning.'

'Lessons first then your comic,' Laura said severely but she didn't have to tell him that. Ronnie would do what was required and quickly.

'Not in your bedroom,' she said as he was preparing to go up. 'It's too cold.'

'No, Laura, it isn't, I'll take off my shoes and go under the quilt.'

She nodded. There were things she wanted to discuss with her father and Ronnie was better upstairs and out of earshot.

Chapter Three

Laura went through to the sitting-room, stood for a moment undecided, then sat down in the armchair that had been her mother's. As she did her father looked up briefly before lowering his eyes once again to the newspaper. The fire was low, in need of attention, but she ignored it for the time being. Soon the weather would be warm enough to do without a fire until the evening.

'Dad?'

'Mmmm.'

'Please put the paper down, we need to talk.'

'Can't it wait? You know I like this time to relax with the news. I work hard all day, you know,' he ended peevishly.

You aren't the only one, she thought, then anger spurred her on. 'No, this won't wait, and like you I've had a hard day and unlike you mine won't end until I go to bed.'

To show his annoyance he dropped the paper to the floor. 'If this is about money you should manage with what I give you.'

'It's not that, I need to know where I stand.'

'Obvious, I would have thought. In your mother's place, I believed you understood that.'

'That won't do,' she said, shaking her head, 'that won't do at all.' Taking a deep breath she added, 'I need something for myself —'

'An increase in your pocket money?' he smiled.

'No, an allowance for my own personal use.'

'Don't be ridiculous.'

'I'm not. Had I left school at fifteen as you wanted I would have been earning a wage.'

'My dear Laura, you have a lot to learn. Once you pay the rent, food, coal, etc. the rest is yours to buy clothes for Ronnie and yourself. The more efficient you become the more there will be left over.'

'No, Dad,' Laura said firmly, 'that works between husband and wife but I am not prepared to stay at home under those conditions.'

'What exactly are you asking?'

'I need some independence and what I propose is to list all the expenses so that you can see where the money goes. As to my allowance, that remains separate and in no circumstances do I dip into it for extra housekeeping.'

He blinked rapidly. 'Words fail me and if your mother could hear you what she would have to say I just cannot begin to imagine.'

'I can, she would be in favour.'

'You have a hard streak in you, Laura. Your Aunt Peggy always said so.'

'Spare me the aunts,' Laura said furiously, 'those two have far too much to say about what is none of their business.'

'All they do is try to be helpful,' he said stiffly.

'Helpful,' she said scornfully, 'what help have we had? Advice, yes, plenty of that. Advice we could do well without.'

'This conversation ends here and now.'

'Just as soon as we agree on a fair allowance for me.'

The sum eventually agreed on wasn't much but at least it was hers. She would have no guilt feelings about putting it into the bank and what was left from the housekeeping would be put aside for clothes for Ronnie. She had to think and plan for Ronnie and herself, for who could tell what another year would bring?

The small victory was hers, or perhaps not so small, and now was the time to apologise.

'I'm sorry, Dad, if I lost my temper.'

The apology surprised and pleased him. 'We'll say no more about it, Laura, we are both under a lot of strain.' He hesitated before adding, 'You have your life to lead and I have mine.'

'Yes.' She wondered what was coming.

'You must get out and see your friends and I must make some effort too.'

'Good idea, but we have to arrange it so that there is someone with Ronnie.'

His brow beetled in annoyance. 'Don't baby him the way your mother did, let him do a bit more for himself and that way you should manage a part-time job.'

'Such as?'

'I don't know, but I imagine shops quite often need assistants for a few hours daily.'

She didn't answer.

Stepping out into the warm sunshine, Laura closed the door and noticed that the knob and letterbox could do with a polish. She promised herself that she would get out the Brasso tin and see to it once she was home and the shopping away.

March had been cold, as cold as in the depths of winter, and that had been followed by an unsettled April with frequent showers of hail then bright sunshine. Here on the first Saturday of May the sun shone from a cloudless sky and Laura felt carefree and happy. How lovely it was to discard thick jumpers and warm skirts, and she congratulated herself that she had had the foresight to wash and iron her summer dresses ready for just such a day as this. In her pink and white cotton dress with its full skirt and narrow belt that accentuated her neat waist, Laura felt both cool and pretty. Over it she wore a fine-knit white cardigan with pearl buttons which were undone. Her long legs were bare and too white but she hoped that the sun would soon change that. Being fair-skinned she usually managed to get a nice tan. Her feet were in sandals that were shabby after having been worn all the previous summer and over her arm was a shopping bag. It held her purse that had been her mother's. A large purse with divisions and in which she kept the house-keeping money.

Her father was in bed, Laura had left him there, his excuse being that there was nothing for him to do and he was better there than getting under her feet. Nothing to do! Laura thought of all the jobs needing to be done but she was learning to swallow her resentment and bite back the words she longed to say. Was he totally blind as well as deaf, she wondered, or just not interested? Life wasn't easy for him and she did try to be fair but didn't he understand that it wasn't easy for her or for Ronnie? Worse for Ronnie, he missed his mother desperately and was clinging more to his sister than he should. It infuriated George Morrison.

'For God's sake, he's not a baby, stop treating him as one,' he'd said on more than one occasion.

'I try not to, but can't you see how lost and bewildered he is and try and make allowances? And you're one to speak. How much have you done to help since Mum died?' And then the rows and the sulky silences and, she had to smile, the cause of it all trying to restore harmony.

If only she could learn to organise her days then she would get through more but she seemed to work back on herself, jumping from one job to another and none of them getting done properly. Perhaps if her mother hadn't been so super-efficient in everything she did, including being good with a hammer and nails, she wouldn't feel so inadequate.

Laura accepted that she wasn't a good housekeeper because her heart wasn't in it. How could it be when hardly a day went by without her thinking of what might have been? She was ashamed of herself because she was sick with envy when she met her friends and had started to avoid them.

She and her father had never been close but until recently she had had an affection for him and made allowances for the grown-up child he was. Now she was fighting not to show her contempt. Other men did jobs about the house and could be seen in the garden at weekends and other times, cutting the grass and tidying up. Not George Morrison, he could be knee-deep in weeds and not notice. Weeds were a problem, her mother used to make a joke about them saying she only had to turn her back and a weed would re-appear. Laura thought she just had to turn her back and there was a whole army of them waiting to be pulled out. Remembering how the garden had looked when her mother was alive, the pride she had taken in it, Laura could have wept.

Since he and Alan were going to watch a school game, Ronnie had been up sharp and he and Laura were about to sit down to breakfast together.

'Before you start, Ronnie, take a cup of tea up to Dad.'

'Why not make his breakfast, Laura, he would rather have that and I'll take it up? I'll be careful.'

'No, he can come down for it.'

The brown eyes were pleading. 'It would put him in a good mood.'

'No, Ronnie.' She handed him a cup and saucer and two Abernethy biscuits. She didn't want her brother to think her hard-hearted but she wasn't going to relent. 'If Dad was ill I'd be only too willing to take up his meals but he isn't and he didn't do this when Mum was alive.'

Ronnie thought breakfast in bed was a small price to pay to keep his dad happy but when Laura had that tight-lipped expression it was a waste of time to try and get her to change her mind.

Opening the door, she watched Ronnie slowly and carefully go up the stairs. She was about to turn away when she remembered the bedroom door would be shut and quickly went up ahead of him to open it, then flew down again.

Sometimes Laura worried about herself, about the kind of person she was becoming, and there were times when she scarcely recognised herself. Once she had been a happy, carefree seventeen-year-old and now at eighteen she felt that all the cares of the world were on her shoulders. To Laura in her narrow world her days consisted of boring, repetitive jobs. Shopping, washing, ironing, mending and in between trying to keep the garden tidy. Cooking wasn't so bad, she quite liked it. As for her social life it was virtually non-existent, with just an occasional visit to the cinema. Not so her father who was out most evenings, with one evening devoted to visiting his sisters, Peggy one week, Vera the next. He went straight from work and each had an appetising meal awaiting him. Laura was happy about that, it gave her a rest from cooking and to the delight of Ronnie they had fish and chips from the Italian's.

Visits from Aunt Peggy and Aunt Vera were few and far between, they much preferred that their brother visit them. At least he was assured of a good, well-cooked meal was what they said to each other, and from what they gathered life at 9 Fairfield Street left much to be desired.

'Laura! Laura!'

Day-dreaming as usual – she was very guilty of it these days – the sound of her own name made her start and swing round. Her face broke into a delighted smile. 'Michael Grayson,' she said, stopping in the street, 'where did you spring from?'

'Just got back home a few days ago—' He broke off and looked uncomfortable. 'Never got the chance to say how very sorry I was – it must have been terrible for you?'

The sympathy in his eyes, in his voice, brought it all back and Laura nodded, unable for the moment to speak.

Michael saw that her eyes were bright with unshed tears and gave her time to recover.

'Thanks, I'm all right now, we're beginning to come to terms with it but as you say it was awful,' she said with a catch in her voice.

'Heard too that you're missing out on college. None of my business but I would have thought something could have been worked out.'

'Something could,' Laura said bitterly, 'but if you remember my dad was never in favour of me going,' She tried to laugh. 'Enough about my troubles, what about you? Tell me how life is treating you.'

'Can't complain, Laura, life is pretty good and the hard work has paid off. I got through the exams, or struggled might be nearer the truth.'

'Nonsense, I bet you sailed through the lot. Does that make you a fully qualified civil engineer?' she asked.

He nodded. 'I'm doing an extra qualification but at least I'm earning while I'm studying and it doesn't come so hard on the parents.'

Although over two years older than Laura, they had been school-friends and she had been thrilled when Michael began to wait for her and they walked to school together. It was a nice feeling to be the envy of her friends and class-mates who had to be content with boys from the same year.

Michael was a nice-looking boy and one of the tallest in his year, just as Laura had been almost a head taller than the others in her year. As they talked she began to study him and note the changes. The extreme thinness that had made him look gangling had gone. Now there was breadth to his shoulders and he held himself well. His grey eyes were just as honest and direct as she remembered and the dark brown hair still flopped over his forehead.

She was under scrutiny too and couldn't fail to see the admiration in his eyes.

'You were always pretty but more so now I think.'

'Thanks,' she said, trying to accept the compliment gracefully but only succeeding in looking embarrassed. She looked down at her scuffed sandals.

'Still go about with the same crowd?'

She shook her head. 'Very seldom see any of them.'

'But surely—'

'My own fault, Michael, not theirs. You see, I feel out of it, we no longer have much in common. All they talk about, and naturally enough, is college and I can't join in.' She stopped. 'You can't understand that, can you?'

'On the contrary, I can understand it very well. Since coming back to Miltonsands I've met up with a few of the school crowd, we chatted for a while but after we'd each said what we were doing there didn't seem to be anything left to say.'

She smiled. She wasn't sure whether to believe him or not.

'Laura, I wish I didn't have to but I've simply got to dash.'

'Of course, it's been—'

'But not before we make a date. I know you are head cook and bottle washer—'

'And a hundred things besides,' she laughed, feeling more like the old Laura.

'Which evening suits you, or better still if you've nothing fixed for tonight how about us going dancing at the Pavilion?'

'Michael, there is nothing I'd like better but I just don't know. Dad goes out most Saturday evenings—'

'That doesn't stop you going out, surely?'

'There's Ronnie.'

'Forgot about your young brother, how old is he?'

'Nearly ten.'

'Couldn't he stay with one of his friends until your dad gets home?'

'Alan goes out with his parents on a Saturday night and I don't know anyone else he could stay with.'

He looked at her strangely. 'You do want to come out with me?'

She looked hurt. 'Very much so. I'll try, Michael, be sure of that, but I can't promise.'

'That'll have to do then.' He was looking at his watch and starting to walk away. 'I'll come for you about eight and hopefully you'll be ready, if not' – he shrugged – 'I'll just have to go along on my own.'

Laura didn't want that, in fact it was the last thing she wanted. Michael had come back into her life and she didn't want to spend the evening thinking about those other girls in Michael's arms. She watched him striding away, unaware that she was smiling. Then she remembered the real purpose of this outing, glanced at the silver watch that had belonged to her mother and gave a start. Where had the time gone? Here she was with an empty shopping bag and if she didn't look smart and get herself to the baker's the bread would be sold out. One had to be early on a Saturday.

Once George Morrison heard the door closing behind Laura he got up and not bothering to put a dressing-gown over his pyjamas, went downstairs and into the kitchen. The breakfast dishes were stacked beside the sink and the teapot was under the knitted tea-cosy. George got himself a clean cup and saucer and carried them to the table. Opening the door of the larder, he saw that, on the marble slab, was the blue and white jug half filled with milk, a plate with butter and a bowl of brown eggs. He could boil himself an egg, three minutes it took if he remembered correctly. The matter received his consideration but in the end he decided he couldn't be bothered. A couple of slices of bread and butter would keep him going until one o'clock. That was when they had their main meal on a Saturday and Sunday and Laura was becoming quite a good cook, he would give her that.

George buttered the bread, poured the tea which was neither hot nor cold but drinkable, and stood while he ate and drank. That over and feeling only marginally better for it, he put the cup, saucer and plate together with the knife and spoon with the other dirty dishes and went into the living-room to see if the paper had come. It was always later on a Saturday, the paper-boy very likely had an extra hour in bed. That made him think about Ronnie, what was to hinder the lad doing a delivery round? It could be a paper round or delivering groceries after school.

The newspaper was on the chair, untouched as he insisted it should remain until he'd read it. Paper in hand, he climbed the stairs and got himself into bed. The extra pillow went behind his head and as usual he turned to the sports page. The news could wait. As he turned the page his hand all but overbalanced the cup on the bedside table and he righted it. Pity he hadn't remembered to take the cup and saucer down with him but Laura could see to that when she came up to make the bed and tidy the room.

These days Laura was often in his thoughts chiefly because she was turning out to be such a disappointment. With her intelligence he had supposed that looking after the house and garden as Ellen had done would have been child's play, instead of which she seemed to be forever in a muddle, and as for his shirts she didn't make a good job of them, none of the collars sat the way they should. His sister was right, when was she ever wrong? Dependable, was Peggy. Ellen should have made Laura do a bit more about the house then she would have been better prepared when she was landed with it. His face darkened in anger. What a nerve she had to suggest that he should be giving her a hand. Didn't she realise how exhausted and drained he was after a day at the office? It was well known, though it had escaped her, that brainwork took a lot more out of one than manual labour. The girl had a lot to learn. For heaven's sake, the weekend should be a time for relaxing and surely it wasn't asking too much to have his breakfast in bed on a Saturday. But no, his daughter wasn't going to oblige and he didn't have to search for a reason. This was her way of paying him back for depriving her of a college education. A pulse in his temple throbbed. Didn't she ever think of anyone but herself? Ronnie got some consideration, far too much by his way of thinking, but as for himself he got none. What an incredibly selfish daughter he had.

Irritably he looked at the sports page and that did nothing to cheer him. Dundee, the football team he followed, had put up a poor show. Pathetic, according to the football news, and there was no excuse for it. They were capable of better and if they weren't careful they would be losing supporters, himself included. Nothing was going right for him either, he thought, and that was more to the point. In disgust he thrust the newspaper aside and began to think about his situation. Six months had gone by since Ellen's death. The pain of loss was less now and there were whole days when he didn't think about her and when he did it was usually in connection with his creature comforts or rather the lack of them.

Looking back, George decided that his marriage had been comfortable. Yes, that was the word. It had been happy too because both Ellen and he had got from it what they wanted. He could see that now and accept that Ellen had mothered him and that he had enjoyed being fussed over. And as for Ellen she had been perfectly content in that role.

He accepted that his life was beginning to change. The quiet sympathy from friends and colleagues was less now. The sympathy was still there but now invitations were coming his way and his male

35

colleagues, who felt they had done their bit, were encouraging him to accept. It amused and secretly pleased him that so many of the unattached females were finding an extra ticket for a show or function. Perhaps he should start to accept instead of refusing as he had up to now. After all, as he was being constantly reminded, one couldn't mourn forever, life must go on.

Certainly life at home held very little for him. His son and daughter had not turned out as he hoped, in fact if he was going to be completely truthful, they were a big disappointment. Why couldn't he have been blessed with a son more like himself, fond of sport and with a bit of life in him? And Laura had him to thank for her good appearance. Ellen had been pleased about that, saying that it was so much more important for a girl. Ronnie would be very ordinary, like his mother had been, but according to Ellen that wouldn't matter. He had a good brain and one day would hold down a well-paid job, she had said proudly.

Putting his hands behind his head, George stared at the ceiling. He was restless and desperate to make a fresh start, to escape from the responsibility of home and family. His heart ached for freedom and he thought longingly of distant shores, Canada or America or anywhere for that matter, just provided it was far away from Miltonsands. He sighed. Just dreams that faded in the light of another dreary day.

Chapter Four

When Laura returned from the shops with a bulging bag there was a smile on her lips and for the first time in a long while she felt happy. Somehow between meeting Michael and getting home she had managed to convince herself that her dad would stay in with Ronnie. How could he refuse when she went out so seldom and he was rarely in? She didn't know where he went, he never said and she never asked. Laura just supposed he had a drink with his colleagues and since she had never known her father to be the worse for drink she had no worries on that score.

Humming happily, she put away the groceries and the large loaf of bread in the bread-bin. It had been the last but one on the shelf in the baker's. That job done, she got out an apron from the drawer in the kitchen and tied it round her waist.

There was plenty of hot water and Laura began on the dishes, noticing as she did that at some stage her father must have come downstairs. An extra cup and saucer had been added to the pile but the white one she'd sent up with Ronnie was missing. Normally that would have annoyed her, that he hadn't troubled to bring it down, but this morning nothing was important enough to irritate her.

She heard him walking about so at least he was up, and fifteen minutes later her father appeared looking smart and fresh. He wore the light grey flannels she had collected from the cleaners the previous day with a fresh shirt, a blue striped one. The top button was undone. Under his arm was the morning paper and in his hand a cup and saucer which he handed to her.

She smiled. 'Thanks,' she said, surprised.

'Did you remember my cigarettes?'

'Yes, on the sideboard.' She didn't think his cigarettes should come out of the housekeeping but he did.

'Where's Ronnie?'

'Told you last night, Dad, that he was going with Alan to see the school team playing.'

'You may have, don't recall, but no doubt I would have paid more attention had he been playing instead of watching.'

'He can't help not being good at sport and I bet many parents would rather their son was clever academically like Ronnie instead of having brains in their feet.'

He laughed and she joined in. It was important to keep him in a good humour and the offer of tea might help.

'Want a cup of tea, Dad?'

'Wouldn't mind.' He went through to the living-room.

Laura had the potatoes peeled and in the pot and the vegetables prepared. She dried her hands, filled the kettle, lit the gas, put the kettle on the ring and took a deep breath. Now was the time. She went through.

'Dad, I've got a favour to ask.'

'What?' He lowered the paper and looked at her.

'I met Michael Grayson when I was out. You do remember Michael?'

'Vaguely.'

'He's done well, got through his exams.'

'What does that make him?' he asked without showing much interest and fingering the paper as though anxious to get back to it.

'A civil engineer.'

'Mmmm.'

'He wants to take me dancing, tonight, to the Pavilion.'

'Tonight?' His brows shot up. 'Short notice, isn't it?'

She chose to ignore that. 'Dad, I want to go, I really want to go and you have to admit that I don't go out a lot.'

'Your own fault, and sorry, but as it happens I've made arrangements for tonight.'

'Not important arrangements though, are they?'

'I consider them to be,' he said coldly.

'That's not fair, Dad,' she burst out, 'you're out nearly every night and what about our arrangements or have you conveniently forgotten those?'

'Not at all, and if you haven't wished until now to take advantage that is hardly my concern. Or are you suggesting it is?'

'No, of course I'm not, but tonight is different,' she said desperately, 'I want to go dancing with Michael, I'm young and I'm entitled to some enjoyment. It wouldn't do you any harm to stay in for a change.' She regretted the words as soon as they were said but she was so angry, so disappointed, that they just came out.

His eyes were icy blue. 'Are you by any chance dictating to me?'

'I didn't mean that and I'm not dictating. All I'm doing, Dad, is appealing to your sense of fair play.'

'Go dancing with your boyfriend by all means and as far as your brother is concerned he can stay with his pal next door or remain in the house on his own. He isn't a baby, Laura, though that is what you are making him.'

'Alan goes out with his parents on Saturday nights and Ronnie can't be left on his own at night.'

'That is just ridiculous, I should be home by ten o'clock at the latest.'

Her eyes flashed angrily. 'Tell me this, were you ever left on your own? No, I'll answer it myself. All through your childhood you were surrounded by doting females who would never have dreamt of leaving you on your own – not at Ronnie's age or even when you were a lot older.'

'That's enough!' He was blazingly angry. 'You'll go too far one day and you'll be sorry.'

Defeated, Laura turned away and as she did became aware of the kitchen filling with steam. The kettle, she'd forgotten it was on!

'Heavens! I completely forgot I had the kettle on,' she said, dashing through to turn off the gas.

'You can forget about the tea too as far as I'm concerned, I'm going out.' A few moments later she heard the front door bang.

Gripping the edge of the table, Laura closed her eyes and clenched her teeth. She wanted to scream with disappointment and rage and the rage was mostly against herself. Why did she have to go and say all that? She might have had a chance if she'd kept her temper, a bit of gentle persuading perhaps. Funny that she'd never thought of herself as quick-tempered or bad-tempered but she appeared to be both.

As she worked Laura began to wonder if she was being unreasonable. Was her father right? He had all but promised to be home by ten o'clock and what harm could come to Ronnie? He would be reading and he always lost all sense of time when his nose was in a book. The time would pass quickly and he wouldn't weary.

Mentally she shook her head. That wouldn't do, she wouldn't be able to relax and enjoy herself thinking of what might happen. The house could go on fire, certainly there was a fire-guard she could put up before she left but she couldn't be sure that Ronnie would leave it there. It kept away the heat and Ronnie liked plenty of heat. She was always telling him he sat too near the fire. No, the risk was too great, she couldn't do it.

Was she still hoping her father would have a change of heart? Perhaps she was, at any rate she was taking a lot of care over the preparation of the meal and her efforts were rewarded when Ronnie beamed across the table to her.

'That was good, the best steak pie you've ever made. Dad, it was, wasn't it?'

'Yes, it was very good, I enjoyed it.' He looked coldly at his daughter as she got up to collect the plates. 'At least your sister can cook.'

'That's not fair, Dad, Laura is good at a lot of things, and do you want to know what Alan's mum said?'

Laura was on her way to take a rice pudding from the oven but lingered to hear what Mrs Brand had had to say.

'Since they are bosom friends, something highly complimentary I imagine,' he sneered.

Ronnie looked at his father uncertainly. 'She said – she said that—'

'Whatever it was you appear to have forgotten.'

'No, I haven't, I was just trying to remember it all,' he said indignantly. 'She said we should be grateful to Laura, that she is the one missing out and that she hardly ever has any fun.'

Laura busied herself with the rice pudding. It had a nice brown skin on it. She divided the pudding between three plates, giving her father most of the skin which she knew he liked.

'Well, Ronnie, you can tell your pal's mother that your sister is going dancing tonight and your father has had to give up his evening to look after you.'

'I don't need looking after,' Ronnie said, going very red in the face.

Laura brought two pudding plates over, then went back for her own.

'I know that, Ronnie, but you see it happens to be illegal to leave a child under twelve alone in the house and we don't want to get into trouble.' Laura didn't know whether it was true or not, and if it was whether the age was twelve, but she thought her father wouldn't know either. The suggestion of possible trouble and that he might be held responsible would be enough to scare him.

'You've made your point, Laura, leave it there.'

'Thanks, Dad,' she said, picking up her spoon, 'thanks very much.'

Little more was said at the table and Laura's thoughts had turned to what she should wear. No one was expected to dress up for the Saturday night dances at the Pavilion but for many of the girls half the enjoyment was wearing what was most becoming, or more important, what would attract the opposite sex. It was a chance to experiment with different cosmetics for that glamorous look that they wanted to copy from their favourite film star.

After a great deal of dithering in her mind Laura finally decided on the dress she would wear.

It wasn't only the girls who were concerned with appearance, some of the young men took a great deal of trouble over theirs. Most would be wearing flannels and sports jacket since it was the summer, but scattered about the dance hall would be a few dark, well-pressed suits worn with a crisp white shirt.

After the warmth of the day the evening was pleasantly cool and the breeze coming off the sea gently ruffled Laura's hair. They left the bus and walked across the wide area of grass that had traces of sand in it. The Pavilion was a landmark and had once been the pride of Miltonsands, catering as it did for all ages. Now it attracted mainly the young. It had a good-sized dance hall and a café that was much frequented in the summer months by visitors where throughout the day plain teas, soft drinks and ice cream were served.

Laura and Michael listened to the music, faint at that distance but steadily increasing in volume as they drew near. Through it they could hear laughter and happy voices and Laura felt a fluttering in her stomach that was excitement. They reached the door and went in.

'You go ahead to the cloakroom, Laura, and I'll get the tickets.'

'All right,' she smiled, and followed others to the cloakroom where a middle-aged, harassed-looking woman behind a table was taking coats and other belongings. The room was very crowded and there was a lot of good-natured pushing and shoving. Laura had to lean against the wall to change into her black patent sandals. Trying to get near to the mirror was hopeless since those at the front appeared to have taken up permanent residence. Being tall, Laura could at least see the top of her head and hurriedly drew a comb through her hair. Taking off her coat, she went across to the attendant and handed over her coat and a string bag that held her shoes and handbag. In return she was given one part of a pink ticket and the other piece was attached by a safety-pin to her coat. As she moved away someone tapped her on the shoulder.

'Good to see you, Laura. Is this you getting back in circulation?'

'Hopefully yes,' Laura smiled. She liked Muriel Galbraith, a nice natured, plumpish girl with lovely glossy auburn hair and a plain, freckled face.

'You look marvellous but then you always did,' Muriel said admiringly.

'You look very nice yourself.'

'Try my best and thanks for those kind words but with the competition around I see myself a wallflower. No fear of you ever being that.' She paused. 'You are not by any chance here on your own?'

'No, I came with Michael. Michael Grayson.'

'Lucky you. I knew he was back, someone saw him. You two had something going at school I remember. Is this it starting up again or had it never stopped? Sorry! Sorry! Sorry!' she apologised as she moved away to let someone through.

'You'd make a good door, Muriel,' a very slim girl shouted.

'Less of that, skinny,' Muriel grinned, 'they could haul you through the keyhole and with room to spare.'

'Very funny.'

There was a lot of laughter and leg-pulling.

'I only met up again with Michael this morning and quite by accident.'

'Lucky accident and he didn't put off much time, did he?' She smiled. 'He's nice and I'm glad for you, you've had a rough time.'

'You aren't here on your own, are you?'

'I'm partnerless if that is what you mean, but Brenda and Ena are somewhere, eyeing up the talent if I know them. Pity it's half past nine before things liven up, it's a long wait.'

Laura knew that that was the time the more sophisticated young gentlemen left the hotel bar and crossed to the Pavilion. One or two drinks would make them moderately happy and they would be careful because the management was strict and no one the worse for drink was allowed in.

Michael was waiting, and seeing him Muriel left with a whispered 'Enjoy yourself and I think he is smashing.'

'Happy hunting,' Laura said mischievously, then joined Michael. 'Sorry, was I a very long time? It was chock-a-block in there.'

'No, you weren't.' His eyes lit up in appreciation. 'I like your dress, the colour suits you.'

'Thanks.' It hadn't been an expensive dress but the fine cotton material had a lovely sheen to it and the different shades of blue shimmered in the dimmed lights. Knowing he liked what she wore helped her confidence. For so long she had done so little mixing that she was out of things. And this very assured young man, smart in grey flannels and navy blazer with brass buttons, was very different to the boy who had carried her books to school.

Other girls had been eyeing up the handsome young man and gazed a little sourly when Laura arrived.

'Michael, would you mind keeping my cloakroom ticket, I've no pocket?'

'Sure,' he said, taking it and slipping it into his top pocket, then as the band struck up a quick-step he led her on to the dance floor. Laura had a reasonably good sense of rhythm but considered herself to be a very average dancer and she had had no practice for months. Would her feet go where they were expected to go? Nervously she hoped so. She needn't have worried. Michael was an accomplished dancer and easy to follow and soon Laura had given herself up to the sheer joy of being in his arms. The pressure of his hand was firm against her back, drawing her closer. The band was good, with the musicians looking as though they were enjoying themselves, and the beat of the drums pulsed through her body. This was heaven, and for the time being her troubles were forgotten. More and more couples were coming on to the floor and before Michael could steer her out of harm's way, a pair of over-enthusiastic dancers careered into Laura's back.

'So sorry, hope I didn't hurt you?' The youth looked concerned, then cheered up when Laura assured him she was still in one piece. The four of them smiled, then danced on.

'Sorry, Laura, that was as much my fault as his, I should have been paying more attention.'

'Michael, he didn't hurt me, not one little bit.'

It was a new and pleasant experience for Laura to feel cherished and she was relishing every moment. The next dance was a dreamy waltz followed by a slow fox-trot and then to the groans of the young folk a group of mature dancers made a special request for an eightsome reel. Michael was for sitting it out but a couple were needed to make up a set and Laura, flushed and happy, hauled him on to the floor and received a burst of applause for her trouble.

After it they were both in need of a cooling drink, and taking her hand Michael drew her through the crowd to where refreshments were served. A number of couples with no liking for set dances had retired to darkened corners and could be seen twined together and oblivious of all but each other. Laura didn't look too closely, knowing if she did that more than likely she would recognise one or two of the girls. She wondered if she and Michael might be doing the same thing before the evening ended. She hoped so and felt excited at the thought.

They settled for a glass of orange and when it came drank gratefully until the worst of their thirst had gone. The remainder they would last out. Laura rather thought that Michael would be on a small salary at present and paying for two would make a dip in his pocket money. Even if he was paying his board to his mother he wouldn't have a great deal left over. Laura, now that she was in charge of the housekeeping, was much more money-conscious. Once she would have been like her friends and expected the boy to pay and thought nothing of it. They were after all better paid than girls, and girls, to attract them, spent more on their appearance.

'Penny for them?'

She smiled into his face. 'I was just thinking how marvellous this is,' she said softly, 'I'd forgotten what fun it is.'

He took her hand in his. 'I'm going to see that you get a lot of fun, you deserve it. Bad enough that you've missed out on a career without—'

'Michael, I'm nearly over that,' she interrupted.

'That I do not believe for a single moment, but you are wise not to dwell on what might have been.' He stopped and made himself look shocked. 'Come to think about it, had you been at college we may not have met.'

'In Miltonsands it would have been difficult not to,' she laughed.

'We were meant to meet again.'

Yes, she thought, perhaps we were meant to meet again, but how long before you tire of a girl who has so much arranging to do before she can accept an invitation?

They were both silent, a comfortable silence, just listening to the music. Then Michael spoke. 'I like being with you, Laura, you're restful. So many girls seem to think it necessary to talk non-stop.'

'Could be I don't have anything interesting to say. My life is pretty dull, you know, Michael, and that isn't a moan it's just a fact.'

He shook his head and smiled. 'We've just met up again and I feel I want to tell you things that I'd normally keep to myself.'

'I'll say this for myself, I'm a good listener.'

He laughed. 'You've asked for it. I did tell you that I was studying to get an extra qualification?'

'Yes, you did. You're ambitious and that's good.'

'With a bit of experience behind me I'll start to think seriously about going abroad. There are tremendous opportunities overseas, Laura,' he said eagerly.

'I'm sure there are, and you are so right to go after what you want,' she said, wistfully wishing her own future wasn't so bleak.

'Go after what I want,' he said, repeating her words. 'Yes, I mean to do just that. By that time I'll be on a decent salary, enough to support a wife.' He stole a sideways glance. 'It would be nice to start married life in a new country.'

Laura knew that he was waiting for her to say something but what could she say? When she didn't respond he seemed disappointed and added, 'If I had to go out on my own then I would.'

'You would soon make friends, Michael, wherever you went.'

'I suppose so but I'd rather the person with me was from Miltonsands.' And when she remained silent, her fingers playing with the glass, he spelt it out. 'You must know I am talking about you, Laura?'

'Michael, we only met a few hours ago and it is far too early to think of a future.'

'For a while we didn't see each other but for me it is as though we had never been apart. Is it like that for you?'

She nodded.

'There are opportunities in the UK but nothing like as good as those on offer in America.'

'Why America?'

'No particular reason, I could go elsewhere but America appeals to me. The pace is faster and it is young men they want, young men full of energy and ambition.'

'That certainly describes you, and you'll be a success I know.'

'Don't you think about the future at all?'

'I have enough to do thinking about the present,' she said a little tartly.

Someone loomed over their table and they drew apart. Laura welcomed the interruption, Michael was annoyed but managed to hide it.

'You two look very serious, must be discussing something very important.'

'No, Alex, just chatting.'

The young man beamed at her and Laura thought she vaguely remembered him from schooldays. He had a girl with him. 'Must make a foursome of it sometime.' He sounded eager.

'Sure,' Michael said with a marked lack of enthusiasm.

The girl smiled thinly. It was obvious that a foursome wouldn't suit her and equally obvious that she considered talking a waste of time when they could be dancing.

'Alex,' she said, pouting her lips, 'that's my favourite tune they're playing and we'll miss it.'

He frowned. 'Oh, all right. 'Bye, Laura, nice meeting you.'

Michael sighed with relief as the girl all but dragged him over to the dance floor.

'You remember Alex Drummond, he was in my year?'

'By sight but I never knew his name. He knew mine,' she said, sounding surprised.

'Alex, let me warn you, has an eye for a pretty girl.'

'Flatterer.'

He drank what remained of his orange. 'Finish yours if you want it and we'll get back before the floor gets too crowded.'

Laura finished hers quickly and got up. They danced three more dances but for Laura much of the joy had gone from the evening. For a while she had managed to forget her responsibilities but they were back. It was going to be hard, very hard, but it would be unfair to Michael to lead him on and have him believe that there could be a future for them. One day when Ronnie was old enough to look after himself, then she could think of herself, but that was years away and no boy would wait that long.

What were her own feelings? Was she in love with Michael? It was too soon to know and that must apply to Michael too. If love was being happy to be with someone and miserable at the thought of losing that person then she was in love.

She couldn't think of marriage for years to come but she wasn't ready for it anyway. Hadn't her mother said not to rush into anything? But there was nothing to rush into and the talk of going abroad made it all the more impossible. Laura didn't see her father ever taking responsibility for Ronnie and in any case would she be able to trust him to put his son's interests before his own? She knew the answer to that and then there was her promise, she must never forget that.

'You've gone quiet all of a sudden, Laura.'

'I'm a bit tired, that's all, don't forget I'm not used to this.'

'I've had enough too. It's too hot in here and the band seems to be getting louder than ever.'

'You don't mind leaving before the end?'

'No, but it is very nearly the end, a couple more dances I imagine.'

'My cloakroom ticket, Michael, I need it.'

'Where did I put it?'

'In your top pocket.'

'Not only beautiful but observant as well.' He fished the ticket out of his pocket and she took it. 'Meet you just inside the door.'

She nodded and went in the direction of the cloakroom to find that others had decided not to wait for the last dance. How easy it was to pick out those who had enjoyed themselves, Laura thought. They had the happy, satisfied, almost smug look that said they had a boy waiting to see them home. The others were silent and glum, the evening that had promised so much had fallen below expectations. All that effort to look nice had failed but by next Saturday it would be forgotten with

47

hope returned. After all, that could be the night that Mr Right put in his appearance.

Laura got her belongings and changed where she stood into her outdoor shoes. Dressed and ready, she went to join Michael. He and Alex were in conversation but broke off when she appeared.

'See Carol in that mob?' Alex asked.

'No, I didn't, but there aren't too many waiting so she shouldn't be long.'

'Thanks,' he said and his eyes were full of admiration.

He was tallish and pleasant-looking but had a good conceit of himself she thought and he certainly didn't appeal to her.

'Alex is smitten with you.'

'Well, I'm not smitten with him.'

'Glad to hear it, I was getting worried.' He put his arm around her. 'The bus doesn't come for another twenty minutes, no use hanging about for it, is there?'

'No, I don't mind walking, in fact I would welcome it.'

'Had a feeling you would say that and we'll be at your house almost as soon as the bus.'

'If we step on it and don't dawdle.'

'You are putting ideas into my head.'

'No,' she laughed, 'they must have been there in the first place.'

Taking her hand in his, they moved away from the Pavilion leaving the noise behind.

'It's such a lovely night,' Laura breathed, 'and Miltonsands is a beautiful place. We are lucky to live here.'

'Privileged people, yes, I think I agree with you but I have to confess I don't think about it, I just take it for granted.'

'We all do. Perhaps it is the night and the silence that make it special.' She had seen this view many, many times but for some reason tonight Laura felt almost moved to tears with the beauty of it. All that sweep of sea fascinated her. Like people it had moods. Moods that changed without warning when the sea would be whipped up into a frenzy as if bent on destruction. After that would come the calm when, like now, the only sound from it was a distant sigh.

'What is it, Laura?' he said softly, watching the changing expressions cross her face.

'The sea.' Her hand took in the wide expanse. 'Wonderful but so cruel, or am I just becoming fanciful?'

'No, it does something to me and I remember when I was just a wee lad and looking away into the far distance. I thought then, and no one could tell me otherwise, that the sea and sky joined up.'

'And as a wee boy where did you think all that water went?'

'It came down as rain, of course.'

'What a clever little lad you were.'

'Still am, only I'm a big laddie now.'

'Seriously though, Michael, doesn't all this' – her arms went wide – 'make us seem so small and insignificant?'

'Insignificant or not we are meant to make the best of our lives and use what talents we are given, or, as my mother would say, we are put on this earth for a purpose.'

Laura smiled. 'That is the kind of remark my mother used to come out with and she could be funny too. If I say my aunts, my father's two sisters, are difficult it is an understatement and to my mother they were a real trial. She often declared that they had been put on this earth for the sole purpose of annoying her.'

'You miss her very much, don't you?'

'Terribly, Michael. I know time is supposed to make it easier but it hasn't, not yet anyway. Each day I think it is going to be better but it just needs something, a trifling something, to remind me of her and the pain is just as bad,' she said unsteadily, biting her lower lip to stop it trembling.

'Believe me, it will get easier,'

'It has to, I know, but I get so angry at times, angry enough to want to throw things about and sometimes I don't even know what I'm angry about.'

'Don't we all – want to throw things, I mean.' He took the string bag from her. 'Sorry, I should have been carrying that, I didn't notice.'

'You don't need to, it isn't heavy.'

'I'll take it just the same. We were talking about anger. We all have a lot of it in us, Laura, and it is perfectly natural when things don't go right to want to lash out.'

'Most people would say that shows lack of control.'

'Have you ever actually thrown anything?'

'No, but I've been very close.'

'There you are then. You didn't let fly, you held back.'

'Michael, you are so good for me, making excuses to make me feel better.'

'I am good for you and you are good for me. In fact we are a well-suited couple.' He stopped and kissed her gently, then with more urgency. The touch of his lips brought tremors of longing but she drew back and immediately Michael let her go. 'Sorry, I'm rushing things and that is the last thing I want to do. I don't want to spoil what we have.'

She shook her head. 'Michael, you don't understand.'

'What don't I understand?' They had begun walking again, Michael swinging the string bag in one hand and holding Laura's hand in his other.

'About me.'

'What about you? I know I want to go on seeing you, or as the folk around here would say, I want us to go steady.'

'Michael, I have to be fair to you and my position is hopeless.'

'Why should that be?'

'Because it will be years before I am free of responsibility.'

'I don't understand.'

'Ronnie.'

'Ronnie is your father's responsibility.'

'Legally he is, but it would never work.'

'You can't know that.'

'I do, and I gave Ronnie my promise that I would always be there for him.'

'We all say things when we are emotional but they are not binding.'

'To me they—'

'No, let me finish. You are too close, Laura, but I can see as an outsider. Your mother was a super person, I remember that, and her loss is terrible for the three of you but worse for you. You are shouldering the burden and that is not as it should be.'

'Dad and Ronnie, especially Ronnie, miss her dreadfully.'

'Of course they do, but it hasn't altered their life the way it has yours. Your dad goes off to work and has his colleagues. Ronnie has school and his friends. And there you are stuck in the house doing something that gives you absolutely no satisfaction. Of course you are resentful, anyone short of a saint would be.'

'I should be making a better job of looking after the house, my father has reason to be disappointed in me, the way I go at it half-heartedly.'

'Well, you were expecting a different kind of life.'

'I should be able to accept what I have but I can't. And that is plain selfish.' She paused. 'I'm not the only girl to have had her hopes wrecked.'

He gave her a hug. 'Never mind, there is one plus in all this.'

'Then I'd like to hear it.'

'One day your housewifely skills will be put to good use. No burnt offerings and a well-run house.'

'Michael, you're hopeless,' she laughed, 'and goodness, we are almost home and I hadn't noticed.'

There was a gas lamp just outside the Morrisons' gate that lit up the path to the door. Michael led her to the side of the house and away from the light. He put her string bag on the ground beside them and drew her into his arms. When he kissed her she felt herself responding and his arms tightened about her.

'It's been a wonderful evening,' he whispered.

'Lovely for me too.'

They kissed again, then Laura moved away. 'I must go in.'

'When do I see you again?'

'That's the trouble, don't you see, Michael, it isn't easy to make definite arrangements.'

'Surely there is one evening you can call your own?'

Was there a hint of irritation in his voice and could she blame him? She sounded pathetic.

'Yes, Michael, you are absolutely right.' She smiled. 'Make it Wednesday if that suits you?'

'It does, and don't you weaken and give in. Mr Morrison needs you every bit as much as you need him.'

Laura laughed. 'I'll maybe tell him that.'

Chapter Five

A routine was established and on Wednesday nights Laura and Michael went to the cinema if it happened to be showing a film they both wanted to see. If it wasn't and the weather was good, they would take long walks, usually along the sea front, and stop at the Pavilion café for a cup of coffee and have whatever was on offer to eat.

The neighbours noticed and smiled. They were pleased to see Laura taking up with such a nice young man. The poor lass, as they said, was too young to have the responsibility for looking after the house but then that was the way of things in this life. It was always the girl or woman who got the heavy end of the stick. Still, things could change for Laura. George Morrison might well take another wife and that sooner rather than later. There had been talk, but then there was always talk in Miltonsands and the problem was knowing how much of it to believe.

If the neighbours were happy about Laura and Michael, George Morrison was not. This friendship was beginning to worry him. When he had last seen Michael he had been a shy, awkward schoolboy but the schoolboy had turned into a nice-looking and very confident young man. Intelligent too and someone who appeared to know where he was going. George had a sneaking suspicion that Laura would be part of those plans. If it should be that the young couple had serious intentions these would have to be nipped in the bud.

The truth was he couldn't afford to let Laura go. He needed his daughter to keep the house and look after her brother.

Laura, too, was having thoughts about her relationship with Michael. They didn't see one another often enough. Wednesday evenings and each alternate Saturday was hardly going steady, Laura thought resentfully. What, she wondered was to stop her asking Michael to the house on Saturday evenings and on other evenings besides? She saw no reason why she shouldn't invite her boyfriend or why her father would object, but he might. It was hard to understand him sometimes. Pity he and Michael didn't get on better. Not that there was any unpleasantness, rather the opposite. They were too polite and couldn't hide their relief when she appeared dressed and ready to go out.

There was another reason for Laura wanting to invite Michael on a Saturday evening and one she tried to hide from herself. The present arrangements seemed to suit Michael very well since they gave him time for study. But hadn't he told her that he could never settle to study on a Saturday night? Any other night but not a Saturday. And if he wasn't studying how did he spend those other Saturday nights? Laura longed to know but could never bring herself to ask.

They were alone and it seemed like a good time.

'Dad, would it be all right if I asked Michael to come here on the Saturdays you are out?'

'I rather think not.'

She couldn't have heard him correctly. 'Sorry, what did you say?'

'I said I rather think not.'

'You rather think not,' she repeated stupidly.

'I believe that to be what I said.'

Laura felt she wanted to throw something at him to take that half-smile off his face. Did she detect a malicious enjoyment in withholding his consent or was he just teasing? No, it wouldn't be that, he wasn't one for teasing.

They were in the living-room where the fire was quite low. Her father was sitting or rather lounging in the armchair with his long legs stretched out before him. A twenty-packet of Capstan sat on the arm of the chair and a cigarette was between his fingers. He liked a cigarette after his meal and before changing himself to go out.

Laura had been standing but the shock of his words had her sitting down abruptly. She was hot and pushed a few stray hairs from her face.

'Would you care to explain that to me? Your objections, I mean.'

He gave an exaggerated sigh and after another puff and inhaling deeply threw the cigarette end into the fire.

'Believe me, Laura, I am only thinking of you and your reputation.'

'What has my reputation got to do with it?'

'Surely that much should be obvious. You know yourself that it doesn't take a lot to set tongues wagging in a small place like Miltonsands.' He paused. 'Laura, it isn't the thing to entertain your boyfriend in the house on your own.'

'Is that your way of saying you don't trust me?'

'You are both young and it is putting temptation in your way.'

'You have a nerve, Dad, saying a thing like that. And what may I ask are we supposed to get up to with Ronnie in the house?' Her face had gone crimson.

'I've embarrassed you?'

'Infuriated, more like.'

'If I know Ronnie he would disappear upstairs. And that's another thing, to my mind he spends far too much time up there.'

'Reading his books in his own room or downstairs, what is the difference?'

'We'll leave that and get back to your boyfriend. Your mother would have been in total agreement with me. No, don't shake your head and look at me with that expression on your face. It is true. In fact,' he put the tips of his fingers together in that infuriating way he had, and Laura was sure it was someone else's mannerism, perhaps his superior's, that he was copying, 'I recall her saying that she hoped you would have sense enough not to rush into marriage.'

'That's right, Mum did say that.'

'There you are then.'

'She said it because she wanted me to have the benefit of a college education and a taste of independence before tying myself down.'

'We are not having that brought up again, are we?'

'No, but try and be honest with yourself. What you're afraid of, Dad, is me marrying Michael and leaving you with the house to look after and Ronnie. Go on, admit it.'

'I'll admit to no such thing and I refuse to be drawn any further into this ridiculous conversation. You asked permission to be alone with your boyfriend in the house and I said no and that is an end to the matter.'

'I see,' she said through clenched teeth.

'You can, of course, disobey me but I don't think you will do that.' He got up, pushing the chair back as he did. 'That fire will be out if you don't do something about it,' was his parting shot.

Laura watched him leave the room, heard him on the stairs and then later leaving the house without as much as saying so. Inwardly fuming, she sat on nursing her wrath until she suddenly realised the fire was down to a few dying embers and she was shivering. The November nights were raw with a damp coldness that chilled the bones and she knew that she had only herself to blame that she'd let the fire go out. It meant starting from scratch and Laura, feeling hard done by, went through to the kitchen for kindling. Selecting the thinnest of the sticks, she placed them in the grate with some rolled-up paper, set a match to it, then added small pieces of coal. Before long a little of the smoke curled back into the room and hastily Laura moved herself back. The chimney badly needed to be swept and it was a job that couldn't be put off much longer. Not easy either to get a sweep. There were only two in Miltonsands and a wait for two or three weeks was not unusual.

Laura dreaded having the chimney sweep, remembering as she did how her mother had been up very early in the morning preparing for him. Old sheets kept for the purpose were used to cover the large furniture and as many as possible of the smaller items removed to another room and the doors kept firmly shut. Even so, soot still managed to find its way through the coverings and under doors and the smell lingered for a long time.

A dirty chimney could so easily go on fire and though there were some folk who welcomed this as a cheap way of cleaning the chimney, Laura knew that there was the very real risk of setting the house on fire. Tomorrow she would book the sweep.

Chapter Six

Suddenly winter had taken its grip and the December night was bitterly cold. A howling gale-force wind had the windows rattling alarmingly and during the darkness a few slates were dislodged and had crashed to the ground in small jagged pieces. By morning the storm had spent itself, the wind had dropped, and George went out to investigate the damage. It wasn't so bad as he feared and coming into the kitchen he announced to Laura that a few slates needed replacing.

'Do I report that to the landlord?'

'Not immediately, this is an emergency. You get someone to see to the damage and the bill goes—'

'To the landlord, Mr Atkinson,' Laura said, relieved. 'For one awful moment I thought you were going to say that we had to foot the bill.'

'No, not our problem. I'll have my breakfast,' he said, blowing on his hands and sitting down at the table.

She put before him a plate on which was fried bread, bacon and sausage.

'Get someone to replace those slates before the rain gets in,' he said as she poured out his tea.

'Is there a danger of rain getting in?'

'A very real danger.'

'Then I'll see about it today.'

'This morning, Laura, and make it early. There will be others in the same boat.'

'Yes, I'll do that.' She was glad that her father was taking an interest in the house and she would certainly do something about the slates.

With a good breakfast inside them and warmly clad, Laura saw her father off to work and a little later Ronnie to school. Her brother had slept through the storm and wondered what all the fuss was about.

Before starting on the breakfast dishes, Laura crossed to the window and looked out at the back garden. What she saw made her heart sink. The place was a shambles, with torn branches everywhere, and those flowers that had withstood the frost and bloomed bravely until now looked tired and bedraggled as they hung wretchedly from broken stems. It was a depressing sight and Laura found herself wishing for a thick blanket of snow to hide the devastation. Not much hope of that, a few flurries perhaps, but the heaviest falls invariably came after the New Year. She would just have to brave the cold and go out and tidy it up.

Christmas was almost upon them and Laura wasn't looking forward to it, in fact she was dreading it. The first Christmas without her mother was going to be an ordeal. An ordeal for the three of them. What was she to do? What would be best? Should she ignore it and treat the day as any other? No, that was impossible, and unfair to Ronnie. Some sort of celebration there must be. A special meal, she could manage that, and she could bake mincemeat pies. Her mother's recipe was some-where, she would search for it.

At the back of Laura's mind had been the thought that the three of them might have been invited to Aunt Peggy's or Aunt Vera's. It was after all a time for family, but there was no sign of an invitation and Laura was relieved. Far better to be on their own and spend the day as they wished. That made her think about presents, she would have to buy her father and Ronnie something. Ronnie would need money to buy his father a gift. He did save regularly from his pocket money but it wouldn't amount to much.

Her thoughts turned to Michael. Should she invite him for Christmas? Would he want to come? She hoped so, it would make the day special for her. She would ask him this evening.

'Looks very festive, doesn't it, Michael?' Laura said as she admired the decorations in the Pavilion café where they were sitting at a small table with a cup of coffee in front of them.

'You look quite festive yourself,' he smiled.

She was wearing her last year's coat, a crimson princess-style coat with a fur collar.

'Ronnie said I look like Santa Claus,' she grinned.

'A very pretty Santa Claus.'

His words and the look on his face brought a warm flush to her cheeks. 'Soon be Christmas,' she smiled.

His eyes went to the ceiling. 'Don't I know it! My mother has been preparing for weeks. She moans about all the work involved but she loves it.'

'I'm sure she does.'

'Everybody, but everybody descends upon us, Laura, and the family gets bigger every year. Mum is marvellous and if this year is anything like the others it will be absolutely great.'

Laura thought of Christmas at Fairfield Street and wondered if it was worth asking Michael. Her expectations hadn't been high that he would want to spend the day with them and now she was almost certain he wouldn't. Almost but not quite. No harm in asking and she was curious as to what he would say.

'I'm sure it will,' she murmured.

'Sorry, Laura, it must be difficult for you,' he said awkwardly, 'but I expect one of your aunts will have invited the three of you to share their Christmas.'

'No, Michael, they haven't, and I have to say I'm relieved.'

'Oh, well,' he said, and unsure what else he could say, Michael lifted his cup and drank from it.

Laura did the same, it gave her time to think, and her thoughts were of Michael's close-knit family. Both his sisters lived in neighbouring streets and Laura knew that hardly a day went by without a visit to their mother. One was expecting her first child and the other had a baby of eighteen months. Michael's dad was a quiet, unassuming man who frequently went about largely unnoticed. His hobby, and it took up much of his time, was making wooden toys, which were good enough to have a local shop stock them. On the few occasions Laura had been there she had admired his handiwork and pleased him by showing a genuine interest. She was at ease with Mr Grayson as she never was with Michael's mother, and that shouldn't be. Mrs Grayson, an attractive middle-aged woman, had been kind, made her welcome, yet Laura felt something was lacking, a slight reserve as though she wasn't the girl she would have chosen for her son.

'I did think of asking you to our house, Laura, but the way you are placed, and Mum agreed with me, that it could only meet with a refusal.'

Laura felt both hurt and angry. How could they be so sure of her refusal, and chance would have been a good thing? Then she tried to be fair. Michael was right, she would have been unable to accept.

'Yes, I am afraid you are right. It would have been lovely but I would have had to say no.' She smiled into his face. 'You could come to us. I don't say the dinner would be as good as your mother's but—'

'Every bit as good,' he said, squeezing her arm, 'but I daren't accept. Mother would be very hurt and greatly offended if I chose to spend Christmas elsewhere.'

Elsewhere! Surely Christmas dinner at the home of his girlfriend wasn't just elsewhere, Laura thought resentfully.

He was watching her face. 'You do understand, Laura?' he said anxiously.

'Of course, think no more about it.'

His hand went into his jacket pocket. 'Might as well let you have this now.'

She took the small, beautifully wrapped package.

'Thank you very much, Michael, I have something for you but I didn't think to bring it.'

'Not to worry, I'll get it anytime.'

Again he was upsetting her. Did her gift mean so little to him that anytime would do to receive it? What was wrong with her? Why was she picking on everything Michael said? She was fingering the small box.

'Don't you dare open it before the time.'

'I won't, but that doesn't mean I'm not dying to know what is inside.'

Her gift to Michael was a tie and pocket handkerchief. She would get Ronnie to take it round to Michael's house on Christmas Eve.

Christmas Day was a success and Laura was grateful to her father for the effort he made to make it so. He was loud in his praise for the meal she had prepared and there was a festive air. No decorations were up but there was holly in a vase and on top of the picture frames. Two days previously, George had attended the office party and at the end had helped himself to a box of crackers left over together with bags of nuts and raisins. There was a lot of laughter as they pulled the crackers, read the jokes and put on the paper hats. Ellen's name was never mentioned yet they all had the feeling that she wasn't far away.

LOST DREAMS

Two or three times Laura had been on the point of opening Michael's gift. He would never know if she didn't tell him but she hadn't yielded to temptation. She opened it in the bedroom on Christmas morning. There was a well-known jeweller's name on the box and inside was a lovely silver bracelet and a card 'With love from Michael'. Her lips curved into a smile. It was a lovely gift. After the work was done she would put on the fine-knitted dress she had treated herself to from her own savings and wear the bracelet.

As had always been done, gifts were handed over when the breakfast was finished. The fire burned brightly with logs on top of the coal and the room was cosy. From her dad, Laura got a scarf and matching woollen gloves which had been chosen by Aunt Peggy.

'Thanks, Dad, very nice and just what I was needing,' she said, dropping a kiss on his forehead. Her own gift to her father was cigarettes, and only later did it occur to Laura that it wasn't much of a present since his cigarettes always came out of the housekeeping. Still, he seemed pleased enough. Ronnie's gift to his dad was a colourful hand-kerchief and a bookmark he had made at school. Hers from Ronnie was a small bottle of Carnation perfume and Laura knew that most of his money had gone on that.

'Ronnie, what a lovely, lovely gift, thank you very much.' She gave him a hug.

He was flushed and happy. 'It's got a nice smell.'

'Carnation is my favourite.'

'I know. You have a bottle on your dressing-table and it's nearly finished.'

'What were you doing in your sister's bedroom?' his father asked but he was laughing.

'Mrs Brand said to find out the scent you liked, Laura, so I had to, hadn't I?'

'Of course you had, Dad is only joking.'

Ronnie's gift from his father was a new ten-shilling note to buy what he wanted and Ronnie's eyes shone. It would go on books.

'Dad?'

'Mmmm.'

'My prize books and *Treasure Island* from Laura and what I buy with your money, can I have my own bookcase – just for my books, nobody else's?'

'We'll see.'

'A second-hand one will do,' he said hopefully.

'Then keep your eyes open and if you see one cheap enough Laura might manage it out of the housekeeping.'

'Typical! Typical!' But Laura was laughing. This was the way it should be all the time, she thought, not just on Christmas Day.

Christmas was over and so were the New Year celebrations. Before long it was back to the bad old days. George was often irritable and difficult to please and Laura was glad to see the back of him when he went out. Ronnie was avoiding his father and this was upsetting Laura. She was in no way to blame yet she did feel some guilt. Her mother would never have allowed such a state of affairs to continue but it had been easier for her to insist on forgiving and forgetting. She had been Mother after all.

Laura saw Ronnie's scowl when his father's back was turned and gave a deep sigh. It wasn't like Ronnie but, poor lad, the hurt had gone very deep.

How happy he had been when he'd rushed home to show her his report card. He was top of his class again and there was a glowing report from his teacher.

'That's splendid, Ronnie,' Laura said, giving him a hug, 'and I'm just very proud of my young brother.'

'You were clever at school too,' he said generously.

'Quite good but not brilliant.'

'Dad is going to be pleased when he sees it, isn't he?' His father's good opinion was very important to Ronnie. Laura hadn't realised just how important.

'He'll be absolutely delighted and very proud of you.'

Ronnie beamed.

Perhaps George Morrison was proud. Perhaps it was just a bad time or work hadn't gone too well. Laura tried to make every excuse but she couldn't forget the wounded look on her brother's face and the battle he was having to hold back the tears.

'Dad, read that and then you have to sign it,' Ronnie said the moment his father entered the living-room.

After sitting down George took the report card and gave it a cursory glance. 'I'll sign it later,' he said, handing it back to Ronnie.

'I'm top boy, Dad, didn't you see that? And I'm getting a prize of money and I've to choose the books I want.' He waited and the glow slowly left his face.

'Dad?' Laura said sharply as she carried the plates through to the table. 'For goodness sake, your son is top of the class.'

'I saw that much, but so he should with all the time he spends over his books.'

'Not school books, Dad,' Ronnie said indignantly, 'I don't spend a lot of time over my homework, do I, Laura?'

'No, you don't,' Laura said, looking daggers at her father.

'I read books because that is what I like doing, I like reading.'

'Pity you don't like other things as well, like kicking a ball around and getting yourself involved in games.'

'I don't like playing football and I don't have to like it.' The words were tumbling out. 'And when I'm grown up I'll get a better job than you and earn a lot of money.' He was shouting by the end and ignoring Laura's warning look.

'Never mind, Ronnie, Dad will see it later. Come and get your soup.'

'Don't want any and I hate him,' he said before dashing from the room and running upstairs. The bedroom door banged shut.

'Impudent young devil,' George said, breathing heavily, and his face had gone a dull red. 'Don't keep anything for him, he can do without.'

'No wonder he is upset,' Laura said as they both sat down at the table. Then she got up again to take Ronnie's soup away and put it back in the pot. Returning, she saw that her father had begun on his. She hoped it would choke him. Taking a sup she put down her spoon, she had no appetite for hers. 'How could you be so – so – unfeeling. Not a word of praise, you just couldn't bring yourself to say "well done".' She paused and swallowed. 'Believe it or not, it was your praise he wanted and he could hardly wait until you got home.'

'I have things on my mind.'

'Don't we all?' She watched him finish his plate.

'That was good. Any more?'

'Not unless you propose taking Ronnie's.'

'I won't, but serve him right if I did.'

'One day you are going to regret this and be sorry for the way you've treated Ronnie. Your son is going to be more than clever, he is going to be brilliant.' She fought the lump in her throat. 'He'll suceed in life not because of you but in spite of you.'

She saw with quiet satisfaction that he was looking decidedly uncomfortable. Getting up, she took the plates through to the kitchen and returned with the meat and potatoes.

'Better get the lad downstairs.'

'He's too upset, he'll come down when he's ready.'

George tut-tutted. 'What a way of doing about nothing.'

'Nothing to you, Dad, you've made that clear enough.' Her voice was shaking. 'You've hurt Ronnie very badly and you've upset me too though I don't suppose that bothers you either.'

'Oh, for God's sake! What I have to put up with! Is it any wonder that I don't want to stay in at night? What pleasure is there for me? I get no consideration from either of you.'

At the sheer injustice of it Laura drew in her breath sharply, and facing him across the table her eyes, so like his, were icy blue.

'Since Mum died I've done my best. Maybe it wasn't a very good best at the beginning but you've nothing to complain about now. Your house is kept clean and tidy, you have a clean shirt every day, your meal is ready for you when you get home and suppose I say it myself, a good, well-cooked meal.'

'Self praise no honour.'

'All I'm likely to get,' she flashed back.

He put up his hands in mock surrender. 'All right! All right! I'm sorry I didn't give your brother the praise he expected but I'll apologise to him before I go out and I'll sign the wretched report card when I get home.'

If her father had apologised and given belated congratulations it would have gone some way to mend relations, Laura thought, but he hadn't bothered. And had Laura known that her father was genuinely sorry she might have been more forgiving.

An apology didn't come readily to George Morrison but he had intended to make one – sometime. The only excuse for his behaviour that he could make for himself was that he had been tired and irritable, and having the record card thrust at him the minute he got in the door had been too much.

When George entered his local, a few looked up from their pint to welcome him, then carried on with their conversation. He got his drink and looked glumly down on it. Right now he wasn't in the mood to talk, wasn't in the mood for anything, come to that. There was a restlessness in him that he couldn't understand. Even at work he was having difficulty concentrating. Being a tax assistant meant dealing with complaints and queries. Thankfully most of those were fairly routine and anything more complicated went up the line to a more senior member of staff and occasionally all the way to the Inspector of Taxes himself.

A complete change of scenery – yes, that was what he needed. His heart ached for freedom and that unpleasantness with his son and daughter had added to his mood. Lifting his glass, he drank some of his beer and nodded to himself. Maybe a change wasn't impossible. From time to time notices were sent round the offices asking for volunteers – London offices in particular were always short of qualified staff.

Financially it was very attractive because for the first month away from home the subsistence allowance was generous, after that there was a sliding scale. Laura would get her housekeeping money but with a deduction since she would have one less mouth to feed. He smiled grimly into his almost empty glass. Who knows, the girl might even take a thought to herself and get a job even for a few hours a day. As for Ronnie, what was to hinder him taking a key and letting himself into the house after school? There were plenty of latch-key children and it didn't appear to do them any harm.

Laura cleared the kitchen table in preparation for its next function. It was where she did the ironing. From the cupboard below the stairs she got out the blanket and sheet. The blanket was folded and placed on the table then the white flannelette sheet went on top. Laura made sure there were no creases. The flat iron had been heating for some time and she checked to see if it was hot enough to begin. Laura liked to do the difficult garments first and shirts came into that category. Once she had almost wept with frustration, unable to work out how it should be done. It had taken time to master but practice was making for near perfection.

The days went in and by now father and son had broken their silence and were talking but there was no warmth in the relationship. Ronnie had got himself a new friend and seemed happier. Laura was particularly pleased about it because Alan Brand's cousin had come to live nearby and the boys, close in age, were encouraged to play together. Mrs Brand had been most apologetic.

'Nothing to hinder the three of them going about together,' she'd said to Laura.

'Three doesn't always work out, Mrs Brand, but honestly don't worry about it. Ronnie has got himself a new friend.'

'Has he now? Well, I'm very glad to hear it.' She did sound relieved. 'Between you and me, Laura, I'd rather it was Alan and Ronnie. They got on fine and I never had to worry about them getting into trouble. This Ian is a bit of a dare-devil and a show-off with it. You know Alan, he'll just follow.'

'Alan might calm him down.'

'Not a chance, but I daren't say too much or there could be trouble. We can choose our friends, Laura, it is just a pity we can't choose our relations.'

Laura laughed. 'You don't have to tell me that.'

'Not still causing problems, are they?'

'The aunts? No, hardly ever see them but advice comes via Dad.'

'Which you ignore, I hope?'

'I do.'

Mrs Brand was moving away. 'Oh, almost forgot and it was what I came out to ask. All right if I use the mangle?'

'Of course, anytime.'

'Thanks, Laura, it's a grand help not having to iron the sheets.'

Washing the clothes and scrubbing them on the washboard was exhausting work and Laura's poor hands suffered from the coarse soap and being so much in water. The mountain of ironing had been a nightmare but gradually it was getting easier and Laura didn't have to spend so long over it. That gave her more time to herself and soon she would make a serious effort to get a part-time job. The extra money would go towards her savings.

She well remembered the drudgery of the wash-house though her mother had seldom grumbled. As she would have said, it had to be done therefore get on with it. Summer or winter Ellen Morrison, with galoshes over her shoes, would go down to the wash-house every Monday morning at half past five to light the fire that heated the water in the boiler. Then, breakfast over, she would hurry down with her loaded clothes basket. Whites got a good boil and were done first.

Coloureds followed and woollens were done in the sink to avoid shrinking. The numerous rinses made it a long process. In fine weather the washing was hung out to dry, but should it be raining they went over the pulley in the kitchen and the remainder went over the clothes horse.

Thankfully Laura was spared all that. Some years ago the kitchens of the houses in Fairfield Street were altered and immediately the rents were increased. Two deep sinks had been provided and in honour of the improvement Ellen treated herself to a small wringer. Then she got the joiner to make a wooden fixture that went between the sinks and on which the wringer was screwed into place. Not having to squeeze out the water by hand was a tremendous help. One sink was used for rinsing and three was recommended. Laura settled for two. Her aunts declared the final rinse had to be in cold water, and Laura agreed to save argument. Her hands went numb in cold water and she saw no harm in using lukewarm.

The disused wash-house had become a cellar and was used to house the mangle. Ronnie helped with this task. It was a job he enjoyed.

'Laura, I help you a lot, don't I?'

'Don't know what I would do without you,' she smiled, as between them they carried the damp sheets in the clothes basket. Laura's first job was to tighten the rollers. That done, Ronnie turned the large handle and she fed through the sheets. Each one went twice through the rollers and the end result was a very professional job.

With most of the ironing done and over the horse, Laura broke off to have a rest, a cup of tea and a glance over the newspaper. But before she could there was a knock at the door and Laura went to answer it. The smallish, pleasant-faced woman standing there smiled. She wore a brown skirt and an oatmeal jacket. A brown beret sat jauntily on her head and showed an abundance of auburn hair.

'You must be Laura, Ronnie's sister?'

'Yes.'

'I'm Jane Turnbull—'

'David's mother? Do come in.'

'I won't keep you if you are busy.'

'I should be but I'm not. This is me having a rest from ironing.'

'Very sensible, I do the same. My day is full of little rests.'

Laura showed her visitor into the sitting-room.

'Do sit down and you'll have a cup of tea?'

'That would be very nice, thank you.'

'Excuse me a minute and I'll bring it through.'

Laura got out a tray, put cups and saucers on it, then a jug of milk and the bowl of sugar. Quickly she got some biscuits from the tin and put them on a plate. Once the tray was on the table she went back for the teapot.

'Milk? Sugar?'

'Neither, just as it comes, please.'

'A biscuit?'

'Thank you.' She paused. 'May I call you Laura?'

'Please do.'

'I just want to say, Laura, how very grateful we, my husband and I, are for the help Ronnie is giving David.'

'Ronnie enjoys helping and if David is benefiting then that's fine.'

Jane Turnbull bit off a small piece of biscuit, ate it and drank a mouthful of tea. 'David is a slow learner, Laura, and unhappy at always trailing behind the others. He isn't stupid—'

'Of course he isn't.'

'Oh, some people aren't so generous and it is very hurtful – never mind that, they probably don't mean to be unkind,' she finished with a sad smile.

'Ronnie is quite a timid boy, Mrs Turnbull —'

'Jane, please, it makes me feel younger.'

Laura laughed. 'As I was saying, Ronnie is timid and my father makes no secret of the fact that he would have preferred his son to be an average scholar and show promise on the sports field.'

Jane shook her head. 'Arthur, my husband, says Ronnie will go far. They talk, you know, and he says the lad has an enquiring mind and a quick grasp of everything he is told. David is just a plodder, he isn't lazy, far from it, but he requires everything explained to him again and again. Once he does grasp it he retains it, I'll say that for him. We have tried to help but he takes it so much better from Ronnie. Your brother has such patience, Laura.' She laughed. 'He won't move on until he is satisfied that David understands.'

'I'm glad, and I'm grateful to you for inviting Ronnie to your home. My brother is a bit of a loner and disappears up to his bedroom to read and more or less just coming down to eat.'

'I hope you won't be annoyed at what I'm about to say, but Ronnie talks quite a lot to us.'

'He misses Mother terribly and it may be that you remind him of her.'

'I take that as a very great compliment,' she said softly. 'Ronnie doesn't say much about his dad but you are the most perfect sister any brother could have.'

'You'll have me blushing.'

'The boy probably understands more than you think. He told me you don't get out with your boyfriend very often. Michael was the name he mentioned,' she smiled.

Laura nodded.

'And I gather the reason is that your father is out a lot and you can't leave Ronnie on his own.'

'He told you that!'

'Yes, and that is part of the reason I am here. You are young and pretty and you should be enjoying yourself.'

'Honestly, I don't do too badly,' Laura protested.

'I'm not so sure. We have a spare bed and Ronnie is very welcome to stay overnight at any time.'

'You are very kind.'

'No, I consider it small payment for what your brother is doing for my son. David is a different boy, Laura. He'll never be clever but at least he is making progress and I can't ask more than that.'

'I really am glad you came,' Laura said and meant it.

'I timed it and it is only a ten-minute walk between our homes so anytime you need a sympathetic ear or just a change of company, please come round.' She got up. 'And now I must go. Thanks for the tea and do let Ronnie stay with us weekdays or weekends, anytime. David is our one and only as you probably know and they will be company for each other.'

Laura was smiling as she saw her unexpected visitor away. Such a nice person and she was sure she had made a friend. Michael would be pleased. Once his studies were over they would be able to spend more time together. After the cinema they could very easily collect Ronnie from David's house and if there was a special dance or a late evening somewhere Ronnie would no longer be a problem.

The announcement when it came was a complete shock. The three of them were at the table enjoying a leisurely Sunday breakfast of bacon, egg, sausage and black pudding.

'London! You're going to London?' Laura said incredulously. 'But you can't, I mean, what about us?'

Ronnie was looking from one to the other in bewilderment.

'Laura, calm down. I'm not going to the other side of the world.'

'I know that, Dad,' Laura said. To herself she was thinking that he might as well be.

'Don't under-estimate yourself, my dear, you are perfectly capable of seeing to things in my absence.' He forked a piece of bacon and put it in his mouth. 'Think about it, you'll have less work to do when I'm not here.' He was smiling.

'There is that right enough.' She smiled back. 'It's just the unexpectedness, I mean you've never even hinted—'

'How could I when I didn't know myself? The reason I am being sent is because of the shortage of staff in London.'

'Why you, Dad? Why pick on you?'

That seemed to have caught him off guard. 'Why me?' he repeated. 'Presumably because I have the necessary qualifications.'

So have some of the others, Laura thought, but she nodded when he looked at her. Later on when she was washing the dishes, Laura wondered to herself if he had been asked or if he had volunteered. She rather thought that he had volunteered.

'When do you have to go?'

'This Friday.'

'As soon as that? Not much notice.'

'One doesn't in an emergency.'

'No, I suppose not.' She smiled. 'The shock is wearing off and I'm beginning to think clearly. Lot to do, Dad.'

'Such as?'

'Getting your clothes ready and two pairs of your shoes need to be heeled.'

'You'll manage and anything I forget you can send on.'

'Yes,' she said absently. Laura was thinking about buttons. Better check for any that were slack. There would be no one in London to look after him and see to his clothes.

Ronnie had been silent all this time but now he spoke and he seemed excited.

'Dad, if you stay in London for a long time me and Laura could come for a holiday, couldn't we?'

'Ronnie, Dad isn't going to be away long.' Laura looked over at her father and waited.

He shrugged. 'Difficult to say. Could be one month or two. It all depends.'

'Since they are sending you I suppose your accommodation must be arranged?'

'Yes, that will be all seen to but if it shouldn't be to my liking I can look around for something else.'

'Isn't London very expensive?' Laura said worriedly.

'I believe so but I get subsistence.'

'What's that, Dad?' Ronnie asked.

'A special allowance for being away from home.' Turning to Laura, he smiled. 'Stop looking so worried. You surely don't think I would leave you both to starve. You'll get your housekeeping with a deduction since there will be one less to feed.'

'Of course,' she agreed readily.

He pushed back his empty plate. 'That was good. And, Laura—'

'Yes?'

'This could be an opportunity for you to get yourself fixed up with a job instead of sitting about doing nothing.'

Laura was stung. It was so unfair and so untrue. When she wasn't working in the house she was tidying the garden. Choking back the words she longed to say, she took a breath and said quietly, 'Yes, I'll see what is available but part-time jobs are not easy to get. I'll try, though.'

With a suitcase in one hand and a Gladstone bag in the other, George Morrison stepped jauntily on to the London train. Laura and Ronnie had come to see him off and watched him claim his window seat. After putting his luggage on the rack and his raincoat on the seat he went back to the carriage door. They went nearer.

'Your sandwiches are in the bag on the top,' Laura said unnecessarily. She had already told him.

'Yes. Yes. I'll get myself tea at the station—'

'Better watch the train doesn't go without you,' Ronnie piped in. 'I heard about somebody—'

'Yes, we've all heard about somebody being left on the station platform holding a cup of tea and watching the train depart. I'm not so stupid.'

'Could happen though.'

'Dad will wait for one of the main stations when it will be a decent stop.' Then she giggled, she couldn't help it. In her mind's eye she was seeing her father returning with his cup of railway tea to see the train disappearing into the distance.

'What is so funny?' he said, irritation in his eyes.

She was spared answering as doors up and down the train were slammed shut, the guard waved his green flag and with a rush of steam the London train began to move.

'Don't forget to write, Dad,' Laura said, running along the platform, 'let us know how you are getting on.'

'Yes, and you look after the house—'

There was more but the words were lost as the train gathered speed.

She stood with her brother until the train was out of sight, then she felt curiously alone, almost as though she had been abandoned. That was ridiculous, she told herself. Her father would be gone one month or two at the outside.

'Come on, Ronnie.'

'Have you any money, Laura?'

'Bad show if I hadn't. Why?'

'Could we have fish and chips when we get home? I'll go for them,' he said eagerly.

Laura watched his face. There was no sadness, no hint of regret when they waved goodbye. He wouldn't miss his father and that was such a pity, a tragedy really. What about herself, would she miss him? Yes, of course she would, a little. She wished it were more.

'Laura?' They were in the living-room. She was sewing a button on Ronnie's shirt and he had just closed his book. Since his father had left Miltonsands, Ronnie did his reading and his homework downstairs.

She raised her eyes. 'What?'

'Do you miss him?'

'If you are referring to Dad then say so.'

He shrugged.

'Why are you suddenly finding it so difficult to call him Dad? You can use Father if you want to be more grown-up.'

'It isn't that.' He paused and looked uncertain.

'Come on, you had better tell me,' she said gently.

'Is it possible to love someone and not like them?'

Laura thought about it. She never spoke down to her brother, not consciously anyway. 'Yes, I suppose so.'

'That's all right then. I have to love Dad but only because he is my Dad, but I don't have to like him.'

'That's not very nice, Ronnie.'

'He isn't very nice and I don't think much of him and I'll tell you why.'

Laura cut the thread, put away the needle and scissors and shut the sewing box. 'I'm not sure I want to hear this.'

'You don't know what I know.'

'And what do you know?' she said with a dangerous calm.

Ronnie looked on the verge of tears. 'You should be angry with him and not with me.'

'I'm not angry with anyone.'

'Dad didn't have to go to London, no one made him go. He went and volunteered. And if you want to know how I know it's because Jimmy Maxwell's dad works in the same office and he told me.'

A sick feeling was erupting from her stomach though she was only having her own suspicions confirmed.

'Aren't you going to say something?' he said, disappointed.

She took a deep breath. 'Yes, Ronnie, I am going to say something and you won't like it.' He was about to get up. 'No, don't get up, just sit where you are and listen. It is time you and I had a serious talk.' She paused to marshal her thoughts. 'Earlier on you asked me if it was possible to love someone and yet not like them—'

'And you said yes.'

'I did, and it is true, but we have to be fair. None of us is perfect, Ronnie. I'm not, not by a long chalk.'

'Only little faults, Laura, like when you get bossy.'

'That is for your own good. You, like me and most other people, have some annoying habits.'

'I'm not saying I don't, but Dad didn't know about them. How could he when I spent most of the time when he was in the house up in my bedroom?'

'Exactly, and that annoyed him. No,' she held up her hand, 'let me finish and get it all out in the open. Everything was fine when Mum was alive, you liked Dad then?'

'Suppose so,' he said grudgingly.

'When she died we were lost. Mum, and I see it now, acted as a sort of buffer—'

'Like an engine buffer.' He grinned, then jumped up. 'You don't have to explain to me, I know what you mean. If we got mad at each other Mum came in between. That's what you were going to say, wasn't it?'

'More or less, and thinking back, Ronnie, I must have been pretty awful, I hadn't a clue how to go about things, and without Mum's loving care and my pathetic efforts no wonder Dad was short-tempered.'

'He never once tried to help you, and I did.'

'That's true, but we just have to try and forget all the bad times and try to be as Mum would have wanted.'

He nodded and she saw his lips trembling. 'Just because I don't talk about her doesn't mean I've forgotten.'

'Ronnie, I know that. We'll always remember but in our hearts.'

'I'll make a promise and it won't be easy to keep because I still feel mad at him, but when Dad comes home I'll try and be nicer.'

'So will I.'

'All the same, it's nice with just the two of us.'

'Go on, away with you and take your shirt up to your room.'

'Did you sew the button on?'

'You must go about with your eyes shut. Of course I did.'

Chapter Seven

The letters began to arrive telling Laura how well her father was getting on and how very busy the office was. She gathered his London colleagues were falling over themselves to make sure that his evenings and weekends were not spent alone. The reason for this, he explained, was because they were just so happy to welcome a qualified person instead of having to make do with the temporary staff who remained only long enough to be trained before tiring of the job and moving elsewhere. Unlike Miltonsands jobs were plentiful in the big city. Laura smiled to herself. She would have good news for him in her next letter.

Once she had seen Ronnie off to school her first move before clearing the breakfast table was to sit down with the newspaper and study the job vacancies. It didn't take long, there weren't very many and so far none that appealed to Laura. She accepted that beggars couldn't be choosers but even so she wasn't prepared to take just anything. One vacancy, however, did catch her eye and she read it again with mounting interest.

> Intelligent young woman, good at figures, urgently required to help out in sub post office. Hours to be arranged. Apply in own hand-writing to Miss Wilkinson, Bridgend Post Office, West Miltonsands.

Laura got up for writing pad and pen and then and there wrote out her application, supplying as much information about herself as she thought necessary. She addressed the envelope, used her last stamp – she must remember to buy half a dozen, she didn't like to be without them – and stuck it on firmly. She would post her letter in time to catch the emptying of the post-box at noon.

Two days later, on the Thursday, she received a brief note from Miss Wilkinson asking her to attend for an interview at ten-thirty on

Friday, which was the next day. Laura was delighted. If she got it –
no ifs about it, she must get it – this would be her first job working
for an employer. The allowance she got from her dad for keeping the
house could hardly be termed a wage. Try though she did, it seemed
impossible to save anything from the housekeeping. As soon as she
had a little aside there was an urgent use for it. Ronnie was stretching
and his arms getting longer. Too much wrist showing, and the buying
of a new coat could not be put off much longer. Shoes were the worst,
as one pair went into the shoe repairer or the cobbler as her mother
used to call him, she collected them and another pair went in. Her
mother had hammered protectors into the toes and heels and maybe
she should think about doing that. The last must be around somewhere.

Miltonsands boasted a main post office and a sub office. Twenty
minutes' smart walking would take her for her interview. Any business
she had, had been conducted at the main office and she had never had
occasion to be inside the sub office.

Ronnie knew but was keeping quiet about it. The only other person
she had told was Jane Turnbull, David's mother.

'Tomorrow for your interview, that's quick.'

'What I thought too, but it did say urgent.'

'I know Miss Wilkinson though not very well.'

'What is she like?'

'A bit straitlaced.'

'I won't mind that, but what kind of person is she? Easy to get on
with, mean?'

'No-nonsense type, very efficient or that was the impression she gave
me.'

'A bit frightening by the sound of her.'

'Not if she is satisfied and I'm sure you will suit her very well.'

'There will be other applicants.'

'Very likely, and may I give you a word of advice?'

'Please do, I'd be grateful and I can do with all the advice I can get.'

'Plain women – and Miss Wilkinson comes into that category – are
usually of the opinion that looks and brains don't go together, so if you
want the job wear the drabbest clothes you possess and flat-heeled,
sensible shoes, preferably laced-up ones.'

Laura laughed delightedly. Jane had proved to be a very good friend and her home had become a second home for Ronnie. 'No problem Jane, I have a wardrobe of drab clothes.'

Jane shook her head. 'You always look lovely and I don't think you appreciate just how lucky you are. Most women spend hours trying to improve themselves and here I am telling you to hide your good looks until the job is yours.'

Laura took Jane's advice and wore her navy trench-coat which had seen better days. Bought for growth, which hadn't pleased her at the time, it had been a reasonable length when she stopped growing and had left school. She unearthed a pair of black school stockings and flat shoes which were too small and pinched her toes. Still, she thought, it was a small price to pay if it helped her to get the job.

On her head was a navy beret and not at the angle she would normally wear it, but straight on. With her hair pushed behind her ears Laura gave a final look in the mirror, made a face and wondered if she'd overdone it.

She shuddered to think she might meet someone she knew but perhaps they wouldn't recognise her. In the event she met no one.

Laura was five minutes early for her appointment. The clock on the wall told her so. There were a few customers waiting their turn and chatting. One was being served stamps by a heavily built woman Laura thought might be the postmistress. A woman in a green overall seemed to be in charge of the shop. There was stationery, jars of boiled sweets, some haberdashery and a shelf of groceries, Laura waited her turn.

'Yes?'

'I'm Laura Morrison—'

'Thought you might be since you are a stranger to me.' The woman turned her head. 'Beccy, keep an eye on the post office.'

'Yes, Miss Wilkinson.'

The postmistress fiddled under the counter, then lifted a section of it and signalled for Laura to come through. She did, and the bolt went back in place.

'We'll talk best away from the counter and Beccy can manage for a few minutes provided it is nothing complicated. By that I mean anything but stamps,' she said drily.

The back room was small, with every inch of floor space taken up with cardboard boxes, obviously stock delivered for the shop. There was a cooker and a kettle on the ring and a small sink with a brass tap. A table held bundles of documents held together with elastic bands.

'Sit down, Miss Morrison,' she said brusquely. 'We are very cramped in here but there are advantages.' She smiled. 'Nothing is far out of reach.' She sat down at the table and moved some documents. 'There is a great deal of work in a post office and rather than leave everything until closing time, I make a start on it when there is an opportunity. The big balance, as I call it, is done once a week and sent off to the head office. There must be no mistakes. That is all just by the way.'

Laura nodded.

'You have a good school record but no experience at all.'

'I did explain—'

'Yes, you did, your letter was very detailed and I appreciated that. At your age it can't have been easy to take the responsibility for the house.'

'It wasn't, but I find it less difficult now.' Laura smiled nervously. 'My trouble was that I had no routine. I have now and that is why I wish to find suitable employment.'

'This is not full-time, you understand that?'

'Yes.'

'Beccy,' she lowered her voice, 'is very dependable in the shop but she has neither the confidence nor the ability for the post office. You are good at figures and quick too?'

'Yes.'

'You were good. Are you still good? From your letter I gather that you have been at home for a year or thereabout?'

'A year, yes, I've been at home a year but I haven't forgotten how to count.' Laura knew she sounded nettled.

'I am going to ask you to prove yourself. You understand I have other applicants, all older and with experience though not necessarily helpful. There you are,' she said, producing a bundle of documents. I have made my calculations, though I haven't as yet checked them. Should you agree with me, that will save me a little work. If we differ, then we shall both have to do our sums again.'

Laura was more at ease now. It was the woman's brusque manner that was off-putting. She wondered how old she would be. Somewhere in her fifties she decided. Her build probably aged her. She had dark hair flecked with grey and secured in a tight bun. Her slightly protruding eyes were muddy brown and her complexion was sallow. Plain she undoubtedly was but the eyes were intelligent and for all her brusqueness there was kindliness too.

She lumbered to her feet. 'I'll go and rescue Beccy and leave you to it.'

Laura picked up the pencil and drew over the scribbling pad to do her calculations. She did them carefully, then checked. Satisfied, she reached over for a bundle of cashed postal orders which she supposed were there for the same purpose. Her pencilled answer was just jotted down when Miss Wilkinson returned.

'Good! We agree.'

'While I was waiting I did these, I hope you don't mind.'

'Most certainly I don't mind.' She went over them very quickly, Laura was amazed at the speed. 'Excellent, Miss Morrison, I think we are going to suit each other very well.'

'Does that mean — ?' Laura began eagerly.

'Yes. I am always businesslike, Miss Morrison. I believe in a written agreement and that way we both know where we are. See if that is suitable to you,' she said, handing Laura a neatly written page. 'I had it prepared.'

Laura read it. 'Very suitable, Miss Wilkinson, thank you.' She liked the thought of an hourly rate and it was higher than she would have expected.

'I would like you to start on Monday, the hours ten o'clock to three-thirty Monday to Friday, but you must be prepared to do extra when required.'

'I would be happy to.' Laura got up and they shook hands. The low shelf caught Laura's beret, lifting it off, and her hair sprang loose.

'Such lovely hair to be hidden.'

Laura didn't know how to answer that. 'Thank you,' she murmured.

There was a thoughtful expression on the postmistress's face and then she frowned. 'Perhaps I was too hasty, perhaps I am making a mistake taking you on and spending time on your training. There must be a young man in your life, you are too pretty to be overlooked.'

Laura was panicking. What if Miss Wilkinson changed her mind even at this stage?

'I am not serious about anyone, Miss Wilkinson, and I won't be for a very long time. You see, I have a young brother to bring up.'

'I'm relieved to hear it.'

They were through in the post office and no customers waited. 'A quiet spell.'

Laura was looking about her. 'This is all very neat and compact.'

'Yes, everything in place and a place for everything. It is irritating and unnecessary to find forms in the wrong section and it is also a waste of valuable time. I've had my share of careless assistants, I can tell you, and they didn't last long.'

'I promise to be careful.'

She smiled. 'I rather think you will. Come and I'll introduce you to Beccy. Beccy,' she called to the other woman, 'come and meet my new post office assistant.'

Beccy came over, smiling broadly. She was of medium height and pear-shaped.

'Thank goodness, Miss Wilkinson. Thank goodness you've got someone. I hate being behind that counter. I just panic.'

'It can't be as bad as all that.' She introduced them and they shook hands.

Laura was uncomfortable with Miss Morrison. 'Please call me Laura.'

'All right, and I'm Beccy, though I can't recall ever getting anything else.' There was a polite cough from the shop and Beccy returned to her duties.

Laura was making her departure and had reached the door when it was opened and she found herself face-to-face with Aunt Peggy. Laura cursed her luck. Living at that end of Miltonsands she had expected to see the aunts at some time but not quite so soon.

'Laura, what are you doing here?'

'I've got a job, Aunt Peggy. I start work in the post office on Monday,' she said, keeping her voice down and managing to get herself outside. Aunt Peggy followed and there was nothing else for it but to stand and talk.

'I have to ask, does your father know?'

'How could he, Aunt Peggy? I've just got the job.'

'You know what I mean. Does he know that you were looking for one?'

'It was his suggestion that I should find myself a job.'

'I'm surprised. Men don't realise just how much work there is in keeping a house as it ought to be kept.'

'I'm inclined to agree,' Laura said, swallowing her mirth.

Her aunt looked at her sharply but Laura's face was straight. 'Don't let standards slip, that would be a big mistake. Vera and I were just saying how much you have improved.'

'Thank you.'

'Any word from your father? Any word when he is coming home?'

'His letter didn't mention anything about coming home.'

'That must be six weeks he has been away. Wasn't it just for a month?'

'One month or two was what he said before he went away. He did say that the work is very far behind and they are desperate to have him stay longer.'

'Too obliging, that is George's weakness, and it doesn't do. People just take advantage. Another two weeks should see him back?'

'Perhaps, we'll have to wait and see.' She wouldn't mention to her aunt that her dad had asked for more of his clothes to be sent on.

'Take my advice, Laura, and write and tell him his place is here. If you don't I certainly will.' She smiled. 'How nice, I'll be able to pop into the post office and see you. That way we can share our news.'

Laura was alarmed. 'I'm only working part-time and I have the feeling Miss Wilkinson won't approve of private conversations.'

'Give me credit for some sense, I wouldn't keep you from your work if you were busy.' Her hand was on the knob of the door. 'I'll get my stamps and a few other things then I must make for home. That's a threatening cloud and I've a big washing hanging out.'

'Give Uncle Archie my love.'

'I'll do that. The wee lad fine?'

'Yes, Ronnie's fine.' She smiled and hurried away.

Chapter Eight

With her father in London and obviously enjoying the life there, Laura saw no reason why she shouldn't occasionally entertain Michael at home. She would see that he left at a respectable hour. Laura reasoned that if he could just up and leave them when it suited him, then she would suit herself too. If she was to be trusted to look after his house and his son, then she could be trusted to have her boyfriend with her to keep her company.

She did feel guilty that with her father in London she was finding life much more pleasant, and certainly Ronnie was happier. It could be that the separation would benefit them all and when her dad did return they would get on better. She promised herself that she would do her best but she would not be dictated to. Michael would continue to come to the house with or without his approval. There was nothing he could do about it.

She smiled at her reflection, knowing that she looked nice. Michael liked her in blue and she was wearing a pale blue lacy jumper with a dark blue pleated skirt. Her feet were in court shoes and on her wrist was the silver bracelet Michael had given her at Christmas. When his knock came she flew to the door to answer it. She had expected him to be casually dressed since they were staying in but he was neat in a dark, well-cut suit with a crisp white shirt and a quiet tie unlike what he usually wore. Laura's heart missed a beat. He looked very handsome.

She held the door open and the minute he was in and the door shut she was in his arms. They kissed, then he drew her away. 'Are we to be on our own or is Ronnie around?'

'He's at David's house.'

'Fine,' he said sounding satisfied. 'I won't have to keep listening for sounds on the stair.'

'Not quite fair, Michael, Ronnie makes plenty of noise before he comes down.' She smiled. 'But it is lovely to be on our own.'

His arm was around her waist as they went through to the sitting-room.

'Any word when Mr Morrison is coming home?'

'Can't be for a while, I've had to send on more clothes. You sit down, I've got something half prepared —'

'You shouldn't have—'

'You want us to go out, that is why you are dressed like that?'

'Not exactly. I was at a business meeting and there wasn't time to change.'

'Then I'll light the oven.'

'Forget about food for the present because right now I want to talk to you.'

Why did she suddenly feel alarmed? Michael just wanted to talk, what was alarming about that? She joined him on the sofa.

'I'm all ears, what do you want to talk about?' she said lightly.

'About us. About our future.'

'Oh!'

His eyes were on her face. 'You must know how I feel about you?'

'Yes, Michael,' she said softly. 'I feel the same way. I love you.'

'I wonder if you really do.'

'What do you mean by that?'

'Is your love strong enough to put me first?'

'Michael, you'll have to be clearer than that. I'm not sure where all this is leading.'

'Don't you? Then you should. I'll spell it out. I want to know where I stand with you.'

'I've already said I love you, isn't that enough?'

'It should be, but with you it might not be. Your father disappearing like that is hardly fair on you.'

'He hasn't disappeared, I know where he is,' she said, sounding annoyed.

'He up and left you and Ronnie, didn't he?'

'Why all of a sudden are you so concerned about my father?'

'I find it strange.'

'I was under the impression that Dad's absence was suiting you.'

'Don't get me wrong, it's been great. It's just—'

'Just what? Come on, tell me what all this is about.'

'You let slip that he volunteered, he wasn't sent.'

'So?'

'He'll be in no hurry to return if his own office isn't complaining.'

'That may well be so.' She smiled. 'Your studying is finishing soon and we'll be able to see more of each other. Incidentally I always meant to ask you—'

'Ask me what?'

'Those Saturday evenings we weren't together, what did you do with yourself?'

Michael looked taken aback. 'What did I do? Does it matter?'

'Not especially. I just wondered since I remember you saying that you could never settle to study on a Saturday evening.'

She saw a spark of anger in his eyes. 'Did I have to stay at home because you weren't available?'

'Not at all,' Laura said stiffly. 'I wish I hadn't mentioned it.'

He pulled himself together. 'No great secret. If you must know I met up with some of the lads and we went dancing. No harm in that was there? It helped to pass the evening.'

'No harm at all,' she said too quickly. She felt the prickle of tears and turned away so that he wouldn't see them. That was it. Michael had gone dancing. Did that mean he had another girl for those times when she wasn't available? A sharp stab of jealousy went through her but she would rather die than let him see it.

'Whatever you are thinking you are wrong.'

'I wasn't thinking anything. Why should I?' Then she looked at him. 'Where did you go?'

'Dundee.'

'You've never taken me dancing there.'

'Better at the Pavilion.' He shook his head. 'Thought you would have worked it out for yourself.'

'Worked what out?'

'Laura, the last bus leaves before the dancing finishes and you must know that. For heaven's sake, how could I possibly be seeing a girl home?'

Laura knew that she had to be content with that.

'I'm sorry.'

'Do I detect a teeny bit of jealousy?'

NORA KAY

'More than a teeny bit. You must take me dancing in Dundee sometime.'

'Maybe,' he said with a marked lack of enthusiasm. 'We are rather straying from what I wanted to talk about. It isn't settled yet but I have a better than even chance of being offered a job in Manchester.'

'Manchester? You've applied for a job in Manchester?'

'That's right.'

'But why? Why, Michael? I thought you were happy here.'

'Up to now it has suited me. Staying with the folks let me save a bit but it was only a stop-gap. This job, if I am lucky enough to get it, is just what I want. The company is well known, with an excellent reputation, and working there would give me the experience I need.' She saw his excitement. 'With that experience, Laura, and my qualifications, I'll be in a position to apply for jobs abroad.'

'I see.'

'Is that all you can say?'

She heard the hurt and disappointment in his voice and tried to make amends.

'Michael, I am delighted for you, of course I am. I'm very pleased.' She swallowed hard. 'I'm afraid I'm just being selfish. I do want you to get on but I am going to miss you dreadfully.'

'If I'm successful I'll be away in a month.'

'You'll get it, I'm sure of it.'

'I have a sneaking feeling I will, you know. When I get my lodgings fixed up you must come through. Manchester is a great city, so I am told.'

'Nothing I'd like better but I'm afraid it is out of the question.'

'If you want something badly enough there is always a way.' His arm had been along the back of the settee but he moved it and brought her to him. Their lips met and then, sighing, she moved away.

'I'll go and put on the oven.'

'Forget the oven. This is our future we are discussing. Laura, listen, a little while to settle into the job then I'll check on the housing position. Find out how much the rent is for different areas. Cheap accommodation may be attractive in some ways but I'm all for living in a good area. You wouldn't mind taking a job to help out, would you?'

'Michael, you are well ahead of me. I love what you are suggesting. You are suggesting marriage, aren't you?' she said mischievously.

'You wouldn't settle for less, would you?'

'Most certainly not, but seriously, Michael —'

'I am serious. I do want to marry you one day, Laura, and that in the very near future. As I said, once I get settled.'

'Michael, if it were only that simple,' she said wretchedly.

'It is that simple. This is our life and we want to spend it together.'

'How can I? You know how I am placed.'

'You have been too soft but now you write and tell your father that we are getting engaged and you'll be coming to Manchester as my wife. He'll have to take responsibility for his son. Could be he has met someone in London and will be getting married himself. That would solve the problem. They would take Ronnie.'

'There isn't anyone.'

'How do you know?'

'It would have come through in his letters, he would have dropped some hint, I'm sure of that.'

'You can't be absolutely certain.'

'When he gets back he must arrange to get a woman in to look after the house and Ronnie,' he said looking hard at her.

'I couldn't leave Ronnie. He would be miserable. You know he doesn't get on all that well with Dad.'

'That is not your problem.'

'I'm afraid it is.'

'The pair of them have had a year of your life.'

'You think I can just drop everything and go with you.'

His eyes had turned cold, a hardness there that she had never seen before.

'I'm beginning to wonder if you just make your brother the excuse. Perhaps you don't want marriage, marriage to me anyway.'

'That is just not true,' she said indignantly. 'It just so happens that I gave Ronnie my solemn promise that I would never leave him. Michael, I can't go back on that.'

He gave a mirthless laugh. 'If you are hoping that Ronnie can come along too you can forget it. I like the lad well enough but he doesn't share our home.'

'I wouldn't expect that.'

'I'm not so sure. At the back of your mind was the hope that I might weaken, but nothing doing, Laura.'

Maybe she had hoped but now she was so angry that she was white with rage.

'I think this conversation has gone on long enough. Thank you for your proposal,' she said stiffly, 'which sadly I am not in a position to accept.'

Michael got slowly to his feet. He looked defeated. 'I'm sorry it's ending this way, Laura, truly I am. I would always have put you first but I see that I would always come second with you. Love isn't like that, Laura, and you have that to learn.' He had been talking quietly but now anger took over or maybe it was frustration. 'You'll end up a lonely, embittered old maid or, if you prefer it, spinster lady. Still,' he said cruelly, 'when Ronnie takes a wife you'll have nieces and nephews to fill your time but no child of your own.'

She was very pale. 'I think you have said quite enough.'

He had walked to the door, then turned when he got there. Was that pleading she saw in his face?

She wanted to go to him, throw her arms around him and almost she weakened but what was the use? She would be pulled in two directions. Ronnie was just a child, he had to come first. If she left him how could she ever know happiness?

'We've both said things we are going to regret, Laura.'

She smiled sadly. 'I know, Michael, I'm sorry, but it doesn't alter anything.' She paused to take a shaky breath. 'Goodbye, Michael, I do wish you well. You deserve success and I'm sure it will come to you.'

'A success you could have shared. Think it over, Laura, don't throw away your – our happiness on mistaken loyalty. I want marriage now, not in years to come. The next move has to come from you, I won't be back.'

The door closed softly behind him and to Laura there was something very final about the sound. For a while she just stood there looking at the door, then she went through to the kitchen. She looked at the food waiting to be cooked. It should have been a cosy meal for two but instead she put it out of sight in the larder. She had no appetite. She clung to the edge of the table fighting her tears and succeeding. Somehow, though her heart was breaking and her whole world shattered, she had to carry on.

When Ronnie got home she was calm and composed.

'Where's Michael?'

'Gone.'

'Already? But he never goes this early and I wanted to ask him something.'

'Well, you can't.'

'What's wrong with you?'

'Nothing, and hang your coat up, don't leave it on the chair.'

'You're in a mood, is that because you and Michael have had a quarrel?'

'Michael won't be back because he is going to work in Manchester.'

'What did he want to go and do that for?'

'He wants to get on.'

'Could he not get on here? I thought he had a good job.'

'This is better and it is Michael's business not ours.'

'Should be yours, you are his girlfriend.'

'I was.'

'Meaning you aren't now?' he said incredulously.

'That's what I mean.'

'Then he won't come and see us before he goes?'

'I don't expect so.'

Laura went through to the kitchen. She needed to occupy herself somehow but Ronnie followed.

'Laura?'

'What?'

'Did Michael want you to go with him?'

'Perhaps, but I couldn't anyway.'

'Is that because of Dad and me?'

Laura didn't want to upset him. 'Partly, but there was more to it than that.'

'If Dad got married it would only be me then and Michael likes me. He wouldn't mind me living with you and I would keep out of the road. I do that when he comes here, don't I?'

'Ronnie, I am not getting married and neither is Dad.'

'How do you know about Dad?'

'Because, nitwit, we would be the first to hear if he was.'

'Some people —'

'Who are some people?'

'Just some people and they think Dad will get married.'

'Gossip, and you shouldn't be listening to it. Want something to eat now or later?'

'Has it to be cooked?'

'Yes.'

'Then it will have to be later, won't it? I'll set the table.'

'Just a minute and I'll get a clean tablecloth.' Laura got one from the drawer and spread it on the table.

'Laura?'

'What now?'

'If it is all off with Michael you'll have to get a new boyfriend.'

'I'm in no hurry.'

Chapter Nine

George Morrison knew that he had been lucky to be sent to such a friendly office and one within sight and sound of St Paul's. Busy though they were, the staff always had time for a cheery smile and an exchange of pleasantries. True, the accommodation arranged for him had come as a bit of a shock, but as it was explained to him there had been a misunderstanding and the more desirable lodging-house was no longer available. Still, it was somewhere until he found a room more to his liking, and since this was cheaper and within walking distance of the office it had those points in its favour.

The house was shabby and was one of a row of early Victorian buildings, all equally shabby. His room was on the top floor, up two flights of stairs which were covered in worn linoleum that had been nailed down where it had sprung apart. It was sparsely furnished but the essentials were there. A bed with a freshly laundered bedspread, a small chest of drawers with each drawer lined in newspaper, the middle one was missing a knob which made it difficult to open. Beside the window was a table with one chair pushed under and another, more comfortable chair nearby. The curtains at the tall, narrow window were of heavy cotton in a cream and brown floral pattern and on the sill sat a flower-pot containing African violets fast approaching their final stage. Dull but clean linoleum covered the floor and two small rugs helped to take away the bareness. George almost laughed out loud when he saw the picture above the bed. It showed a cottage with roses round the door and the words 'Home Sweet Home' embroidered at the top. How had it got there? Had it been a parting gift from a former occupant with a sense of humour?

Heating when required came from a gas fire which had to be fed with coins, and should George wish to make himself tea there was a gas ring and a kettle provided. It was a far cry from his comforts in Fairfield

Street but this was London and he would put up with a lot for his freedom. In any case he didn't expect to do much more than sleep in his digs. His landlady, Mrs Butterworth, a blowsy woman of indeterminate age, was brisk and businesslike and produced a good, well-cooked breakfast for her lodgers, and most important of all the place was clean. For his other meals the office had its own canteen and there was an inexpensive restaurant nearby which never seemed to close. George wasn't grumbling.

After those first bewildering days he got used to the crowds and the roar of traffic that never seemed to stop. He had wondered how anyone could sleep through it but of course they did. Like everything else it was just a case of getting used to it, and that proved to be true for him. In a remarkably short time the noise ceased to bother him and became no more than a background hum.

George had expected to do his own sightseeing at weekends and in the evenings but a few of his colleagues had taken it in turn to show him the main tourist attractions. He duly admired Westminster Abbey, was impressed with the Houses of Parliament, looked up like so many others at the face of Big Ben and gazed with interest at Buckingham Palace. So much to see, so much magnificence, but sadly not enough time to fully appreciate anything before having to move on. He would have liked time to stand and stare but there was always someone urging him on to other places that simply had to be seen. Perhaps he would return on his own. George had considered buying postcards to send to Laura and his sisters, then decided against it. Postcards made one think of holidays and he didn't want the folk back home getting the wrong idea.

How quickly he had settled in and how contented he was! Tax work was much the same as at home but instead of taking his turn at the desk and face-to-face interviews he remained behind the scenes dealing with queries and complaints that had come with the post. That was a relief to George as he had difficulty in understanding Cockney, especially at the rate most of them spoke. Best of all he had no responsibilities, only those at a distance which for the present could be dismissed from his mind. Laura, to give her credit, wasn't making a fuss about his lengthening stay. She was coping and appeared to be enjoying her few hours working in the post office. No, Laura wasn't the problem, it was Peggy and Vera. Why had he never noticed how bossy they were? He was angry, very angry indeed, that they should write to remind him of his responsibilities. The cheek of them to tell him that it was high time that he was home to keep an eye on things. According to them, and they had got it from a reliable source, Laura was having her boyfriend to the house and at times when Ronnie wasn't there. What was George thinking about to give the girl that kind of freedom? Didn't he realise the dangers? His daughter wouldn't be the first to get into trouble.

So Laura was disobeying him? Well, he could hardly blame her for that. He had left her in charge and she would see it as a licence to do as she wished. In spite of what he had said, and unlike his meddlesome sisters, George did trust Laura. His worry at the time had been that she and Michael would get married and leave him with the house and Ronnie. He now thought that fear groundless at least for the foreseeable future. His trouble was that he hadn't thought it through. There was too much of Ellen in Laura for her to go away and leave Ronnie since it was always Laura the lad clung to whereas he and his son had never hit it off.

How wonderful life would be if he could only stay in London and break free from Miltonsands, he thought. A permanent transfer would be a simple matter and as for his job at home that would be quickly filled. In the provinces Civil Service jobs were eagerly sought after, not so much for the remuneration, but because it meant security. Once in it was a job for life.

The contrast between this and his life in Miltonsands could not have been greater. Londoners were forever on the move as though every minute of every day was too precious to waste in idleness. Compared to this the life at home had two speeds – dead slow and stop.

Nevertheless it was time he packed his bags and George was finally coming to terms with it when the totally unexpected happened and he fell in love. Never before had he felt this strange excitement and certainly it had never been like this with Ellen, not even at the beginning. The times he spent with Connie were magical and the days when he didn't see her were just days to be got through.

In the office his mind kept wandering and the change in him was noticed. It meant him being teased mercilessly but he didn't care and, of course, it was kindly teasing. They were pleased for him since what could be better than the getting together of a beautiful young widow, perhaps not young but youngish and a handsome widower. And to think but for a last-minute change of mind they would never have met.

The invitation, which he had so nearly turned down, was given casually, but that was the way they did things down here. His immediate superior, Richard Morton, had stopped at his desk to put down some papers.

'George, we are having a few friends in for drinks this evening and if you have nothing better to do, come along about eightish. Gwen and I will be delighted to see you.'

'I'm not sure if I'll manage but thank you very much.'

He should have said a firm no but by the time he thought of it his boss had moved away. Still, he didn't have to go and he had promised himself faithfully to sit down this night with pen and paper and write to Laura and long overdue letters to his sisters.

George's good intentions lasted just until he returned from the office and climbed the stairs to his digs. What a waste it would be to sit in his shabby room when he could be elsewhere enjoying himself. After all, what was to hinder him from coming away early and scribbling a few lines before he got into bed? Nothing at all, he convinced himself. One task, however, could not be put off. It had to be done or he would be without clean clothes.

Spare laundry lists were in the drawer and he took one out. At the top George put his name and address, then ran his eye down the column. He put a number in the boxes opposite the articles to be laundered.

Sheets – here he marked (l). Not two, since the top sheet went to the bottom. He seemed to remember Ellen doing that and possibly Laura did it too.

Pillowcases   (2)

    Shirts   (7)

    Socks   (6 pairs). One pair had a huge hole in the toe and since he had no way of getting it darned he would either keep it to take home or throw it out. He hadn't made up his mind. George completed the list, then as instructed pushed the dirty washing inside one of the pillowcases and took it down to Mrs Butterworth. She in turn would give it and the other bundles to the man on the laundry van who collected weekly.

Shaved, washed and looking smart in his light grey suit, George left his digs and in the warm sunshine walked quickly to the bus stop. After five minutes one came along and he climbed up to the top deck. Since the bus made so many stops it was a slow journey that took almost half an hour. Having been to the Mortons' home once before, George remembered where to get off. The house was in a quiet residential area and five minutes took him to Ashville Terrace where the Mortons lived.

Even if he hadn't remembered the actual house he would have been drawn to it by the sound of voices and laughter. All the downstairs windows were wide open with the gentlest of breezes moving the curtains. George went in the gate and his feet crunched up the drive. He rang the bell and stood back. In a moment or two it was opened by Richard Morton in his shirt-sleeves and obviously feeling the heat. His face broke into a smile.

'There you are, George, glad you could make it. Come in! Come in!'

George stepped into the spacious hall where brass ornaments gleamed on a table. He followed his host through a door and into a very large, high-ceilinged room from which much of the furniture had been removed. Guests, most holding a glass, were engaged in animated conversations in their groups and didn't notice George's arrival. Richard was about to break into the nearest group to introduce George when he caught his wife's eye or maybe her eye caught his.

'Sorry, George, I'll have to leave you for a few moments, that was Gwen looking as though she wanted my assistance.'

'That's all right.'

Feeling slightly self-conscious but not wanting to show it, George took a few paces and began to study the paintings on the wall.

'You look lost.' The voice was low and husky and he turned quickly, a denial on his lips.

'I'm waiting for Richard, he'll be back in a moment or so, he said.'

'Then let me suggest you get yourself a drink.' With her free hand she pointed in the direction of a tray of drinks.

George went over, took a whisky and added water. The woman had joined him.

'I was expecting to see a kent face, someone from the office.'

'You work with Richard?'

'He is my superior.'

'What a quaint expression. He's your boss.'

'Yes, Richard is my boss. I'm George Morrison and at present I am on loan to the office.'

'Lucky office,' she smiled. 'I'm Connie Taylor.' She held out a slim hand and George took it in his. She was very attractive, he thought, with her blue-black hair swept up and her face a perfect oval. She had very dark, intelligent eyes and well-shaped eyebrows. Now that he was studying her he saw the tiny lines about her eyes which made him think the woman wasn't as young as he had at first thought. She was tall but not too tall. He didn't go for very tall women. He would rather look down than have eye-to-eye contact. Her figure was good and showed what she wore to advantage. The dress she had on was of fine geor- gette and in delicate autumn shades. It fell in soft folds to calf length.

'Well?' Her eyes held a hint of mischief. 'Will I do?'

George went red with embarrassment. 'Forgive me. Was I staring? I'm so sorry.'

'Don't apologise, I was only teasing.'

'Even so, it was rude of me. Are you – are you a friend of the Mortons or are you family?'

'A near neighbour and we are good friends.'

Richard bore down on them. 'Thanks, Connie, you're looking after George and you both have a drink?'

'We are fine, Richard.'

'George is a colleague but just a temporary one I'm afraid. We'd love to hang on to him but – oh, heavens,' he said turning his head. 'That's Gwen after me again. What can it be this time?'

'Better go and find out,' Connie laughed.

'Safer anyway. Food will be along directly.'

'Should I not be helping?'

'No need, just you keep George happy.' He left them.

'Such a nice couple, I do like them. Richard, I imagine, would be easy to work for?'

'I've no complaints but I do know that if the work isn't up to stan- dard he can come down on the culprit like a ton of bricks.'

'So he should, that is what he is being paid for after all.' She grimaced. 'This is tiring, especially in these high heels. I'd love to kick them off but I had better not. In any case I don't see the point of standing when we could be sitting.' She looked at him questioningly.

'If you would rather circulate please say so, you don't have to be tactful. I never am, tactful, I mean. I see it as a mild form of dishonesty.'

George was completely captivated by this woman. He had never met anyone like her. He nodded as though in agreement with her. If tact was a mild form of dishonesty he had never thought about it that way.

'I would much prefer to be with you, but how about you?'

'I'm quite happy.' She smiled into his face. 'I do so love to hear you speak. You don't rush your words the way we do.'

'I have to confess that I used to miss a lot of what was said but not so much now.'

'When the eats come there is going to be a mad rush for the chairs so come on.' She led and he followed her to the far end of the room where there was a round, glass-topped table with an ash-tray on it and chairs against the wall.

'Be a dear and bring two chairs over to the table and I'll see what Gwen has produced in the way of food.'

She returned with a plate of dainty sandwiches and a selection of savouries which she put down on the centre of the table. Then she picked up the ash-tray. 'I'll put this on the floor meantime. Do you smoke?'

'Yes. I'll have one later but only if the smoke doesn't bother you.'

'It doesn't. I don't mind at all.'

'A lot of women enjoy a cigarette these days.'

'I'm not one of them.' She nibbled at a savoury. 'Here's hoping you had a meal before you came. These are delicious but hardly filling.'

'I did,' he smiled. He'd had bacon and egg in the restaurant he most often frequented. It had used to amuse him that they served bacon and egg all day. To him it was purely a breakfast dish.

'This on loan to Richard's office, what does it mean?'

'Just that. From time to time notices are sent round for volunteers to help out at the busier offices. There is difficulty in getting qualified staff down here. Plenty of vacancies and not enough people to fill them.'

'You volunteered?'

'Yes.'

'Forgive me, but was that to get away from home or a need for change?'

'Both.'

'Are you going to explain that or am I to remain curious?'

He took another sandwich. 'I wouldn't want to bore you.'

'Try a savoury after that and you won't bore me. If you start to do so I'll tell you.'

'Things were difficult at home.'

'Where in Scotland is home?'

'Miltonsands on the east coast. It isn't the home of golf but it does have a good golf course.'

'Are you finding life hectic with all this noise and rushing about?'

'Not now. The noise can be a bit much at times but I am enjoying my stay and there is so much to see. Perhaps you don't appreciate what you have.'

'Or perhaps I would appreciate a bit of peace and quiet and the slower pace of where-did-you-say?'

'Miltonsands.'

'Sands, that means beach, you can go swimming?'

'We do have a lovely beach but apart from a few weeks in the summer it is only the hardy souls who venture into the sea.'

'Are you a hardy soul?' she laughed.

'No, absolutely not.'

'When do you have to return?'

'I can't put it off much longer.'

'Sounds as though you are not anxious to go home.'

'I'm not.'

'Poor you. Is your wife reading the riot act for being away so long?'

'My wife is dead.'

'Oh, dear!' Connie shut her eyes as though in pain, then opened them. 'Forgive me, I am so very sorry. That was unthinking.'

'You weren't to know and I'm over the worst. It's over a year since it happened.'

'At the risk of sounding flippant, could I say that I am in the same boat?'

'You mean you are a widow?' Why did his heart give a leap?

'My husband died over two years ago.'

'I'm sorry, you must be feeling very lonely?'

'No, George, I have not been lonely and I am not going to sin my soul by pretending otherwise. Don't look so shocked. I was only nineteen when I married Philip and he was forty-two.'

George was certainly surprised and wondered if he dared risk the question, then decided he would.

'You are a very beautiful woman, Connie, and at nineteen you must have been a lovely girl. Why did you throw yourself away?'

She made a face. 'Usual reasons. Philip offered security and a good life-style. A man in his forties when he is good-looking and sophisticated is very attractive to a young girl.'

'The age difference didn't bother you?'

'Not to begin with. It did when his hair thinned and his waistline spread. Had it been more gradual it would have been easier to accept but it happened so quickly and Philip hated growing old. He became bad-tempered and difficult to live with. I had never been unfaithful, George, though that isn't to say I wasn't tempted. Philip, however, was convinced there was someone and would hardly allow me out of his sight. Poor Philip,' she sighed, 'was ill for a long time and suffered great pain. When the end came it was a relief I think for both of us.'

'You haven't had an easy time.'

'I chose it. Looking back I see now that I saw Philip as a substitute father. I never knew mine, he was killed when I was a baby and my mother had a hard struggle bringing up the pair of us. My sister is two years older and we both couldn't wait to leave home. There you have my life history and not many can say that.'

'I'm flattered.'

'Ships that pass in the night, that's what we are. It is easier to talk to strangers.'

'Meaning we'll never meet again?'

'Highly improbable, isn't it, since you are shortly to be back in Scotland and I expect to be going to New York.'

George was devastated and he couldn't understand himself.

'New York?' he said in total disbelief.

'Yes, New York. New York in America,' she said, sounding amused.

George got himself together. 'Why New York?'

'My sister Lottie and her husband are there.'

'You would go and live with them?'

'Until such time as I found my own place.'

'It is a very big step.'

She shrugged. 'Not when I have someone to go out to. I do have a little money and more when the sale of the house goes through.'

'Will that be soon?'

'Yes.'

'Am I asking too many questions?'

'I'll let you know when you are.'

'What will you do when you get out there?'

'Find myself a job in due course but there will be no urgency. Something in the fashion world would suit me. My brother-in-law Harry Lambert has good connections. For your information Harry is an American and holds down a very responsible position.'

'Good for him,' George said a trifle sourly.

'Lottie and Harry are very happy. They have a family of three and lively children from all accounts.'

'Have you any family, Connie?'

'No, and I don't feel deprived, not in the very least. It isn't that I dislike children, I don't, and I'll probably dote on my American niece and nephews.' She fiddled with some crumbs on the plate, gathered them together and popped them in her mouth. 'Contrary to popular belief, George, all women are not cut out for motherhood.'

'Perhaps I wasn't cut out for fatherhood,' he grinned.

'A reluctant father, is that what you are? How many?'

'Two. A son and daughter.'

'May I offer you something else to eat?'

'No, thanks.'

'I think I've had enough too. Good! Here is Gwen with the coffee.'

'Coffee?'

'Please, Gwen.'

Gwen served them coffee, said a few words, smiled and moved on to fill other cups.

'We were talking about you having a son and daughter?'

'Were we?'

'Yes, and don't try and wriggle out of it. You know my family history, now I am entitled to know something of yours.'

'Not a lot to tell.'

'Tell me what there is,' she said impatiently.

'Laura is eighteen and coming up for nineteen.'

'I was that age when I got married.' She paused. 'I'm sure she is pretty.'

'So everyone says.'

'Like her mother?'

He shook her head. 'No, not like Ellen. My late wife would have been the last to lay claim to beauty. She wasn't plain, just—'

She smiled. 'Ordinary.'

'Yes, I suppose so.'

'She gets her good looks from you?'

'She is supposed to be like me,' he said awkwardly.

'If it wouldn't upset you to do so, tell me about your wife.'

'I don't get upset, not now.' He leaned back in the chair and chose his words carefully. 'Ellen was very capable. She was a good wife to me and a good mother to our two. Added to that she was a first-rate house-wife and could turn her hand to anything.'

'Frightening.'

'No, not in the very least. She was just there and did all that was necessary.'

'And when you lost her the three of you didn't know which way to turn? Am I right?'

'Yes, you are right. Laura was pretty useless, she hadn't had it to do, you see.'

'You, I imagine, would be equally useless, or are you not including yourself?' she said, frowning.

'No, I'm not.' He was frowning too. 'I was working, remember.'

'Even so, but never mind, instead tell me about your son. Does he resemble you?'

'He does not,' he said shortly.

'How old is the boy?'

'Ten.'

'Poor boy,' she said softly, 'I'm sure he must miss his mother dread-fully. Boys try to hide it but they need a mother perhaps more than girls.' She smiled. 'Eight years between them, that was bad planning, wasn't it?'

'No planning,' he laughed, 'they just arrived. From the very begin-ning they were Ellen's children and it was always like that.'

'Did you resent that?'

'No, it suited me very well.'

'George, if you will forgive me I have a mental picture of Ellen mothering the three of you.'

His brow puckered. 'I'm not at all sure that I like that.'

'Don't be offended. Whether you like it or not you are the type that women like to mother.'

'Including yourself?'

'No, excluding me.'

'Glad to hear it.' Their eyes met and suddenly the air was electric. They were both aware of it. Connie was the first to drop her eyes and when she spoke there was a slight tremor in her voice.

'Who is looking after the house in your absence?'

'Laura, of course. She is looking after the house and Ronnie.'

'Poor Laura, not a lot of fun for the girl.'

'What else could I do? I was working all day and Laura was of an age to leave school.'

'If her mother had lived what were her plans?'

'To go on to college.'

'Brains and beauty. Poor girl, was she very disappointed?'

'She made a fuss to begin with which is probably why she made such a rotten job of looking after the house. My sisters tried to help, point out her mistakes, but she didn't take kindly to that.'

'Few of us do,' Connie said drily. 'Incidentally, did your sisters give actual help or just advice?'

'Advice, they have their own homes. It's all right, Connie, Laura is managing all right now.'

'And I am asking too many questions?'

'The answer to that would be yes to everyone else.'

'Not many more to ask. Does Laura have a steady boyfriend or as the saying goes is she playing the field? That is the saying, isn't it?'

'I wouldn't know, but Michael comes about the house.'

'Your son now and that is the last, I promise you.'

'The lad is very bright but a dead loss when it comes to any kind of sport.'

'You should be proud to have a clever son with a good future ahead of him.'

'I am, but I would much rather that he were average in both, it makes for a more rounded person.'

'No it doesn't, you couldn't be more wrong. Many, many people are mediocre and only a gifted few are brilliant. You were a good all-rounder, I take it?'

'Nothing wrong with that is there?' he said huffily.

'No.'

'Give him every encouragement, George. Clever children are usually very sensitive and I'm sure your good opinion means a great deal to him. Heavens! Where has the evening gone?' she said as there was a general move among the guests. She glanced at her watch. 'Gracious, I had no idea.'

George had looked at his own watch and was equally surprised. 'Believe it or not I just intended staying for an hour then going back to my digs to write long overdue replies to letters.' He moved away to stand in line to shake hands with his host and hostess and thank them for an enjoyable evening. He could say that in all honesty, it was an evening he would long remember.

Before making for the door his eyes searched for Connie and then she was beside him. 'We didn't get a chance to say goodbye,' she said.

'Does it have to be goodbye? And are you leaving just now?'

'No, I'll give Gwen a hand with the clearing up and Richard will see me to my door, I live quite near.'

'Could we meet?' he said urgently.

'That should be possible,' she smiled.

'A meal somewhere? You choose time and place. You know your London, Connie, and I don't.'

They met as often as they could. The theatre on two occasions and several times to the cinema. Walking was something they both enjoyed and it allowed Connie to introduce George to a London seldom seen by the tourist. She proved to be a good, knowledgeable guide. They ate in restaurants tucked away in side streets where the food was good and not ridiculously expensive. Hand-in-hand they would stroll along the Embankment, steal a kiss perhaps and no one bothered. How different from Miltonsands, but then he would never have behaved like this in Miltonsands.

With the passage of time it was now taken for granted that George Morrison was on indefinite loan to the London office but it also meant that he was down to the basic subsistence. He had been forced to reduce Laura's allowance but as he had carefully explained to her in his letter she now had her wages and the time to take on a full-time job. Letters between them were short, Laura's as short as his, but at least, Laura consoled herself, they corresponded. As to Peggy and Vera, he couldn't bring himself to write to either of his sisters. He had nothing to tell them. All they seemed interested in was the date of his return to Miltonsands.

The strain was becoming unbearable for George, and Connie, he thought, was feeling it too. Like young lovers they walked with their arms around each other. They said very little but they were both deep in thought.

'Connie, shall we stop here for a coffee?'

'Yes, that sounds like a good idea, I could do with a drink.'

They went inside. A few of the tables were occupied and they settled for one some distance from the others. A waitress took their order and a few minutes later returned with two cups of coffee.

George added sugar, stirred it, then put down the spoon. Each action was slow and deliberate.

'Connie,' he said softly as he covered her hand with his. 'I love you and I can't bear the thought of you going away.'

'I love you too.'

'Then why go away? Why can't we just get married and stay in London?' he pleaded.

'George, we've been through all this before.'

'I know, but your reason for leaving doesn't make sense to me.'

'You don't want it to.'

'If you really loved me you would give up all thought of New York and stay here in London.'

'Make no mistake about it, George, I do love you but I know myself. I can be incredibly selfish and if I've set my heart on something—'

'Like going to America?'

'Yes. If I let you persuade me to remain here it is just possible that sometime in the future I would blame you. That is a risk I am not prepared to take. In any case the sale of the house has reached its final stage.'

'You have made up your mind,' he said in a clipped voice that couldn't hide his hurt.

'Yes, George, I have made up my mind.' She paused and looked at him steadily. 'There is a solution to this but I doubt that it would appeal to you.'

'It might, I would have to hear it first.'

'Come to New York with me.'

He blinked rapidly. 'Connie, how on earth could I do that?'

'Very easily I would say. Give up your job. We can get married here and make a good life for ourselves in America.' Her eyes were dancing. 'Think seriously about it, George.'

'You don't know what you are asking.'

'I am only asking you to come with me. No, don't interrupt, let me finish. Your daughter has managed all this time on her own and by your own admission you are not a close family.'

'Even so, but I couldn't just — '

'At this moment you are not capable of serious thinking but I have done a great deal of it. According to you, Laura and this boy Michael are serious about each other and he gets on well with Ronnie.'

'It is possible that they could get married and possible too that they would give Ronnie a home,' he said thoughtfully.

'There you are then and, of course, you would have to send money for Ronnie's keep. He would still be your responsibility.'

'You have given a lot of thought to this,' he said admiringly.

'I am a good organiser, George.'

George was out of his depth. Connie was going much too fast for him. This needed a very great deal of thought. Indeed until a very, very short time ago he would not have even considered giving up his job. One didn't, especially a Civil Service position. Although he couldn't see Connie persuading him otherwise he still wanted to hear what this fascinating and remarkable woman had to say.

'Connie, what about my job? I'd be taking an awful chance chucking it in.'

'You would get a better one out there.'

'You can't be sure about that.'

'Almost sure,' she said, looking hard at him. 'No one can say more than that, there is nothing absolute in this life.'

'Exactly, and that is what worries me.'

'Forgive me saying so, George, but you don't earn a vast amount, do you?'

'No,' he said slowly and with obvious reluctance, 'nevertheless it is a decent salary and I could be in line for promotion.'

'You are not one for taking chances?'

'I'm afraid not. Not when it comes to my job.'

'I see.'

'Connie, apart from the enormity of giving up my job I have to confess that I have very little savings. Having to send money home to Laura means it is impossible to save.'

Connie was looking both thoughtful and disappointed but managed a smile before she said, 'Listen, my dearest, I've told Lottie and Harry about you and Harry appreciates that you hold down a responsible position, that you are honest and reliable. Employers are looking for those qualities and Harry will fix you up with a job, a suitable job. If it isn't exactly what you want you can take your time to look around for something else. New York, my dear George, is a city of opportunity and I just know that you will be welcomed with open arms.'

'So you say.'

She threw up her hands. 'I've done my best but if you find the risks too great, and it has to be your descision, then so be it.'

'It isn't that.' It was, but George wasn't prepared to admit it.

'Don't you want to see a bit of the world? I know I do and for me a degree of risk makes it that bit more exciting.'

Was the risk so very great? There would be a job waiting for him, so shortage of money wouldn't be an immediate problem. It needn't be a problem at all, George was thinking. Added to which Connie would be his wife.

Connie had been watching his face, seeing there both uncertainty and longing. She kept silent.

He smiled as though coming to a decision. 'I've often thought how marvellous it would be to throw up everything and travel, but it is so much easier for you, you know.'

'Not necessarily, it is a big step for me too.'

'You don't have a family to consider, I have Laura and Ronnie. What about them? How do I break it to my son and daughter that their father is marrying a clever and beautiful woman and departing for distant shores?' He said it lightly, jokingly, but he was anxiously awaiting her reply.

'Laura is a young adult,' Connie said slowly and clearly, 'she will understand that you want to make a new life for yourself. Ronnie is a problem, I admit, and I do feel guilt if in some way I am responsible for breaking up the family. On the other hand brother and sister seem to belong to each other and you were never all that close to either.'

He nodded. Connie was telling him what he wanted to hear. His smile was broad. 'Connie, my darling, I am becoming more excited by the minute.'

'Meaning that you are coming round to marriage and New York?'

'I was always in favour of marriage and if that means New York then America here I come.'

She laughed delightedly and leaned over the table to kiss him just as a rather bored-looking waitress came over with the bill.

George was his most charming. 'Two more coffees if you please,' he said, smiling into her face.

'Very good, sir, and you can sit as long as you like, until we get busy, that is.'

'Thank you.' He must leave her a tip, he didn't usually unless in the evening, but George was feeling generous.

They waited until two fresh cups of coffee were placed before them before taking up where they left off.

'I'll write to Lottie and Harry and get things moving.'

'And I'll write to Laura and tell her about us and our plans.'

'Has the poor girl any idea?'

'Probably guessed, I've mentioned a special friend and being in her company.'

'Won't come as such a shock then.'

'Being Laura she'll take it in her stride, or at least I'm hoping so.'

'Do you mind the registry office for our marriage?'

'No, that suits me very well.'

'Just the two of us and a couple of witnesses or whatever is necessary?'

'Again that suits me.'

'You won't mind not having someone of your own? Be honest.'

'Not if it is the same for you?'

'It is, but then I have no close family here.'

'That's true, but I don't think I want anyone from my side.'

Chapter Ten

The letter dropped on the mat and Ronnie, dressed for school, picked it up and went into the kitchen with it.

'Laura, it's a letter from Dad.' Before putting it on the table Ronnie examined the envelope. As always it was addressed to Miss Laura Morrison. Why couldn't it, just for once, be addressed to Master Ronnie Morrison? He wasn't blaming Laura, she always let him read the letters. But it wasn't the same just getting a read of it. It didn't have to be a long letter, he wasn't asking for that, even a postcard would do. In fact a postcard would be better. One of the Tower of London or Big Ben or anything, he wasn't asking a lot. Looking glum, he sat down at the table and waited for Laura to bring his breakfast.

'Just one letter?' Laura called through as she turned off the gas under the porridge pot. She couldn't help sounding disappointed though it was stupid of her to expect Michael to write, not after the way they had parted. She had, though. She had thought he would have let her know how he was getting on in Manchester. One of his sisters had let drop that he had got the job. The hot tears were at the back of her eyes and she blinked them away before facing her brother.

'Yes, what were you expecting?'

'Nothing, just wishful thinking,' she smiled. She put down his porridge.

Ronnie poured in milk to the very brim and she frowned.

'I keep telling you, Ronnie, not to put so much milk in or you'll spill some on the tablecloth.'

'Forgot, that's all,' he said sulkily. His eyes kept straying to the letter. Laura was taking her time about opening it. If she wasn't interested he was. Ronnie wanted to know when his dad was coming home. He wasn't in any particular hurry for it to happen, the two of them were getting on nicely, but some people were getting curious about Dad's long absence and kept asking him when he was coming home. He couldn't be forever saying he didn't know. 'When are you going to open it?'

'In a minute.' She picked it up and fingered the envelope. A lot thicker than usual, she thought, surely Dad had some news for a change. 'That's the kettle boiling,' she said, getting up quickly, 'I'll make the tea.' A few moments later she returned with the teapot covered with a multi-coloured knitted tea-cosy made by her mother from left-over wool and now badly tea-stained She had considered washing it, then decided against that since it would probably shrink. She would buy one at the next church sale of work, usually there was quite a variety on the stall. The Guild ladies were always busy knitting or sewing.

Laura took a spoonful of porridge, then slipped her finger under the flap of the envelope and brought out the pages. Three pages, two of them written on both sides.

Ronnie was growing impatient. 'Well?' he demanded. 'Is he coming home or is he not?'

Laura didn't answer, she hadn't heard him. Shock had widened her eyes and there was a loud drumming in her ear, and Ronnie, sensing that something was wrong, pushed away his porridge and got up to stand beside her.

'What does he say? And why don't you answer?'

Still she didn't reply and he pushed her arm. 'He's my dad too, I should know what is happening,' he was almost shouting. 'Is he dead or something?'

Laura had recovered slightly. 'Dad would hardly be writing to tell us he was dead.'

'I only said that because you wouldn't answer.'

'Sorry, Ronnie, the news is just so unexpected, such a shock.'

'Is he staying in London for good and we have to go and live there?' There was a gleam of interest in his eyes.

'No, I think I was prepared for that possibility.' She paused and looked at her young brother. 'Ronnie, Dad is getting married to an English lady called Connie and they are going to make their home in New York.'

'New York in America?'

'Yes.'

'Can he do that, Laura?' Ronnie sounded scared.

'He appears to be doing it anyway.'

'That means he is never coming back to Miltonsands? He is never going to live with us any more.' He sounded incredulous.

'Sounds like it,' she said gently.

'What is going to happen to us?'

She mustn't let him see that she was as scared as he was. 'We'll manage.' She smiled brightly. 'Ronnie, how long have we been on our own? Come on, clever clogs, how long?'

He thought. 'Dad left in March, didn't he?'

'Yes.'

'Next week we'll be into August so that makes it nearly six months.'

'And no disasters?'

That had him giggling. 'Some little ones.'

'Nothing we couldn't cope with.'

'Should be all right then but what if —'

'If what?'

'If he forgets to send money.'

He was voicing her own worries. 'Dad wouldn't do that.'

'Just supposing though that he didn't or it got lost. We wouldn't have enough money then, would we? You don't earn a lot, you said you didn't.'

'Ronnie, stop worrying, everything is going to be all right, and if you don't get a move on you'll be late for school.'

'Do I get to read Dad's letter when I get home?'

'Of course, it is to both of us.'

'I won't go to David's, I'll come straight home.'

'No, Ronnie, just do what you always do. I know you aren't likely to, but make no mention of this to anyone. Obviously it can't be kept a secret—'

'The people in Dad's office must know.'

'Yes, I hadn't thought of that, but we'll keep it to ourselves meantime.'

'You know what I bet?'

'Ronnie, the time,' Laura said warningly, pointing to the clock.

'I know I'm not blind, bet you anything if Aunt Peggy or Aunt Vera have had a letter from Dad one of them will be down at the post office at the double.'

Laura groaned. 'You could have spared me that.'

With Ronnie gone and on her own Laura picked up the letter and read it once again. This time she went over it slowly and carefully as if afraid of having missed something important. The address at the top of the page was the same. The scruffy digs he had complained about couldn't have been as bad as he made out or he would not have stayed all this time. She began reading.

Dear Laura,

This is a very difficult letter to write but you are adult enough to understand the loneliness of my life since your mother died. I tell myself that with my long absence you may already have guessed the news I am about to give you. Laura, my dear, I have fallen in love with a very charming and lovely lady called Connie. We met at a colleague's house and the attraction was immediate. Connie has been a widow for two years.

She was in the midst of selling her house and preparing to go and live in New York where she has a married sister. This is still to happen but now we are going out together as man and wife. There will be no wedding, just the ceremony at a registry office. Very soon after our marriage we leave for America. The date of our departure I shall give you later.

Giving up my civil service job gave me a few sleepless nights I can tell you but love for Connie won. She is very beautiful and two years younger than I. As to a job out there, that is taken care of. Connie's brother-in-law has a lot of influence and a clerical position awaits me I understand. No worries about being unemployed.

Connie won't settle for the little housewife role, not with her sharp intellect. She rather fancies something in the fashion world and she does have excellent taste in clothes. She goes for the understated look. I'm learning you see! Knowing how capable you are, Laura, I have no fears about you managing, after all you have done it up to now. You haven't mentioned Michael recently but knowing the attraction between you, I imagine he will be popping the question before long if he hasn't already done so. As regards your house-keeping this will continue until I leave the UK then other arrangements will have to be made.

With me gone the house may well be too big for you and Ronnie and perhaps it would be a good idea if you were to think of taking in a female lodger or perhaps a couple during the holiday season. There are some who would prefer to do for themselves and have the use of the kitchen but I don't see you objecting to that since you have your post office job.

Your aunts are going to be very shocked and I must confess that they have become a trial to me. Perhaps you were right all along, Laura, you always found them too interfering. I won't let them dictate. This is my life and I have every right to enjoy it.

The sad part is that after a lot of careful thought I have decided not to come through to Miltonsands to say farewell. It would be too painful for all concerned. Letters must do instead. You must continue to write to me at the usual address until I tell you otherwise. Before I forget please dispose of what remains of my clothes. I have all I need thanks to you sending on that parcel.

Since your mother's death you have been like a mother to Ronnie and for that I'll always be grateful to you. Even if Connie, who is childless, were willing to take on a stepson, which she isn't, your brother would never leave you.

[Blackmail, Laura muttered to herself.]

Please try not to think badly of me and be understanding. Had I not met Connie when I did and had we not fallen in love, then by now I should be in Fairfield Street with you both. How true it is that we never know what is ahead of us.

When word gets round there will be talk and I won't come out of it too well. Perhaps that should bother me but it doesn't. I have known great sorrow and surely it cannot be wrong to grasp a second chance of happiness. I'm still young.

Once I have the final arrangements for our departure I shall be in touch.

My love to you both,
Dad

After the shock and disbelief came the anger. He had a nerve, a diabolical nerve, to just up and away with this Connie woman. Running away from his responsibilities was what he was doing and it was so selfish and cruel of him. Didn't he ever think of anyone but himself? Why should his happiness be so important? Why should it come before all else? She fumed and banged the table. The explosion of temper helped, then despair took over as she wondered about the future. In his absence it was true she had managed perfectly well but that had been because it took only a train journey to bring him back. Now he wouldn't be coming back at all and Laura felt her panic rising. What if once he was in America with his new wife, he decided to forget about his son and daughter and the money dried up? That would suit this Connie for as he had more or less said she had no interest in a stepson or a stepdaughter. How would they live? And what would become of her clever little brother? Would he have to leave school at fourteen and take just any job? Was he to lose out just as she had? Was there anything she could do about it even at this late date? Could she beg him to stay in this country and think of them? No, she wouldn't, she wouldn't beg.

Tempting though it was to write and tell her father what she thought of him, she wouldn't. She couldn't afford to be too outspoken and she would have to be careful what she said in a letter. The money that came from him made the difference between managing and not managing. It was as simple as that.

Of course he was expecting her to look after Ronnie, and she would. She would do it because she wanted to and because it was what her mother would have expected of her. Even so, Laura couldn't help but think of the chance of happiness that she had thrown away. She wouldn't mention Michael to her father, what was the point? Instead she would give them her good wishes for their future happiness. Her weak father needed someone and this Connie sounded a very managing person.

With only herself to consider she would have gone to Manchester with Michael and then perhaps it would have been New York for them. How strange if she had met up with her father and stepmother-to-be.

Goodness! She was forgetting the time. In fifteen minutes she would have to leave the house and she couldn't afford to be late, Miss Wilkinson depended on her. Instead of getting on with the housework she had been sitting there with the letter in her hands. The beds were unmade and the breakfast dishes unwashed and they would have to remain that way. There was no time for anything but getting herself ready. Laura wasn't in the least bothered. No one would be in to see the mess and she would clear it up when she got home.

Situated as it was in the midst of a heavily populated part of Miltonsands, the post office was always busy and especially so on Thursdays and Fridays when it went like a fair. Laura was glad it was a Thursday. She wanted to be busy, to have her mind occupied, and with cash transactions she couldn't afford to let her mind wander. She managed very well. None of her customers could have guessed the turmoil of her thoughts as she smilingly served one after the other.

'Laura?'

Laura recognised the voice before she raised her head.

'Hello, Aunt Peggy, more stamps? You must be writing a lot of letters,' she smiled.

'I don't want anything,' she said in a voice a little above a whisper. 'I've had a letter, have you?'

'From Dad, you mean?'

'Of course from your father. How you can stand there and smile is beyond me.'

'For the simple reason I have to work, Aunt Peggy,' Laura said through clenched teeth. 'Please let me get on. Miss Wilkinson doesn't approve of chatting when customers are waiting to be served.' She beamed. 'Just put your parcel on the scale, Mrs Cochrane.'

'Is it well enough tied up, Laura?' the woman asked anxiously.

'A bit slack but I'll keep it aside and make it more secure.'

'Thanks, you're a nice obliging lass.'

'When do you finish?'

'Half past three, Aunt Peggy.'

'Come round and I'll have a cup of tea waiting for you.'

'All right,' Laura said resignedly. It was as well to get it over.

Like the previous two days it was coolish and dull when the sun cheated and came out in the evening. Aunt Peggy lived in a quiet street and the houses were very similar to those in Fairfield Street. The difference was in the size of rooms. Aunt Peggy's living-room was small and the heavy furniture gave it an overcrowded appearance. The surface of the table and sideboard shone, the result of much elbow grease, and there was the lingering but pleasant smell of furniture polish.

'Come away, Laura, I've infused the tea and your Aunt Vera will be here in a minute or two. I told her to come round.' As if on cue the outside door opened and closed and Aunt Vera with a tight smile came in and put down her shopping bag. She sat down on the horsehair sofa.

'A fine kettle of fish this is, Laura,' she said, sitting bolt upright.

'Don't the pair of you be starting until I have the tea out. Bring that small table over, Vera. There was no time for baking so it will just have to be a biscuit.'

'A biscuit is fine, Aunt Peggy, you didn't need to bother with anything.'

'I find a cuppie helps when we're upset.' She poured the tea, handed round milk and sugar and then a plate of biscuits.

'What on earth has come over our George?' Vera said in a strangled voice.

'Yes, what has come over the man?' Aunt Peggy added.

'Your brother has fallen in love.' Laura knew it wasn't funny, there was nothing to laugh about, but she was in danger of exploding with mirth. Maybe it was nerves.

'Some designing English besom got her clutches on him. I'm very much afraid that is what it is,' Vera said as she rattled her cup on the saucer.

'That's what I'm afraid of too,' Peggy said. 'Right from the start I said that no good would come of him going down there. Nothing but fast women and poor George would be like putty in their hands.' She crashed down her cup, spilling some in the saucer.

'Calm yourself, Peggy.'

'Calm myself? How can I calm myself when we are never going to see George again? Fancy not even coming to say goodbye.' The tears rolled down her cheeks.

'Don't let it upset you, Aunt Peggy.'

'We are both upset, Laura, but I can't say the same for you. Don't you care?'

'Of course I do.'

'Then do something.'

'Such as what, Aunt Vera?'

'I don't know, but I wish you looked more concerned.'

'I'm not going to dissolve in tears if that is what you are waiting for.'

'It's so out of character,' Peggy moaned.

There was silence apart from the munching of biscuits. A grain of biscuit was causing Aunt Vera some discomfort and she excused herself to go along to the bathroom to remove her bottom dentures and the offending crumbs.

'Sorry about that,' Vera apologised on her return. 'I should know better and keep to a soft biscuit.'

'I wouldn't blame the biscuit, more likely it's the plate getting too slack and needing some adjustment.'

'Nothing of the kind, my teeth are in perfect order, thank you very much.'

Aunt Peggy raised her eyebrows. 'More tea, Laura?'

'No, thank you, that was fine.'

'I'll get the table back to its own position.' She did so and came back to join her sister on the sofa. 'Going to London was a mistake. I tried to tell George at the time but they were so short-staffed down there and desperate to get him. Said himself he just couldn't refuse.'

'Not a word of truth in it,' Laura said quietly.

'I beg your pardon?'

'Dad didn't have to go to London, Aunt Peggy. No one tried to persuade him, he volunteered.'

'Volunteered? I don't believe it. You should be careful what you say, Laura,' Aunt Vera said sharply.

'I was taken in too until by pure chance I heard from someone in a position to know, that everyone was very surprised when George Morrison requested a transfer to London.'

That kept them both silent as they looked at each other, then Aunt Peggy turned on Laura angrily. 'It's all your fault.'

Laura was taken aback. 'How do you make that out?'

'You drove him to it.'

'I did no such thing, how dare you?' Laura had got to her feet and her eyes were flashing dangerously.

'Peggy put it rather harshly but I'm afraid I have to agree.'

'Do explain yourself and tell me where I have failed.'

'Your tone is impudent and yes, I'll tell you, you little madam.' Tiny drops of spittle were at the corner of her mouth. 'You drove him away.'

'How did I manage that, Aunt Peggy?'

'You and your never-ending grumbles. What kind of home-coming was that after a long hard day? A man needs a bit of peace and quiet and you should have been seeing to your father's comfort instead of feeling sorry for yourself and complaining to him that he did nothing to assist.'

'You get a lot of help from Uncle Archie.'

'All men aren't the same,' she blustered, 'and I'm not as able as I was.'

Laura took a big shaky breath. 'I admit that my first efforts at house keeping left much to be desired but I don't remember being over-whelmed with help from you or Aunt Vera. What I did get and could have done without was advice, there was plenty of that.'

'Your mother made a poor job of your upbringing, that becomes more evident every day,' Aunt Peggy said with a sniff.

'Leave my mother out of it. She was the best mother any girl could have and God only knows how she put up with you two all those years.'

Aunt Peggy gasped. 'Such language and taking God's name in vain.'

'I'm sorry, I don't normally talk like that but you make me so angry.' She took a deep breath. 'Before I go let me tell you something about your precious brother. If you hadn't mollycoddled him all his early life he might be a stronger person today.'

'Are you suggesting—' Aunt Vera seemed unable to go on.

'You spoilt him rotten, that's what I'm telling you.'

'You've said too much, my girl, now will you kindly leave my house?'

'With the greatest of pleasure,' Laura said, getting to her feet.

Her head held high and flushed with triumph, Laura walked to the door, opened it, went along the narrow lobby to the front door and let herself out. When she had calmed down she would no doubt regret saying so much but just now she felt that she had fought and won a war.

'Laura, you didn't!' Ronnie was rubbing his hands together and there was admiration in his eyes.

'I did, and I've given it to you more or less word for word.'

'Wish I'd been there. Wish I could have seen their faces.'

'I'm glad you didn't.' She grinned. 'Aunt Peggy was nearly purple and I thought Aunt Vera's eyes were going to pop out of her head.'

'You know something, you don't need to worry about Dad finding out because I've read his letter and he doesn't like them as much as he used to.'

'True. I wonder if she'll come into the post office or get someone else to buy her stamps.'

'Or go in when you're not there,' Ronnie added. 'Do you think she'll ever speak to you again?'

'Once she cools off she won't be able to resist asking about Dad because I don't see him writing too often to them.'

'He'll write to us, won't he?'

The worry was back in his voice and hearing it she grew more worried herself. 'Of course he will, didn't he say so in his letter?'

'I didn't like what he said about a lodger. I don't want anyone else in the house.'

'I'm not keen on it either.'

'It wouldn't be like our own house any more, that would be the worst of it.'

'We could manage to keep ourselves separate.' She smiled at her brother. He was trying hard to be grown up and she was proud of the effort he was making.

'Summer visitors wouldn't be so bad, Laura. It would only be for a few weeks.'

'We are too far away from the beach. Attracting lodgers wouldn't be easy, certainly not so easy as Dad seems to think.'

'Laura?'

'What now?' She looked up from darning a stocking, then snipped the wool with the scissors. 'If you cut your toe-nails shorter you wouldn't be so hard on your stockings.'

Ronnie chose to ignore that. 'You wouldn't do anything without telling me, would you?'

'Nothing important.'

'I might think something was important that you don't.'

'Don't worry, we'll talk everything over.'

'David's mum said I was the man of the house and I had to do everything to help you.'

'You already do.' Laura smiled as she saw him puff out his chest. Poor boy, he was having to grow up before his time. The physical changes were there too and the awful thinness had gone. His face had filled out and there was some flesh about his shoulders. He would never have his father's build nor be half as handsome, but he would be better equipped for life. Already there was a determination about the chin and the intelligent eyes missed very little.

Disappointing summer weather meant buckets and spades bought especially for the holidays being left in the boarding-houses and parents searching for other ways to entertain their children. Then the clouds would lift, the sun come out, and smiles replace the sulks. There would be a mad rush to collect buckets and spades and all the other paraphernalia necessary for the beach. Those who, minutes earlier, had been secretly wishing themselves home now lay contentedly on the warm sands with eyes closed and hearing the excited shrieks of the little ones as they played in the sand building castles or running down to paddle in the sea.

There was no Sunday School during the summer months but Ronnie declared himself finished with Sunday School. He'd had enough and wouldn't be going back, he was too big, he said and his friends weren't going back either or so he said.

'I won't make you.'

'You can't.'

'You must go to church though.'

'You don't always go.'

'I don't always have the time.'

'You said there is always time to do what you want to do,' he said cheekily.

Laura had to laugh, she had said it a number of times. It was what her mother used to say. 'All right, we'll both go.'

'Every Sunday?'

'Nearly every Sunday.'

The hot weather had been slow to come but it was lasting. Laura was in the garden doing some weeding. She wore a faded sleeveless summer dress and her fair hair was tied back. Cropped hair was all the rage and she was thinking of having her own cut short. She would have gone for the new look sooner but Michael hadn't approved. Michael had nothing to do with her now, she could please herself. Laura sighed as she tugged at a particularly stubborn weed. She had lived in hope that Michael would get in touch but he hadn't and he wouldn't now. In a fit of loneliness she had nearly persuaded herself to get his address from his sister and write. Just a friendly letter, but she hadn't and she wouldn't now.

Ronnie had been at church and changed out of his Sunday suit.

'Good turn-out?'

'Not bad.'

'Sermon interesting?' she asked.

'Not very and it was too long.' He started to laugh. 'Mr Skinner, you know—'

'Yes, I know who you mean.'

'He gave a mighty snore and his wife gave him such a dig with her elbow that he nearly fell off the seat.'

'I don't believe a word of it, you are making this up, Ronnie Morrison.'

'No, honestly, he was nodding and Mrs Skinner—'

'Gave him a gentle push, that sounds much more like it.'

'Oh, well.'

'That sounds like someone at our door, go and see who it is.'

Ronnie returned with David and his mother.

'Hello, Jane. Hello, David,' Laura said, getting up from her knees. 'I shouldn't be doing this on the Sabbath day. My mother would have had a fit.'

'See no harm in it. The better the day, the better the deed, isn't it?'

'What does that mean?' David asked.

'You tell him, Ronnie.'

'Laura, my dad's working in the garden. He's cutting the grass and Mum said he won't go to heaven.'

'I said nothing of the sort.'

'Yes, you did and Dad said he didn't have much chance of going there anyway.'

Laura laughed. 'We'll all be together.'

David was a nice-looking boy, sturdier than Ronnie with a healthy complexion and thick brown hair. His eyes were brown and soft like a spaniel's.

'Were you helping your dad, David?'

'No, Dad says I don't know the difference between a flower and a weed.'

'Your pal doesn't either.'

'When is a weed not a weed?' Ronnie asked.

'You answer the professor, Jane.'

'A weed is a weed, Ronnie, because, well, it just is.'

'But why? Lots of them have pretty flowers.'

'Dandelions are not pretty,' Jane said as though grasping at a straw and appealing to Laura.

'We think dandelions are pretty, don't we, David?'

'No, but I think daisies are.'

'Daisies aren't weeds, that's why,' Laura said, then tried to change the subject, but she might have known her brother wasn't satisfied.

'Why do you pull them out when they just start to grow again?'

'If we didn't the whole garden would be overgrown.'

'You two,' said Jane going into her purse, 'go and buy yourselves ice cream and don't hurry back.'

They went away grinning.

Jane picked up the hoe.

'No, Jane, I don't want you working, we'll go inside and I'll put the kettle on.'

Jane shook her head. 'Never refuse help. Thirty minutes' gardening, then inside for tea and a gossip.'

At the end of thirty minutes the earth had been turned over and the weeds removed. 'Thanks, Jane, I'm very grateful. You get through twice as much in the same time.'

'I like gardening, it's when I do my thinking,' she smiled. 'The roses look healthy, I like that deep red.'

'They don't need much attention, that's what I like about them.'

Jane followed Laura indoors. 'You wash your hands in the bathroom and I'll use the sink.'

Laura got out an old card table and put it at the back door where it was cooler. She set the cups and cut some sultana cake.

'I'm glad you came,' Laura said as they drank their tea, 'I felt in need of a bit of company.'

'You can always come round to me,' Jane said gently.

'I know, but there never seems to be the time, or more truthfully I don't organise myself properly.' She paused. 'You've heard?'

'Yes, but not from Ronnie.'

'What did you hear, if you don't mind telling me?'

'That Mr Morrison was marrying an English woman and going off to Australia.'

'Apart from the country being wrong that is about it. They're going to live in New York, Jane. Dad is married now,' Laura said in a small voice, 'and they leave for America next week.'

'How do you feel about it or is that a silly question?'

Laura shrugged. 'It's not a silly question and I don't know how I feel about it. To begin with I was just too shocked to feel anything except perhaps anger. Jane, when I think too much about it I just get scared.'

'No need to be scared. You've managed very well all this time. In fact I would say you have been absolutely wonderful.'

'It was different before. You see, anything too difficult for me to handle Dad was near enough to come and take charge or tell me what to do. I didn't worry too much because at the end of the day the responsibility was his. Am I rambling on or does that make sense to you?'

'Yes, it does,' Jane said thoughtfully. 'Thinking about it I'm not sure how I would cope on my own with David.'

'You are a manager, Jane, you would be all right.'

'Perhaps, one doesn't know until one is faced with it. There is nothing to be scared of though. I mean, nothing awful is going to happen.'

'I know, it's just my overactive imagination.' She couldn't tell Jane or anyone of the fear that haunted her day and night. Far, far worse during the night when she would waken from a dream drenched in sweat. In the dream that was a nightmare she and Ronnie were alone with no house and no money and nowhere to turn.

'You aren't alone, my dear, you have your friends and those awful aunts.'

'Those awful aunts and I have fallen out.'

'Now that is a pity. Relatives, I know, can be a trial but when it comes to the bit blood is thicker than water. They would want to help, I'm sure.'

'They'll come round in their own good time. Not because they have much love for me but they'll be desperate to know about their brother.'

'Won't he write to them?'

'He didn't bother much when he was in London. They wrote regularly but only once or maybe twice did he send a short note. The second note would be giving them the news about his forthcoming marriage and his plans.'

'Don't be angry if I ask one more question.'

'Ask anything.'

'What has gone wrong between you and Michael?'

'We parted company because Michael has moved to a job in Manchester.'

'Am I right in thinking that he wanted you to go with him or have an understanding and you refused?'

'Yes, something like that.'

'Was there no way round it?'

Laura felt a spurt of anger. Even Jane didn't seem to understand.

'Try putting yourself in my position but make it a younger you and David your young brother.'

Jane was silent. When she spoke there was sympathy in her voice. 'Very difficult, I do understand that.'

'You do see that I just couldn't leave Ronnie?'

'Yes, but it is so unfair. Your father just waltzes off and leaves you with the responsibility for his son.'

'Jane, Ronnie must never get to know.'

'That you lost Michael because you had your brother to look after?'

'Yes.'

'Probably Ronnie will have worked that out for himself.'

'No, I don't think so. He suggested in all seriousness that since Michael had gone to Manchester I should find myself a new boyfriend.'

'Why don't you?'

Laura smiled. 'I wouldn't object to the occasional night out but I am not going to get serious about anyone. It would be unfair.'

'Are you heartbroken about Michael?'

'Was I in love with him? Yes, I loved Michael very much, he was part of my life and I still miss him dreadfully.'

'First love, was it?'

'Yes, started when I went up to senior school, then he was away and we didn't see each other. When we did meet up we just seemed to pick up where we left off.'

'This may not help but I'll risk saying it. If what you shared was real love, Laura, somehow you would have found a way of being together.'

'There was no way, Jane, unless Ronnie came too.'

'That was asking a lot of Michael.'

'Too much as it happened.'

Chapter Eleven

With her duty in the post office over, Laura was back home and catching up with some housework when she heard the knock. Wondering who it could be, she put down the duster and went to answer the door. Standing on the doorstep was Uncle Archie and she gave him a surprised but delighted smile.

'Uncle Archie, come in, come in. Ages since I saw you.' Then a little warily as she remembered her quarrel with Aunt Peggy, 'Oh, dear, you are speaking to me then?'

'Och, lass, yon's what I've come about.'

A joiner to trade, Uncle Archie wore his brown overalls over his everyday clothes and carried a large bag of tools. He was of medium height, reduced by his slight stoop which had developed in spite of his wife's repeated scoldings to straighten himself up unless he wanted to look an old man before his time.

'This you knocking off early?' Laura said as she got him seated.

'Something I'm not guilty of, lass, but I had a mind to come here today. Someone has to sort this out.'

'I'm blaming no one, least of all you. Peggy's tongue has a habit of running away with her but she has her good qualities and she's a good wife. That said I'm not blind to her faults but then who amongst us hasn't some?'

'I do know that, Uncle Archie, and I'm not making out—'

'She's upset, lass, real upset and missing sleep over it.'

'That makes two of us. She upset me, Uncle Archie.'

'I don't doubt it and I'm not here to plead her case.'

Laura had drawn her chair close to his and she was leaning forward with her fingers locked together.

'Maybe I lost my temper and said more than I should—'

'You both lost the heid, woman-like, and said things you didn't mean.'

Laura couldn't go along with that. She had meant them, meant every single word, but she wouldn't say so to Uncle Archie. He was trying to be the peacemaker so she nodded her head.

'Yon crack about spoiling your dad went home. By jove it did, Laura, and I'm telling you this, I had a quiet smile to myself. You'll no' mind my outspokenness but your mother, bless her soul, carried on where they left off.'

'I know, and I had no intentions of doing likewise.' She grinned. 'Poor Dad, I used to get so mad at him sitting about feeling sorry for himself. He could do something about the house I used to tell him and that made him crosser than ever.'

'He could have given you a bit of help but he's your father and I'll say no more.'

'I muddled through.'

His grey head nodded. 'You got there and believe it or not Peggy is coming very near to admitting that they let George off with too much.'

'No kidding?'

'No kidding. She's had her eyes opened. Found it hard to believe that George lied about having to go to London.'

'Maybe I shouldn't have said anything about Dad volunteering—'

'Better you did.'

'Maybe he wanted to go to London to get away from me?'

'No lass, it was to escape his responsibilities. Never could see it myself what folk saw in London.'

'Have you been in London, Uncle Archie?'

'Years ago I was there for two days and that was long enough. I'll grant you there are some fine buildings and it is a city we should visit once in our lifetime but to live there – all that noise and bustle, couldn't be doing with it.'

'I hope to go one day for a lengthy stay.'

'Could be it's improved since I was there but then you see, Laura, I was never one for city life.' He paused and had a look around the living-room. 'You've everything looking grand.'

'Thanks.'

He patted her hand. 'Still miss your mother as bad?'

'Yes, Uncle Archie, but not in a tearful way. I just feel so sad and then I feel angry that she was taken.'

'She was a good lass was Ellen.'

'I wish I were more like her,' Laura said wistfully.

'No two folk are alike. You are a fine lass yourself, I see nothing wrong with you. You've good spirit and it'll see you through all your troubles. We all have them, troubles I mean, but that is life.'

'The aunts – sorry, I mean Aunt Peggy and Aunt Vera – don't think much of me.'

'I wouldn't say that, just a wee bit of resentment more like.'

'Why resentment?'

'I never said this, remember, but you and Ronnie have a lot on top and ours are very average. School for them was a place to get away from as quickly as possible. Mind, that's a true saying that you can take a horse to the trough but you can't make it drink.'

Laura thought about her cousins. They were older but seemed contented enough and she said so to her uncle.

He nodded. 'They had the sense like their old man to accept their limitations and settle for what they could do and do well. Peggy, like many a mother, set her sights too high.'

'My extra years at school didn't do me much good.'

'You liked school and you enjoyed learning?'

'Yes, I did.'

'Then it wasn't wasted, education never is. Missing out on college was a pity, a great shame I would say, but it is possible to succeed and you are going to make a success of your life. That said tell me about the young lad.'

'Not so little now, Uncle Archie, he's stretching and filling out too.'

'Your good cooking,' he winked.

'Could be,' she smiled. 'I'm glad though that he can stick up for himself now. Instead of running away from bullies he faces up to them.'

'I'm glad to hear it. Bullies are cowards. Clever bairns, particularly boys, don't have it easy, they have a lot to put up with but in the end they reap the benefits.'

Laura jumped up. 'What on earth am I thinking about? I'll go and put the kettle on this very minute.'

'You won't.' He put out a restraining hand. 'Just sit yourself down. I didn't come to drink tea. I really came to ask a favour.'

Laura's heart sank. She knew what the favour would be. Uncle Archie wanted her to apologise to Aunt Peggy and she couldn't. She just couldn't. The words would stick in her throat.

'Lass, you have to remember this. Peggy was more like a mother to your dad than a sister and all this carry on, him pretending he had to go to London and taking up with an English woman—' He stopped and shook his head. 'She's taking it bad. One minute angry then bursting into tears and my Peggy isn't the tearful kind.'

'I am sorry, Uncle Archie, and I can't understand Dad. He must have changed because he would never willingly have hurt his sisters.'

'There are times I could wring his neck, Laura, but we are family and we have to forgive and forget.' He smiled. 'We don't have to like our relatives but we have to pull together because at the end of the day we have to help one another.'

'You talk a lot of good sense, Uncle Archie.'

'Think I was meant for the pulpit,' he twinkled.

'Not so many nodding off if you were. Uncle Archie, if it is any help to Aunt Peggy, Dad didn't write home all that often and I only replied to the ones I got.'

'Sensible of you. Peggy wrote far too often and I told her that. I have to confess that I am no great correspondent and George probably couldn't be bothered when he got back to his digs which from all accounts were very grim.'

'Can't have been as bad as he made out or he wouldn't have stayed there so long. If all he did was sleep in his digs and eat out I suppose he could put up with it.'

'This new woman in his life will be taking up most of his attention. I was about to say that there is no fool like an old fool but then George isn't that old and besides he is a fine-looking man.'

'A few around here were casting their eyes in his direction.'

'Likely made it too obvious and scared the man away. The English female would have known better.'

'Connie is supposed to be lovely and very intelligent.'

'No photograph or snapshot?'

'Not as yet.'

'How do you feel about having a stepmother?'

'I don't think of her as that, just the woman Dad is married to.'

'You must be curious about her?'

'Not very.'

'Laura?'

'I know. You want me to apologise to Aunt Peggy, don't you?'

'I do not. I wouldn't ask that of you. Let Peggy make the first move and believe me that will be as hard for her to do as it would be for you.' His eyes were pleading. 'When she does you will go half-way to meet her, won't you?'

'More than half-way I promise you.'

He got up. 'I'm glad I've got all that off my chest and now I'll be getting on my way.' He looked at the clock. 'That the right time?'

'A minute or two fast.'

'Good! I'll be arriving home about my usual time.' He picked his bag up from the floor. 'We'll keep this visit a secret. Mind now, any wee job that needs doing let me know. No use having a joiner in the family and not making use of him.'

'Thanks, I'll remember that.'

'Your mother could turn her hand to anything. I used to tell her she should have been a laddie and she would have made a first-class joiner.'

'I can't even hammer in a nail straight.'

'You have other talents. Tell Ronnie I was asking for him and tell him to stick in at school. The day will come when we will all be very proud of him.' He patted her on the arm. 'Cheerio, Laura, and see and take care of yourself.'

'Cheerio, Uncle Archie.' She watched him go and felt a lump in her throat. Her mother used to say that Archie was the salt of the earth and she could only agree.

About three weeks after Uncle Archie's visit, Aunt Peggy came into the post office. It was a quiet spell and Laura was taking the opportunity to check the postal orders and mark down on the requisition pad those that were running low.

'Busy, are you?'

Laura stopped her counting and looked up quickly. She had recognised the voice.

'It's you, Aunt Peggy.'

'Yes, it's me.' She was smartly dressed in a herring-bone coat with the collar turned up and a pink chiffon scarf at the neck. Her head was uncovered and her hair looked as though it had just had a marcel wave which turned out to be the case. 'I'm just out of the hairdresser's and I didn't want to flatten it with a hat.'

'Looks very nice.'

'The new lass is coming on,' she said, patting her hair. 'I hope she stays longer than the last one but I doubt it. She's a bonny girl and all her talk is of her young man.'

Her aunt was talking for talking's sake, Laura thought. She was obviously ill at ease and Laura surprised herself by feeling sorry for the woman. Surely it wasn't beyond her to make the first move. In a sense Aunt Peggy had already made it by coming into the post office.

'Aunt Peggy—'

'Laura—'

They spoke together, then both laughed. Aunt Peggy got in just ahead.

'I'll say this for myself, I'm not one to harbour a grudge. If you are prepared to forgive and forget, Laura, so am I.'

'Happy to, Aunt Peggy. I've been hoping you would come in, and Uncle—' Laura clapped her hand over her mouth. 'I mean—'

'You mean you weren't supposed to let me know that Archie had been to see you?'

'I didn't mean to say that,' Laura said wretchedly, 'it just came out.' She wondered what Uncle Archie would think of her.

'That I gathered, but no harm done since I already knew.'

'You did?' Laura said faintly.

'Lass, you don't live with a man as long as I have without knowing when they are trying to keep something from you. Archie has never been able to hide anything. Two or three times he has given himself away but I never let on.'

'I thought a lot of him for coming.'

'My man speaks his mind when he feels it necessary and holds his tongue when he thinks that will do more good.'

'Very sensible, pity more of us weren't like him.'

'Oh, he has his annoying habits and there are times he just about sends me up the wall.' She smiled at Laura. 'There's a saying that the shoemaker's bairns are the worst shod and as for a joiner – I wouldn't like to tell you how long I've been waiting for an extra shelf in the scullery. When I've time, when I've time is all I get or else he goes conveniently deaf.'

Laura giggled. 'He offered to do any small job.'

'So he would and you would get them done too. Very obliging is Archie until it comes to his own house. That said, maybe I wouldn't have him different.'

Two women with bulging shopping bags came in.

'Better let you get on with what you are paid to do but before I go —' She stopped.

'What were you going to say?'

'Mind if I come round to Fairfield Street? Sometime when it is convenient but I must be home in plenty of time to prepare your uncle's meal.'

'Come about four today, I'll be home by then.'

'That'll do champion.' She turned to apologise to the two women waiting patiently. 'Don't blame my niece, I kept her talking.'

'No harm in having a wee blether and we're in no hurry.'

'I'll be round the back of four.'

Laura nodded and smiled, feeling light-headed with relief. The first meeting between aunt and niece since the exchange of angry words had not been the ordeal she feared. In fact it had gone remarkably well. Neither of them had taken back anything and it wasn't a case of forgiving and forgetting. What had been said couldn't be unsaid and for her part Laura wouldn't take a word of it back. She had only spoken the truth and she knew that from now on there would be a wariness between them and that included Aunt Vera. Laura told herself that she didn't mind, that it was probably better that way.

She didn't linger and left her work sharply, wondering what it was her aunt wanted. Once home, she threw her coat over a chair and hurried to put the kettle on. After that she brought over the small table and gave it a quick dust since it didn't get one every day. On it went an embroidered cloth then the tea things. The Madeira cake didn't appear to be too dry and she cut it into slices before placing a doyley on the plate and arranging the cake. The biscuit tin was empty, Ronnie was making a habit of raiding it when he got home from school. She made a mental note to remind him that biscuits were too expensive and he would have to make do with bread and jam in future.

When Aunt Peggy arrived everything was ready.

'I didn't mean you to go to all this trouble,' she said, slipping her costume jacket off and having it taken from her and put on a chair.

'No trouble at all. I like a cup of tea when I get in.'

'The lad not home yet?'

'He usually is but Ronnie said he was staying behind to do something for his teacher.' Laura fervently hoped that Aunt Peggy would be gone before her brother put in his appearance. Ronnie wasn't very good at hiding his feelings.

Laura poured the tea and handed her aunt the plate of Madeira cake.

'Thank you.' She put it on her plate and cut it in two. 'This marriage, what are your feelings on it?'

'I'm just accepting it. What else can I do?'

'Nothing at all, but you must have feelings on the matter?'

'To be honest I'm finding the marriage easier to accept than him going off to New York.'

'Terrible that, not coming to say goodbye. You would have thought they would both have come but then again maybe George didn't want us to meet this Connie woman.'

'Probably Dad said much the same to you, that he had fallen in love and Connie has connections in New York to help them. He's gone, Aunt Peggy, and we are better to keep our thoughts to ourselves.'

'You are being very sensible I must say. This is a nice piece of cake. Madeira gets that dry sometimes.' She drank some tea then spoke again. 'Mind, I did expect George to marry again but not so soon, and when he did we, Vera and I, thought it would be to someone from these parts.'

Laura smiled. 'Those available didn't appeal.'

'This is none of my business but Archie thinks I should ask. How are you managing financially?'

'I'm managing. Dad gave me a bit extra to tide me over until he can make arrangements to send money.'

'That's fine. I told Archie that your father would see you all right.'

Laura hid her worry. She didn't doubt but that the money would come eventually but the extra she spoke of had been very little and would be swallowed up since the landlord had decided to up the rents.

'More tea?'

'No, but I enjoyed that.' She smiled. 'What about yourself? Is it still on with this Michael?'

'No, it's all off, Aunt Peggy, Michael is working in Manchester.'

Her aunt noted the bleak expression. 'You'll miss him?'

'Yes, I do but I'm getting over it.'

'Life is full of disappointments.'

'Michael wanted me to go with him to Manchester,' she said in a rush.

'You mean he proposed marriage?'

'Yes.' What else could she have meant?

'You weren't ready to settle down?'

'I was ready but I have Ronnie to consider.'

'From all accounts and I don't see that much of him, but being a quiet laddie he wouldn't be any bother.'

'Aunt Peggy, be fair. How many young men would be prepared to start married life with the added responsibility of a young boy?'

'Many have landed with a crabbit mother-in-law.'

Laura laughed. 'Never thought of that but you could be right.'

'How is the lad taking his father's desertion?'

'He doesn't say much about it but you have to remember they were never close.'

'More's the pity. Still clings to you?'

'Not in the way you mean,' Laura said sharply. 'Ronnie does everything he possibly can to help me and we had better stop talking about him because I hear the door.'

'Hello, Ronnie,' Aunt Peggy beamed.

Ronnie stopped dead, opened his mouth, saw Laura's warning look and closed it again.

'This you being kept behind at school?'

'I wasn't kept in,' he muttered, 'Miss Ingram wanted books transferred from one cupboard to another and she asked two of us to help her.' He dropped his schoolbag on the floor.

Laura saw Aunt Peggy look at it.

'Take your schoolbag up to your bedroom as you always do, then once you have washed your hands come and get some tea.'

Ronnie looked at his sister in amazement. He never took his schoolbag up to his bedroom, he did his homework on the kitchen table. Picking it up, he went to the door and with Aunt Peggy's back to him he made a face and put out his tongue.

'My word, he is stretching and probably eating you out of house and home.'

'Sometimes I wonder where he puts it all.'

'I'll get on my way now if you don't mind. Not once has Archie come into an empty house, not like some I could mention. Thanks for the tea, lass, and well, it's fine that all that unpleasantness is behind us,' she said awkwardly.

'Thanks for coming and give Uncle Archie my love.'

Ronnie came running downstairs when he heard the door shut.

'What did she come for?'

'To make peace.'

'Pull the other.'

'No, really, and I'm glad, Ronnie. She is family and we are better to be on speaking terms.'

'If you say so. That cake is like sawdust, is there nothing else?'

'No, and you'll have to go easy on the biscuits.'

'Why?'

'Because money doesn't grow on trees. See that,' she pointed to a letter on the mantelpiece, 'that is notification of an increase in rent.'

'What a cheek. How much?'

'More than we can afford. Read it yourself and that way you'll understand how essential it is to economise.'

'I don't see why, Laura. Dad will get more money in America than he got here. You'll have to write and tell him to send more because the rent has gone up.'

'If only it were that easy. We don't know that he is working, Ronnie.'

'He said there was a job waiting for him.'

'He said a lot of things.'

'You could write and tell him though, couldn't you?'

'Not until I get an address.'

'Why don't you have one?'

'You read the letter yourself. Remember he said that they were to be staying with Connie's relations until they found somewhere of their own.'

'No address for those relations either?'

She shook her head. 'No.'

'Why would he not give you their address?' He was looking worried.

'Must have forgotten.'

'Who else would know?'

'No one.'

'Somebody must, Laura.'

'All we have is the address of his digs and he won't have left a forwarding address there.'

'Nobody knows where they are?' His eyes were round in disbelief.

'Connie will have left word with someone but that isn't any help to us.'

'Maybe he just wants to forget about us.'

'Don't be silly,' she said sharply. 'The letters have been delayed, that's all. It does happen, it's not unknown.'

'I know that, I'm not stupid,' he said angrily as he carried the cups through to the kitchen.

Laura closed her eyes, she hadn't meant to snap. 'I'm sorry, Ronnie, I didn't mean to take it out on you but Dad is the absolute limit. He must know that I'll be hard pressed for money and he could have done something about it before now.'

'I won't eat any more biscuits, I promise.'

She gave him a quick hug. 'Just go easy on them that's all.'

'Maybe I'll manage to get a job. Mr Thomson said there was a chance he would need a boy after school. And if I don't get that I might get a Saturday job.'

A few short weeks ago and Laura would have said that it was unnecessary but not now. Every little helped and it would go towards clothes for him.

Chapter Twelve

Wearied after tossing and turning and unable to sleep, Laura got up and in her bare feet padded over to the window. She parted the curtains and gazed out at the night sky, her brow pressed to the cold pane. An aspirin might have helped to ease the throbbing in her temples brought about by worry. They were in the bathroom cabinet and she didn't want to risk disturbing Ronnie. Not that it was very likely, he usually slept soundly, but he sensed that she was more worried than she made out and that uneasiness had transferred to him.

Even the aunts had gone quiet on the subject and no longer enquired if Laura had received a letter. They all waited and hoped but slowly hope was fading. She kept her financial worries to herself. Pride wouldn't allow her to seek help but clearly something would have to be done and soon. She was seeing her small savings dwindling away.

Sometimes Laura's anger was so great that she wanted to scream and felt an urge to hurl articles about the room. What right had her father to heap those worries on to her? Didn't he care what happened to them? Had his new wife such an influence on him that he could conveniently forget the other life he had left behind? In calmer moments Laura knew that she was being unfair blaming her stepmother but she had to blame someone and it was easier to blame Connie, the stranger, than put all the blame on to her dad. In a strange sort of way that made no sense she felt protective of him.

She had made all the enquiries she could. The ship had docked safely with its passengers and listed were a Mr and Mrs George Morrison. Only when it could no longer be put off did Laura take a bus to her father's old office and ask to speak to Mr Hart.

He came. A kindly, middle-aged man with greying hair and she saw his bewilderment.

'So completely out of character, Laura.' He shook his head. 'Indeed his wish to take a temporary transfer to London surprised us though we accepted that after his sad loss he felt the need of a change.' He smiled at her. 'He did say how well you were coping.'

Laura clutched at the 'completely out of character'. It gave her an opening. 'As you say, Mr Hart, it isn't like my father and that is why we are all so worried.'

'I can fully understand your concern but what I cannot understand is George not leaving an address with you. Somewhere where he could be contacted.'

'He – I mean they were to be staying with my stepmother's relations until such time as they found their own accommodation. My father was promised a job, he wouldn't have gone otherwise. Everything was arranged and the only explanation is that he thought he had given me an address,' she ended lamely.

Mr Hart was tapping the top of his pen on the desk and looking thoughtful. 'He could be ill, but then surely your stepmother would have written.'

William Hart saw the dark shadows under the lovely eyes and felt outrage that any father could do this to his daughter. He had found George Morrison a pleasant and conscientious worker but not a lot of backbone about him. His good looks had a lot to do with it, he thought. His kind always had willing slaves.

'You would have thought so.' She looked down at her fingers locked together. Until recently she hadn't done that. It was another sign of stress. She unlocked them.

'There should have been a few letters by now and I can't be forever blaming the post office,' she smiled. She got to her feet. 'It was good of you to see me, Mr Hart.'

He sprang to his feet. 'Not at all, I'm just sorry I can't be more helpful. Perhaps there is one other approach we can try?'

Laura felt a small surge of hope. 'There is?'

'If you wish I'll get in touch with the London office and see if anyone there can throw some light on the mystery.'

'I would be very grateful,' she said quietly.

Laura left the building. The talk hadn't been particularly helpful though Mr Hart had done his best. She didn't expect much help from the London office. Her father hadn't been there long enough to make close friends and Connie, as far as she was aware, had no association with the office.

She would keep her misery private. No one liked a gloomy face. It was far better to look on the bright side. At this very moment there could be a letter lying on the mat, a letter with an American stamp.

Why was Michael so often in her thoughts these days? Could it mean that he was thinking of her? It was a nice thought.

The end of a busy day with the last customer served. Laura was on her way home when she saw him. She blinked and looked again, unable to believe her eyes. It was as though all her lonely longing had conjured him out of the air. Was she imagining it? Would he disappear? No, it was Michael and he had seen her. She saw his start of surprise then that remembered smile and she was almost running.

'Michael, it is you? I thought I was imagining things. What are you doing here?' she babbled.

'A short break. Arrived last night.'

'For how long?'

'A week.'

'A whole seven days, that's not short, it's wonderful.' Her eyes were shining. 'Is Manchester all you hoped it would be?'

'That and a bit more—' He broke off as a girl came out of the shop and walked over to stand beside him. She was petite and dark and very, very pretty. She glanced quickly at Laura then turned to Michael.

'They didn't have what I wanted, Michael,' she said, smiling into his face.

'Never mind, I'll show you where else to try.' He put an arm round her shoulder. 'Alice, I want you to meet a very old friend of mine. This is Laura and she and I were great friends at school.'

Laura's lips felt stiff but she forced them into a smile. 'Alice, just in case you are adding years to my age,' she said quickly, 'let me tell you that Michael is three years older.'

Alice pouted prettily. 'Cradle snatching, darling, I always kept to the boys in my own year.' She broke into a laugh, a surprisingly loud laugh for such a small girl. Michael, Laura was remembering, hated loud laughter in girls.

Inside she was weeping but she wouldn't rush away and give

Michael the satisfaction of seeing her upset. Maybe she spoke too quickly, laughed too often, but on the whole she was pleased with her performance. She chose the time to part, showing the right degree of regret and saying how simply delightful it had been to see them. Then she was walking away and putting the distance between them. The silly smile she wiped off her face and with tears nearly blinding her Laura took the road to the beach. Few people would be down there, it was too chilly and the grey sky promised rain.

The lonely beach stretched for miles and on the shore a few sea-birds pecked about the sand. Far out where it would seem that sky and sea met was the faint outline of a ship. She watched until she could no longer see it. What a fool she had been to believe that Michael would come back into her life. It had all finished before he went to Manchester and now he had a new love. She had learnt something. She was on her own.

So many calculations but always the same result. Another scrap of paper went into the fire. It was no use, she couldn't make ends meet. Her job, even with the extra hours she worked and Ronnie's small contribution from his Saturday job, did not cover their expenses. With ever more scrimping and saving they might have managed to hang on but not with the steep rise in the rent. Soon she would have no savings. She wouldn't beg, borrow or steal, so what was left? A card in the newsagent's window offering a room to a lodger, male or female, with or without attendance, had yielded nothing.

'Sorry, Laura, if it is any consolation you are not alone. Those other two cards have been in the window longer than yours.'

'No one is interested?' She gave a sad smile.

The shopkeeper shrugged. 'Could be the summer will bring something but then again it might not. We're at the wrong end of the town and folk don't want a walk to the beach, not with bairns they don't.'

'Thanks anyway, Mr McKenzie.'

'Leave it. You never know your luck and it's not doing any harm where it is.'

Or any good, Laura thought as the all too familiar depression took hold. Back in the house she considered what her next step should be. The house was too big for them since no one wanted the spare room. She could try for an exchange to a smaller house but that could take a long time and there would be the removal expenses.

She picked up the newspaper and went over the situations vacant but with little hope. She had a fair wage from Miss Wilkinson for the hours she worked and with her lack of experience in office work, even if she was taken on the likelihood would be less money than she was getting now. Her eyes went down the page. Not many vacancies and hardly any in Miltonsands. These were hard times. Domestics wanted, she made a face and wondered if she could hold down two jobs. One might be worth another read. She took a mouthful of tea that she had allowed to get cold and then went back to the paper.

Kindly woman urgently wanted to look after
small child. Comfortable accommodation for
right person includes own sitting-room. Apply
giving full particulars.

It was obvious to Laura that they were seeking a mature woman, a motherly type. Had it not been for the mention of accommodation Laura wouldn't have given it another thought. A bedroom and a sitting-room for one's own use. Could she see a single bed in that sitting-room? The bedroom for Ronnie, a quiet boy who would give no trouble and a bed-sitting-room for herself. How marvellous to have a roof over their head and no worries about rent and coal and all the rest of it.

Some hope! Her imagination running away with her again. She put down the paper and went through to the kitchen to peel the potatoes and prepare the vegetables. She had another read of it. Nothing ventured, nothing gained. Where was the harm in applying? None that she could see. Before she could change her mind she sat down and wrote out her application. Then she addressed the envelope and stuck on the stamp. A waste of a stamp, that was all it would be.

'Laura, there is a letter for you and it isn't a bill, at least I don't think it is. It's typed though.'

'It had better not be a bill,' Laura said, coming through and taking the letter from him. 'Pour the tea, will you?'

Ronnie poured tea into both cups.

'Wonders will never cease, I've got an interview.'

'For a job?'

'Yes.'

'What kind?' he said, spreading butter on his toast and not too thickly since they could no longer afford to be extravagant.

'Looking after a small child and doing light housework. I won't get it.'

'You wouldn't want to do that.'

'I might.'

'What did it say in the advert?'

'There it is, I cut it out.'

'What about me?'

'I don't accept unless you can come too.'

'Not a chance.'

'I know.'

'Why did you bother to apply?'

She put her head in her hands, then looked up. 'Desperation.'

Ronnie shivered. 'Will the landlord put us out in the street if we can't pay the rent?'

'It could come to that.' There was no point in hiding their troubles and she was too tired to go on doing it.

'Dad should be shot,' he said and burst into tears.

'Saying he should be shot won't solve anything,' she said sharply and pointedly ignored the tears. 'We don't know what has happened in America. And look at the time, you're cutting it fine again.'

'I don't care if I am late. I don't care about anything and why should I work hard when I'll have to leave school when I'm fourteen!' He scraped back his chair, wiped his eyes with the back of his hand and went to get his blazer. Laura couldn't let him leave like that and she went after him.

She put an arm round his shoulder. 'You won't be leaving school at fourteen, Ronnie, I promise you that.'

'You can't promise anything, Laura, and I'm not mad at you but I'm mad at everybody else.'

They were both smiling, with the tears very close.

'I'm mad too and when I am something nice happens.'

When he had gone she went back to the letter and had another read of it.

Braehead
Albany Terrace
Miltonsands

Dear Miss Morrison,

Thank you for answering the advertisement, Please call for interview on Friday first between 2 pm and 4 pm or should evening be more convenient between 6 pm and 8 pm.

Yours sincerely.

It was signed Fergus Cunningham.

Chapter Thirteen

If she was going for that interview it was high time she was getting a move on. What on earth had possessed her to apply for a job she knew she had no hope of getting? Still, it would be the height of bad manners not to turn up, she thought, and she didn't want this Mr Cunningham to think badly of her. Laura put on her coat and collected her gloves and bag. All the time she was aware of Ronnie's eyes on her.

'Promise you won't take it unless I get to come?'

This was the third time in the last hour that he had asked the same question. What more was there to say to convince him?

'Ronnie, listen and listen carefully because I think there is something wrong with your ears. I'm almost one hundred per cent sure that I won't be offered the position but in the unlikely event that I am then rest assured that my acceptance depends entirely and absolutely on being able to have you with me. I can't make it plainer than that, now can I?'

'No. It's just – just that I'm frightened you'll forget.'

'I won't.'

'You won't get it. Nobody is going to give you a job if it means taking me.'

'You never know, they might be desperate.'

'Need to be,' Ronnie said with a touch of humour.

Laura could only agree.

'You look nice in that red coat. Bet you look better than all the others.'

'Thanks for those kind words,' she grinned.

'I could come with you and wait outside.'

'In a freezing November night? The last thing I need is you in bed with a chill. I could be in and out in five minutes or this Mr Cunningham may not be ready for me and I'll have to wait.'

'You know what Miss Wilkinson told David's mum?'

'No, and hurry up if you're going to tell me.'

'She said you were a find and she wouldn't like to lose you.'

Laura was pleased. 'That was nice of her.'

'She won't be pleased if you leave.'

'I wouldn't be happy about it myself.' Laura fastened her coat up to the neck, then crossed to the door. 'Don't answer the door to anyone.'

'Don't be daft. You're treating me like a wee kid. I can look after the house as well as you.'

'Of course you can. Cheerio.'

The rain, spasmodic during the day, had cleared. Laura walked to the bus stop where a few people were waiting and stamping their feet to keep the circulation going. After about five minutes the bus came into sight, stopped and they all got on. Albany Terrace was on the outskirts of Miltonsands and was where the better-off families lived. The houses were tall stately buildings set well apart from each other and each one given added privacy by the mature trees and shrubs. The terrace itself was well lit by gas lamps. One was positioned just outside Braehead and lit up the gate and part of the drive leading to the house. Lights shone from the windows and the house had a welcoming look.

The drive was on a slight slope and Laura stopped before the imposing front door. There was a bell-pull and she pulled at it, hearing the ring as she did. The thought then struck her that perhaps she should have gone to the back door. Too late, someone was coming. The door opened, there was a flood of light and a homely-looking woman in a tweed skirt and Fairisle twin-set smiled.

'I'm Laura Morrison and I have an appointment with Mr Cunningham.'

Laura saw the look of surprise before it was quickly hidden.

'Please come in.'

Laura stepped into a wide, very spacious hallway where Persian rugs were scattered on the polished parquet floor. Her eyes were drawn to the hall table with its beautiful carving and the huge Indian vase on its centre. A grandfather clock struck the hour, booming out six chimes. On the opposite wall was a smaller clock of similar design and Laura took that to be a grandmother clock. The woman smiled. 'They both chime but they never quite get it together.' She opened a door and ushered Laura in. 'Please take a seat and I'll tell Mr Cunningham you are here.'

'Thank you.'

The door closed quietly and Laura looked about her before deciding where she should sit. It was a beautiful room, large and high-ceilinged, furnished with taste though not without comfort in mind. The embossed paper was deep cream and there was a very long sideboard with a string of elephants from a tiny baby elephant to one that stood about a foot high. There were other ornaments that made Laura think that the family, or some member of it, had spent many years in the East. After the cold of the November night the brightly burning fire was a welcome sight. At the side of the Adam fireplace was a square-shaped brass box filled with logs.

The leather armchairs were shabby but looked very comfortable and inviting. Laura could imagine sinking into their depth but she wouldn't. Instead she would sit in one of the upright chairs and look more efficient and business-like for her interview.

Laura was sitting with her long, shapely legs crossed neatly at the ankles when the door opened quietly and a tall, finely-built man entered. He wore a dark business suit, the jacket of which was slightly crumpled, and Laura imagined him sitting at a desk all day. Her father's jacket had looked like that when he got home. This man looked very distinguished and when he was nearer she found herself looking into intelligent eyes. She thought him to be in his early thirties but that was a guess, he could be older or younger. There was no trace of grey in his thick brown hair.

'Good evening, Miss Morrison,' he said pleasantly.

'Good evening,' she smiled.

'Are you comfortable there?'

'Yes, thank you.'

He sat down near her in one of the leather armchairs and while he settled himself and crossed his long legs, she studied his face. A nice face with regular but strong features and the hair was worn slightly longer than was fashionable. He looked kind.

'Miss Morrison, I very much regret having brought you out and on such a cold night. The advertisement should have been better worded.'

'I thought it perfectly clear, Mr Cunningham. You wished someone to look after a small child. A kindly person and I consider myself that.'

His lips twitched. 'A mature woman. I am looking for a replacement for Mrs Mathewson, the lady who showed you in.' He smiled. 'She has been very good with my small daughter but sadly she is having to leave us.'

'A grandmotherly type,' Laura said quietly and they both turned as after knocking Mrs Mathewson put her head round the door.

'Sorry to disturb you, Mr Cunningham, but a Mr Archibald Scott is on the phone.'

'Thank you. Will you excuse me, Miss Morrison, I'll only be a moment.'

'Of course.'

A child, a pretty fair-haired girl, wriggled free from Mrs Mathewson and rushed to grab one of the long legs.

'Daddy! Daddy!'

'No, poppet, out you go and stay with Mrs Mathewson.'

'Don't want to. Want to stay here.'

Laura saw her chance. 'I'll look after the little girl if you wish,' she said quietly.

'Well— '

'Please, Daddy, and I'll be good.'

'That'll make a change. Just leave her then, Mrs Mathewson.'

The older woman shook her head, then left them.

The child looked at Laura with the unblinking stare that some adults find so uncomfortable. It didn't worry Laura. They both looked at each other, then the child giggled.

'What is your name?' she lisped.

'Laura. What is yours?'

'Sylvia.'

'That's a pretty name.'

'I'm three and a half and when I'm five I'm going to school.'

'You'll like school. I did when I was a little girl.'

'Sorry about that,' Fergus Cunningham said as he came in.

'Daddy, is the lady going to live here?'

'Out you go, dear, come on now and no nonsense, I want to talk to Miss Morrison.'

'It isn't Miss Morrison, it's Lau–Laura. She told me her name and I told her mine.'

'Shoo,' he said, picking her up and putting her outside the door where Mrs Mathewson was waiting. They heard a small protesting voice then silence as another door closed.

'The child, you will have gathered, is my small daughter.'

'Yes. A very friendly little girl.'

He nodded. 'Now, where were we? Ah, yes, the question of age and you are very young.'

'Is that such a disadvantage?' Laura said, stung by the dismissive tone.

'Far from it but in this case it is I am afraid, Miss Morrison. My wife died when Sylvia was a baby and Mrs Mathewson, who is really my housekeeper, has looked after the child since then. She wanted to and has been quite wonderful. It is going to be very difficult to replace her and the child will be heartbroken to see her go.'

Laura did some quick thinking. She had nothing to lose. 'May I speak freely?'

He looked a little taken aback but gave a grave nod. 'Please do.'

'I'm quite sure that Mrs Mathewson has been wonderful but in a grandmotherly way.'

'She is getting on a bit which is why she is leaving us.' He was frowning.

'A younger woman—'

'Someone like yourself?' Was it amusement or sarcasm she heard in his voice?

Her head went a little higher. 'Yes, Mr Cunningham, someone like me. A younger person would have more energy to play with the child, take her to the park, feed the ducks in the pond and do all the things that little children enjoy.' She saw that she had his attention.

He gave a small nod and at the same time raised an eyebrow.

'May I ask if you are employed at present? You made no mention of it in your application.'

'I have a part-time job but I need more than that.'

'And the nature of that employment?'

'The post office, I am an assistant,' she said quietly.

'There is a very great difference, Miss Morrison, between post office work and caring for a small child.'

'I'm aware of that and it is quite possible to be accurate with figures and understand the needs of a child.'

'May I ask your age?' He smiled. 'You are young enough not to resent the question.'

'I'm nineteen.' She was still short of her nineteenth birthday but nineteen seemed a lot more mature than eighteen.

'Hardly old enough to have much experience of anything.'

That angered Laura. 'How wrong you are, Mr Cunningham, to assume that I have no experience of life,' she said, unaware of the bitterness that had crept into her voice, and determined to have her say. There was no chance of being offered the job, he had made that clear enough, but then she hadn't expected to be successful. Nevertheless she wasn't going to let it go there. She wanted to give him something to think about before she departed. Laura took a deep breath. 'I was seventeen when my mother died and I had gained a place at college which hopefully would have led to a teaching post. That fell through. My father decided that my place was at home looking after his house and my young brother. Ronnie, to let you understand is eight years younger than I am. She had been talking fast and when she stopped to get her breath back he spoke.

'A great deal of responsibility to put on very young shoulders.'

'Yes, it was. I didn't exactly excel in the first months but I improved. I must have improved quite a lot and showed that I could cope because my father – he was a civil servant – decided to take a temporary transfer to London.' Laura looked to see if Mr Cunningham was growing impatient but if he was it didn't show. 'We weren't exactly hitting it off, nothing seemed as though it would ever be right again after my mother died.' Her lips were trembling and she paused briefly to compose herself. 'To be honest, Mr Cunningham, life was easier with Dad away and I applied and got a part-time job in the post office. With what I earned and the allowance from my father I was managing well enough. Then I got the shock of my life when he wrote to say that he was getting married and they were going to make a new life for themselves in America.'

'I can see it must have been a very great shock,' he murmured.

'Worse was to come,' Laura said bitterly. 'Dad hasn't written. Not a single letter. He even forgot to give me an address in New York where he could be reached.'

'You are saying that you have no way of contacting your father?' he said sharply.

'That's right. I've been in touch with everyone I can think of but without success.' She paused. 'I'm sure Dad will get around to writing one day but by then it will be too late.'

'Why do you say that?' He knew, or had a good idea, that the girl was in financial difficulties. His law experience put him one jump ahead.

'This is not a sob story, Mr Cunningham,' she said with a quiet dignity, 'and I'm afraid I've made a fool of myself and said too much.' Suddenly Laura felt weary of it all and wished that she had just accepted that she was unsuitable, gone home and saved all this.

'I know it isn't a sob story,' he said, 'I can tell those a mile off. What I do think is that you are a very brave and remarkable young woman. Since you have gone this far perhaps you should let me hear the rest.'

'The rest?' she said, surprised, 'you can't want to hear more?'

'If it wouldn't upset you?'

'I'm beyond that.' She gave a half-smile. 'All right, here it is. My allowance has stopped. To be fair to my father he did give me a bit extra before he left. It was meant to tide me over until he could make arrangements, with the bank, I suppose.'

'Only he hasn't?'

'No.'

The man was nodding thoughtfully. 'You mentioned a young brother.'

'It's far, far worse for Ronnie. He's so bewildered by it all and his confidence has gone. I'm not just saying this but he is an exceptionally clever boy and it would be dreadful, sinful even, if circumstances forced him to leave school at fourteen.' She got up abruptly. 'Forgive me for taking up so much of your time.'

'Please sit down, Miss Morrison, I may have been hasty and perhaps I need to think again.' He paused and strummed his fingers on the arm of the chair. 'Life can be the very devil, can't it?'

'I couldn't agree more.'

'Now that I know your position, Miss Morrison, let me try to explain mine. My wife, as I said, died when Sylvia was little more than an infant. We had a young woman, a nursery maid was how she described herself, and she was a friend of my wife's. She looked after the baby and I expected that to go on. It did but only for a very short time. She didn't wish to continue with my wife no longer there. I was left with the problem of a replacement.'

'Upsetting for a baby who had already lost her mother.'

'Yes, she cried a lot and Mrs Mathewson seemed the only one who could settle her.'

'I can understand that. She would have grown very attached to the child and the child to her.'

'I may be a reasonably good lawyer but when it comes to household matters I'm the first to admit I'm pretty hopeless. Unfortunately my parents had retired down south or they would have been a big help. Friends and neighbours were very supportive but that only goes on so long. Anyway,' he smiled, 'we struggled on and have managed so far. Your grandmotherly remark may have some truth in it.'

'I'm sorry, I really am, I should never have said that. Grandparents are usually marvellous with children and I only meant—'

'I know what you meant. An older person is short of the energy to keep up with an active, enquiring child and Mrs Mathewson has reached that stage. She did have the run of the house and my permission to engage whatever staff was required for the smooth running of Braehead. Her own duties, apart from seeing to Sylvia, were only supervisory and she did the household accounts.' He smiled. 'You would have no difficulty there?'

'No,' she said, hardly daring to believe that she might, just might, be being considered for the position.

'Forgive me bringing your tender years into it again—'

'You are thinking of discipline, Mr Cunningham. I would be firm but kind. It was how my mother was with us. Children don't mind discipline, it makes them feel more secure. Someone cares, you see.'

'I agree, but it wasn't discipline I was going to mention.'

'I'm sorry, I should think before I speak.'

'Not at all. We are back to your tender years. You see, Mrs Mathewson issued orders to the staff, she had that authority as my housekeeper. How would they accept orders from a nineteen-year-old?'

Laura did some quick thinking. 'So long as they weren't issued in a bossy way I see no problem and in a well-run house very few would be necessary.'

'You do have an answer to everything,' he smiled.

'Am I being seriously considered, Mr Cunningham?'

'It would appear so.'

She flushed. 'You would have no cause for regrets.'

'I sincerely hope not. A young child, Miss Morrison, is a very great responsibility and unfortunately I cannot be with my daughter as often as I would wish. Do you think you can keep her happy and at the same time instil a little discipline into a rather spoilt little girl?'

'Yes,' she said confidently. 'I can promise that.'

'Good.'

Now was the moment of truth, the worst moment. She swallowed nervously. What would he say? Very little. Just a quiet withdrawal when he knew about Ronnie. A kindly but firm shake of the head to show that it was out of the question. 'Mr Cunningham, there is something I haven't mentioned—'

'A problem?' He pushed up an eyebrow.

'That depends, I don't know. It's about my young brother. Ronnie is a very quiet, well-behaved boy and for most of the time he has his nose in a book.'

'He could do worse.' He paused. 'This brother you mention is eight years younger which by my calculation makes him about eleven?'

'Yes.' Laura was surprised, she hadn't expected him to remember a small detail like that.

'I take it he can't be left with a relative?'

'No.'

'He must accompany you?'

'I promised him that we would never be separated.'

'And one cannot go back on a promise like that?'

'No, I couldn't do that.'

He nodded thoughtfully. 'You have no objections if I ask some questions? This is not idle curiosity, you understand, but I need answers.'

'I'll answer any question you care to put to me.'

'Your home, is it rented or does it belong to your father?'

'It's rented. Had it not been I should have been able to carry on. The rent went up recently and by quite a lot. The landlord,' she said bitterly, 'was quick enough about putting up the rents but it is a different story when it comes to seeing to repairs.'

'A common complaint, I'm led to believe.'

'I did try to get a lodger, you know.'

'A female, I hope.'

'I couldn't afford to be choosy, I would have welcomed male or female.'

He was frowning heavily. 'Dangerous. One can be too trusting even with references.'

Laura laughed. 'I would never have thought of asking for a reference and remember, Ronnie would have been in the house. Anyway it didn't happen, no one was interested.'

'If you were to come here your house would require to be given up and there would be the disposal of the furniture.'

'Yes, I had thought of that, but I'll manage. It might have been upsetting once but not now.' She looked at him and he was struck by the beauty of her eyes. Deep blue, clear and honest. 'No, that isn't completely true. It will be upsetting, how could it be otherwise? I was born there and seeing my mother's things going to the saleroom—' she faltered.

'Sad but necessary,' he said kindly.

'Sad, yes, but a lot easier than being put out of the house and finding Ronnie and myself homeless.'

'Could it come to that?'

'Landlords don't have hearts, Mr Cunningham.'

'A few of them do. Perhaps you have just been unfortunate.'

'Maybe I am making him out to be worse than he is. Mum said he wasn't bad but he had a nagging wife who was always wanting more money. No doubt we would have had a few warnings. We do have two aunts who would have come to our assistance but most reluctantly.'

'Not a happy situation to be in.'

She didn't answer.

'That was a stupid remark of mine. What I wanted to say was, don't break your heart. Those possessions you cannot bear to part with, bring them here.' He reached over for his pipe, appeared to have second thoughts, and put it back.

'You are very kind.'

'My late wife had an extension built on to the back of the house. This was to give the housekeeper her own separate accommodation and more importantly keep the other rooms for guests. My wife liked to entertain but there is very little of that done now. Mrs Mathewson will let you see your rooms but I can tell you there is a bedroom, bathroom and small sitting-room. As to where your brother could be accommodated—' He frowned.

Laura didn't want that to be a stumbling block and it mustn't be, not when everything was working out so well.

'Would it be possible for Ronnie to have the bedroom and the sitting-room become a bed-sitting-room for me?'

'Out of the question. That suggestion does not meet with my approval. The sitting-room remains what it is – a sitting-room.'

Laura felt her heart drop like a stone.

He must have seen the light go from those lovely eyes and there was the same look of defeat he had glimpsed earlier on. It made him hasten in with, 'We can come up with something I am sure. And I seem to recall a bedroom now used as a store. All that stuff could go up to the attic and with the rubbish out and a lick of paint it should do a young boy very nicely.'

'Thank you very much,' she said gratefully.

'We haven't discussed remuneration or a starting date.'

'Whatever the remuneration you had in mind there must be a deduction made for Ronnie.'

'Poor little lad, am I to charge him board and lodgings?' He was laughing. 'My dear Miss Morrison, that was very charmingly said but totally unnecessary.'

'Then you must give Ronnie some jobs to do,' she said firmly.

'Like dusting my books and putting them in proper order,' he teased.

'Ronnie would love to do that.' Laura was quite unaware that he was only teasing.

'That should be about everything for the present,' he said, getting to his feet, and Laura got up too. Her hand was shaken and then he was opening the door. 'Mrs Mathewson will take over now and answer any questions you have. As to a starting date we had better leave that open until you finalise arrangements about your home but to take no longer than four weeks.'

'I'll get started on it right away.'

He smiled. 'Don't be hasty, get this all in writing first. We do like to feel we can trust people but we all feel more comfortable with written confirmation.'

'Thank you again.'

'Feel free to come at any time and see Mrs Mathewson. She will be delighted to see you. As to your young brother, bring the boy along so that we can be introduced.'

Seeing her daddy, Sylvia came running over and took his hand.

'Mrs Mathewson, I have decided to engage Miss Morrison. Perhaps you would be good enough to show her the accommodation.'

'Of course I'll do that.' If Mrs Mathewson was surprised, and it turned out she was, she hid it well.

'Goodnight, Miss Morrison.'

'Goodnight, Mr Cunningham.'

'No, Sylvia, you would be in the way but if you are a good girl I'll read you a bedtime story.'

'It isn't bedtime,' she said, outraged.

'It soon will be.' Putting her over his shoulder, Fergus Cunningham carried his small daughter back into the sitting-room.

'She's a delightful bairn but getting too much of a handful for me. You are young and maybe that is what the lass needs. My joints are too creaky and I'm too old to be running about.'

'You must have mixed feelings about leaving Braehead?' Laura said.

'I do but for all that I'll be glad to get away. A body needs a bit of peace and quiet at my time of life and a chance to do the things there never was time to do. It is a good position, you will be all right here, Miss Morrison.'

'Call me Laura, please.'

'A slip of a lass like you doesn't want a title. Laura it is then. He's a gem, a proper gentleman is Mr Cunningham.'

'Yes, he's very kind.'

'He's a lawyer as you might know. Senior partner in the family firm now that old Mr Cunningham has retired. Mrs Cunningham, his mother, belongs to Devon and that's where they have retired to.' She walked ahead. 'This is where the extension begins, hardly know, would you? Beautifully done it is. I've been very comfortable I must say and I felt privileged to have a place of my own and away from the family.'

'Poor child to lose her mother when she was just a baby.'

'It was a tragedy all right.' She added nothing more and something in the woman's face stopped Laura from enquiring further. 'Here we are. This is to be your bedroom. Not as tidy as usual but then I wasn't expecting to be showing it to anyone.'

'It's lovely and I would say very tidy.' The room was of generous proportion and the wallpaper was beige with pink and blue tiny flowers. There was a single bed with a blue and white striped cover and beside it a bedside table with an alarm clock. Against one wall was a double wardrobe and to the side was a dress hanging on a coat-hanger.

'A job I promised myself. It needs to be shortened. Mind, the shop would have done it but at a price and though I'm no dressmaker taking up a hem isn't beyond me.'

There was a kidney-shaped dressing-table with a glass tray on which rested a tortoiseshell comb and brush set. Next to the bedroom was the bathroom. Laura saw it from the door.

'Lovely.'

'No shortage of hot water,' She closed the door and went over to open another. 'This will be your sitting-room, Laura, some pieces are mine and will be going with me. You'll likely be bringing a few bits and pieces yourself?'

'Yes, I'd like to.'

Laura was well satisfied with everything and in particular with the sitting-room. It was charming, nicely decorated and comfortable. Floral curtains were at the window and Mrs Mathewson pointed to the plants on the sill.

'Those will be left for you. Don't be killing them with kindness. Some folk can't resist giving plants drops of water every now and then. Once in a while give them a good soak and that is all that is needed. We have a good gardener and a lad to help him. Come spring there will be a grand show and speak kindly to him and he'll keep you supplied with flowers.'

'My mother was a good gardener but I'm afraid I haven't got her green fingers. She died two years ago,' Laura added.

'I'm sorry to hear that, lass,' Mrs Mathewson said gently, 'it isn't easy to come to terms with the loss of a mother.'

'No, it isn't.'

'We'll leave it there for the night, I think,' she said, moving away. 'You'll be anxious to get home?'

'Yes, I've left my young brother on his own.' Laura did want to go home to see Ronnie's face when she told him the news. That made her think of Miss Wilkinson and she was saddened. The postmistress had been more than kind and it was a bad time to be left in the lurch with

Christmas only a few weeks away. Not much time to train someone else but Laura determined to do all she could to help.

'Pop in any spare time you have. I'm seldom far from the door and it'll be a chance for you to get to know the wee lass. Don't be bothering Mr Cunningham, he's a busy man and we can manage this between us.'

'I'm sure we can.'

'You'll get a look around the house when you come back. Were you told about the domestic arrangements?'

'Not really, I was to hear them from you.'

'Poor soul, he does his best but it isn't a man's job and you can see he just wants to put the responsibility on to other shoulders. I looked after the bairn, took her mother's place as best I could.'

'Yes, Mr Cunningham is very grateful to you.' She paused. 'Wasn't it a lot for you holding down two jobs?'

'It was hardly that. I wasn't overworked. I looked after Sylvia and gave the occasional check to the house to see that all was as it should be. There is Mrs Barclay, the cook, and Annie who does the housework and Jean Fairley for the heavy work. All good conscientious workers who know what is expected and get on with it.'

Once out in the street Laura saw the outline of the bus through the gloom and sprinted to the stop. She made it and was thankful for the next wasn't for another fifteen minutes.

Ronnie had the door open when he heard her step.

'I was almost coming to look for you,' he said half angrily.

'Sorry, the interview took longer than I expected,' she said breathlessly. 'Ronnie, I got the job.'

'And—'

'There is a bedroom to be made ready for you.'

'You mean it is all fixed up?'

'Yes, I get confirmation through the post. Put the kettle on, Ronnie, I'm dying for a cup of tea.'

'It's on and everything is ready, has been for ages.'

'Good. Make it and I'll be down in a minute.'

He had the tea made and poured out when she got back.

'Is it all right?'

'Yes, fine,' Laura said, looking at the coloured water and wishing she had reminded him to give it time to infuse before pouring it in the cups.

'What is this Mr Cunningham like?'

'Very nice and I'm sure you are going to like him.'

'Will we never be on our own?'

She drank some weak tea. 'Of course. We are to have our own sitting-room. It is in a new part that has been built on to the house.'

She saw his face brighten. 'Like our own house but without having to pay the rent?'

'Couldn't have put it better myself.'

'Where will we eat?'

'In the kitchen, I expect.'

'That's good because I wouldn't want to eat in a posh dining-room.'

'You wouldn't get the chance. Mr Cunningham will dine there.'

'What does he do?'

'He's a lawyer.'

'And what is it? A boy or a girl you have to look after?'

'A little girl. She's called Sylvia and she is three and a half.'

'Will she be a pest?'

'I shouldn't think so but remember she is the daughter of the house.'

'Meaning she can be a pest if she wants to be?'

'She won't bother you. You can be in our sitting-room and you'll be able to visit David, it is still walking distance.'

'I wasn't going to tell you this but I can now. You know what I thought?'

'No, what did you think?' she asked.

'I thought if we had to get out of the house and you couldn't keep me with you then I might have to go and live with Aunt Peggy.'

'Where was I going to be?'

'I didn't know but I didn't think we would get to be together.'

'What makes you think that Aunt Peggy would take you?'

'If Uncle Archie told her she had to then she would have to.'

'I'm lost. You'd better explain this.'

'Uncle Archie thought you might get married to Michael, that he might not want me and if he didn't then I was to stay there. I would have hated it, Laura.'

'It wouldn't have happened, you silly. Your trouble is you don't have enough confidence in me.'

'This place is going to be all right, isn't it?'

'I think myself very lucky to have got it, and Ronnie—'

'What?'

'The little girl lost her mother when she was a baby. Wasn't that very sad?'

'Worse than us. She won't remember her mother.'

'No, poor little thing.'

'Still, she's got her dad.'

Laura had no answer to that.

'What about time off? You won't have to work all day, will you?'

'No, I won't but my hours weren't discussed. There will be a letter in the post detailing everything.'

'You look happy.'

'Ronnie, I'm just so relieved and you and I deserve a treat. How about the pictures tomorrow night?'

'Great! One of the boys in my class said it was good and not much lovey-dovey stuff.' He grinned. 'You mean we can really afford it?'

'No, I don't suppose we can.'

'You aren't going to change your mind?'

'Of course not. When do I not keep my promise?'

'Not very often and Laura—'

'What?'

'I want to keep on my Saturday job.'

'You don't have to.'

'I like it and I like to have money of my own.'

'Then you hang on to your Saturday job but you save some of the money.'

'I know that and I want to save. It's good having money, sort of makes you feel important.'

'I'm not sure that that is a good thing, feeling important, but I agree it is comforting to have a few coins to jingle.'

Chapter Fourteen

Two days after her interview at Braehead the letter arrived. She picked it up from the mat at the front door and took it with her into the living-room. Ronnie had already left for school and a glance at the clock told her that she had time to read it. Sitting down, Laura slit open the envelope and drew out the typewritten page. First of all she admired the layout. It was well spaced and very clear, just as she would have expected from a lawyer's office. She read it over twice then put it in the envelope and tucked it behind the clock on the mantelpiece. All very satisfactory.

Beyond the window the November fog swirled over the buildings, all but obliterating the houses opposite. It was a dull, bleak morning, the kind she detested, but Laura hardly noticed. For her the sun had come out from behind the clouds and chased away her worries. Not that she was completely happy, how could she be in such circum-stances, but at least for the foreseeable future their lives would be settled.

Mr Cunningham had stated her duties and the hours she would be expected to work. These were to be flexible to suit both parties. Laura would have a day off each week and most Sundays she would be free after midday. The annual holiday entitlement would be fourteen days. A two-week paid holiday and a day off each week was generous, Laura thought, until she remembered that she would be tied most evenings. Still, she wouldn't grumble about that, rather she would count her blessings.

Leaving the house, Laura was suddenly struck by the enormity of what she was doing but she wasn't going to resort to panic. The day would come, surely it had to, when she would hear from her father. When she did, what would he have to say when his daughter had to write and tell him that she had given up the house, his house, and disposed of the furniture? Without seeking advice, too. She was doing it on her own.

A better relationship with Aunt Peggy meant that the matter could have been discussed. Advice there would have been but that wasn't what was required. It was financial assistance and that was something she wouldn't ask. In all probability it wouldn't have been forthcoming and she would have cringed to hear the excuses.

As to what her father would say when he found out Laura didn't much care. By his callous, uncaring treatment of his son and daughter he had forfeited any right to consideration. In any case what it boiled down to was the plain fact that she couldn't afford the increased rent and it would only have been a matter of time before a notification arrived from the landlord requesting her to vacate the house. Ronnie and she would have been out on the street, begging-bowl in hand. She wasn't being fanciful, it did happen. It had happened to others.

She would allow herself no regrets. What had to be done would be done. There was no other way out of their difficulties and this job she had landed was heaven-sent. Stop thinking and prepare for the way ahead, that was what she must do. With so much to do where did she begin? She would start by listing the jobs and in order of priority. Then she would work through the list systematically. Three weeks, which was roughly what she would allow herself, wasn't so very long. Not when she had a demanding job to do during the day and it was essential that she hung on to her post office position until the last minute. She owed it to Miss Wilkinson and she needed the wages.

Miss Wilkinson's name had gone to the top of the list. Laura was dreading handing in her notice but the sooner she did the sooner the post mistress could advertise for a replacement. The landlord would be next. No pleasantries there, just a bald statement informing Henry Atkinson that she was giving up the house. That would no doubt receive an acknowledgement by return of post together with a demand for the rent outstanding. Serve him right if she did a 'moonlight'.

Mrs Brand, next door, was going to be surprised and probably very upset to learn that they were leaving the district. Not moving all that far but it wouldn't be the same, no longer would they be neighbours.

The aunts – heavens! She wasn't looking forward to telling them but she daren't put it off too long in case it got to their ears from another source. Unlikely but then again one could never tell, not in a place like

Miltonsands. Jane would have to be told though Ronnie would probably break the news.

How did one organise a removal? Surely it was just common sense. It wasn't a complete removal since most of the furniture was going to the saleroom. This very day when she got back from the post office she would make a start on the drawers and throw out what wasn't worth keeping. That shouldn't take long.

As Laura expected, Miss Wilkinson was shattered, no other word could have described the expression on her face.

'Laura, you can't mean this?' They were sitting in the back premises. She had delayed her announcement until the last customer had been attended to and the door shut.

'I'm so very, very sorry, Miss Wilkinson, I feel dreadful about it. You've been so good to me and I have enjoyed the work.'

'I have to understand your reasons but I feel sure something could have been worked out,' she said unhappily.

Laura shook her head. 'I haven't taken this decision lightly, Miss Wilkinson. You must believe me there was no other way. I even tried to get a lodger, had a card stuck up in the newsagent's window, but nobody was interested. Getting this live-in job and Ronnie being made welcome was the answer to my prayer.'

'You could have borrowed from me to tide you over.'

'That is very good of you, Miss Wilkinson, but I could never have done that. My mother warned me often enough to live within my means and never to borrow money. She said it could be habit-forming and to be avoided at all costs.'

The postmistress smiled. 'I can't see you making a habit of it.' She paused and looked a bit uncertain. 'Forgive me asking but haven't you had any word—'

'From my father?' She shook her head. 'Nothing.'

'It seems so strange but I'm sure you've tried every avenue.'

'I have. I've made every possible enquiry and so have my aunts.'

'Oh, dear, this has really upset me. I was depending on you so much, even to the weekly balance. You were getting into the way of it and I was seeing myself easing off.'

'I enjoyed doing it and got a real thrill when everything balanced.'

'Yes, it is a nice feeling, one of satisfaction to get it balanced first time and not to have to check and recheck.' She sighed. 'I must advertise and do it right away but you will be very difficult to replace. When must you leave?'

'In three weeks. I'll work to the last minute and Miss Wilkinson—'

She raised her eyes, tired eyes that showed the strain of working with figures, sometimes far into the night when the books didn't balance.

'I am to have a whole day off each week and with Christmas coming and if you need assistance, I'll be only too willing to help out.'

'I may hold you to that although I don't imagine your new employer would approve.'

'He needn't know and I suppose I can do as I wish on my day off.'

The postmistress gave another sigh. 'We shall just have to wait and see how things turn out.'

In the event they turned out better than either of them could have dared hope. A well-written reply arrived in answer to the advertisement. The woman, a widow, had come to live in the district, wanted part-time employment and had post office experience.

Mrs Brand was in carpet slippers that bulged in places where the cloth was stretched to accommodate the painful bunion she had on each foot.

'Laura, come away in. Excuse the slippers but my feet were killing me. I was toasting myself at the fire. Bad for the legs but I'll risk it.'

'Don't blame you.'

'Sit yourself down,' she said, moving the other armchair nearer to the fire.

Laura braced herself for what she had to say. 'Mrs Brand, I don't know how to tell you but we are leaving Fairfield Street.'

'Never! You're not?' Her eyes widened in astonishment.

'Yes. I'll tell you the reason but I don't want anyone else to know.'

'No danger of me spreading it around.'

'I know.'

'Wait! If this is going to take a while we'd be the better of a cup.'

Laura heard the kettle being filled, the rattle of cups as they went on the tray. In a remarkably short time the small table was cleared of odds and ends, the tray placed on it and the teapot put down beside the fender.

'We'll give it a few minutes.'

'I wish Ronnie would remember to do that. Coloured water is what he serves but he's always so chuffed that I haven't the heart to tell him.'

'Time I was showing Alan how to do something for himself.' She paused. 'Still no word?'

'From Dad? No, nothing, and that is the reason we are having to move. To put it bluntly, Mrs Brand, I needed the money Dad sent and now that it has dried up I can't afford the rent.'

'Yon was a hefty increase but complaining to that landlord of ours is a waste of breath. Greed, pure and simple, is what it is. That window,' she pointed, 'rattles like the dickens but will Henry Atkinson do anything about it? Not him.' She frowned. 'Here I am blathering on about very little. You get on with your story, lass.'

By the time Laura had finished her tale she was feeling just the teeniest bit disappointed. Mrs Brand seemed genuinely sorry that they were leaving Fairfield Street but hardly devastated.

'Had you given me your news this time last week I would have been more upset but since we are moving ourselves, only just settled, so I couldn't have told you before—'

'You are? Where are you going?' Laura couldn't keep the amazement out of her voice.

'Montrose. Bert has seen the writing on the wall for a while now. Short time to begin with then the dole staring him in the face. This job he has managed to get means a drop in wages but a house goes with the job so all in all I reckon we'll be neither better nor worse off.'

'Will you be sorry to leave Miltonsands?'

'In many ways, yes, but I'll tell you one thing, Laura, I'll be glad to get Alan away from that cousin of his. Nephew or not I don't like the lad and if the truth be known I think Alan only follows where he goes because he's scared not to. You wouldn't get him admitting to that but I know and he seems happy about going to Montrose. Is your cup empty? More tea?'

'Just fill it up, please.'

Mrs Brand filled both their cups and pushed another sponge cake on to Laura's plate.

'The thought of all that packing, I don't know about you, Laura, but I confess I don't know where to begin.'

'That makes two of us.'

'You won't have heard about the other removals?'

'No.'

'But then you wouldn't. You don't take much interest in what happens around here, do you?'

'I have to plead guilty.'

'You are young, it's not to be expected, but in the years I have lived in Fairfield Street there have been very few changes and now here we are. You leaving and us. The McDonalds at number 12 are moving to a smaller house now that Janet has got herself a man. Then the folk at number 15 are going but I couldn't tell you where. No one will mind their departure, noisy lot and impudent with it.'

'My mother used to say that everything went in threes but that is four. Thanks for the tea and I'm glad if we have to leave that we are doing it together.'

'Strange how things work out. Don't be afraid of change, Laura, and in your case this could be a very good move and a happy one too.'

'I hope so, I get butterflies in my stomach thinking about it.'

'Only natural. It would be a pity not to keep up and I would like to hear how you are settling in, and Ronnie.'

'I'll let you know, I promise, and you must do the same.'

'Must remember to exchange addresses. Just a thought, we had better get ourselves organised with boxes and tea chests for the flitting. Get in quick too for I see a rush.'

'Thanks, I never thought about that.'

As she let herself into the house Laura was doing some organising in her mind. Ronnie would help her with the boxes and they would need a place to store them. That would obviously have to be her father's bedroom. Most of his clothes had already gone and what was left could be given to the ragman. Or if the ragman didn't appear then to some poor soul who came to the door begging. One beggar made regular appearances in Fairfield Street and if he had had a good day they would be treated to a song and he had a surprisingly good voice. The furniture in her father's room could go to the sale-room first and come to think about it, the heavy furniture from the front room could be cleared out at the same time.

Most tenants when they moved left the rooms bare, even to removing the linoleum. She wouldn't do that since she would have no use for curtains and flooring and whoever followed might be glad of them. How kind it had been of Mr Cunningham to suggest they bring a few items of their own to Braehead. Those she would select carefully.

As to the room that was to become Ronnie's she would be better able to decide what to take once she had seen it. Her own bedroom furniture was in better condition than her brother's and she would probably take hers. Ronnie wouldn't bother just so long as his bookcase and his precious possessions went with him.

So far so good, she had that clear in her mind and she would start on the drawers before Ronnie got home. Be ruthless, no dithering as to whether something was worth keeping or not. If she didn't have a use for it then out it would go. Sadly it wasn't turning out to be as easy as she thought. What was rubbish? Here she was kneeling on the floor surrounded by an assortment of knick-knacks. Of little use but each one bringing back a memory of a holiday or day trip. Souvenirs that had been bought with precious pocket money or given to her by her parents. She felt the lump in her throat get bigger. Such happy times they had been with no inkling of what the future was to bring.

She blew her nose and dabbed at her eyes when she heard the back door. Ronnie came in blowing on his hands.

'It's perishing cold out there and you can see only a wee bit in front of you.'

'I know, the fog hasn't lifted all day.'

'What are you doing?'

'What does it look like?'

'You never clean out drawers. Why are you doing it now?'

'Necessity. I never had the time before.' Nor the inclination, she added silently.

'What are you looking for?'

'Nothing.'

'Then why have two piles?'

'I'm trying to decide what to keep and what to throw out. You'll have to have a clearing out of your room and put out the rubbish.'

'I don't have any rubbish,' he said indignantly.

'Of course you have, you're a hoarder.'

'You won't throw anything away when I'm not here, you wouldn't do that, would you?' Ronnie asked anxiously.

'No, I'm leaving it to you.'

'You said I was getting a bedroom.'

'I know what I said.'

'Then I don't see why everything in my room upstairs can't go into that room at Braehead.'

Laura sighed. She wasn't going to win this one.

'I told David about us moving, that was all right, wasn't it?'

'Yes, I expected you would. After I see the aunts I'll go and see David's mum. Thought I'd go over to Aunt Peggy's tomorrow after work. Aunt Vera is sure to be there so that will kill two birds with one stone. You could come and give me some support.'

'You must be joking and anyway I wouldn't be home in time.'

'Meaning you'll make sure you aren't?'

He grinned. 'It might not be too bad and you get on better with Aunt Peggy now.'

'I have a feeling that when she hears what I have to tell her we'll be back to square one,' Laura said gloomily.

Yesterday's fog had lifted and a pale wintry sun was making fleeting appearances when Laura set out for her Aunt Peggy's home. She was expected. Laura had decided it wise to half prepare her for what was coming.

'It's important,' she had said, 'but I can't possibly tell you more than that just now.' She couldn't either because a few customers waited to be served.

'I'll expect you between half past three and four and I'll have your Aunt Vera there. It's her day for coming.'

'I remembered that.'

Warmly clad in her winter coat with a woollen scarf round her neck and a beret on her head, Laura left the office and set out for her aunt's house.

They were both waiting and she got a smile from each of them.

'Get your coat off, lass, and come and get a heat.'

'Thanks,' Laura said, taking it off and handing it and scarf and beret to her aunt. 'Lovely and cosy in here.'

'Perishing cold it might be but mark my words this is just the beginning and we are in for a severe winter. Have to pay for a good summer, you know.'

'Was it? A good summer I mean?' Aunt Vera went closer to hold her hands out to the fire. 'Didn't seem that to me.'

'No matter. I made the tea when I saw you turning the corner, Laura, so it should be just right for drinking.'

The tea things were on a low table and covered by a cloth. Aunt Peggy whipped it off and under were home-baked scones already buttered and triangles of shortbread. Laura was getting more nervous by the minute and wondering how to begin.

'Is what you have to tell us to do with George?' Aunt Vera asked as her sister finished pouring the tea and put the teapot down on a tile beside the fender.

'No, it isn't.' Laura sipped at her tea then plunged in with her news. Both looked equally scandalised but managed to keep quiet until Laura had finished.

'What right had you to even contemplate such a thing?' Aunt Vera burst out.

'Every right I would have thought,' Laura said quietly.

'In the first place the house wasn't yours to give up.' Aunt Peggy's face had the dull flush of anger.

'And the furniture wasn't yours to dispose of,' Vera added. 'Really, this is outrageous.'

'I agree with Vera that it is outrageous and as to what your father is going to say —'

'It is Dad's fault that it has come to this.'

'That is beside the point and doesn't alter the fact that what you have done is wrong. The house is not in your name.'

'No, but I am paying the rent which for your information, Aunt Peggy, the landlord saw fit to put up.'

'I accept that things were getting difficult for you but to take such a drastic step without talking it over with us is beyond me. Words fail me, they really do.'

Laura was in danger of losing her temper but she had promised herself that she wouldn't. She almost choked on a piece of shortbread and had to drink some tea to clear it from her throat.

'How quick you are to blame me when Dad is the real culprit.'

'Some of the blame is undoubtedly his,' Aunt Vera conceded, 'but knowing my brother he would have given you a generous housekeeping allowance from the time your mother died. That was your chance to put some by for a rainy day. But with you it would be easy come, easy go and no thought for tomorrow.'

Laura was stunned by the unfairness of it.

'It most certainly wasn't easy come easy go. Dad gave me enough to keep the house but it couldn't be described as generous.'

'Adequate though?'

'Yes, Aunt Vera, adequate. You should know that when Dad went off to London my allowance was greatly reduced.'

'As you would expect. Of course he had to keep something back. We all know how expensive it is to live there.'

'Which was why he was given a generous subsistence allowance for the first month.'

'Then nothing?'

'No, reduced but still adequate to use your own expression.'

'Laura, you and I have come to understand each other better and it would be a pity to lose that.' She took a deep breath. 'Nevertheless I have to say, and I know your Uncle Archie would agree, that what you have done is quite appalling.' She straightened her spine. 'Your trouble is that you haven't budgeted, but that only comes with practice.'

'I know how to budget, I've had plenty of it to do.' Laura smiled grimly. 'I must have expected something like this because I came prepared.' She opened her handbag and all but slammed a page of a jotter on the table. It was neatly lined. In one column Laura had entered her post office wages and as an afterthought Ronnie's pittance for his Saturday job. In the other column she listed their expenses. 'Before either of you say another word cast your eyes over that.'

Aunt Peggy, her lips pursed, read it first then wordlessly handed it to her sister.

'You will see from those figures that I have not included clothes. I can manage with what I have but Ronnie has to be decently turned out for school.'

'In such an emergency you could have used a little of your own savings,' Aunt Vera said but she seemed a little less sure now.

'My savings are gone,' Laura said bitterly, 'all my hard-earned savings.'

'This new job you are going to, tell us about it.'

'I was very lucky there. For me it has been like the light at the end of a very long tunnel. You know,' she said shakily, 'there are still good people. My new employer is one such person. Knowing the circumstances, he is willing to have Ronnie and we are to have our own accommodation and by that I mean our own bathroom and sitting-room.'

'Don't you feel some guilt at leaving Miss Wilkinson in the lurch?'

'Yes, Aunt Peggy, I do. Miss Wilkinson has been marvellous to me and I hated handing in my resignation but she has been very understanding. If it had been possible to give me full-time employment she would but even with that I would have had a struggle to make ends meet.'

'Too impulsive, that is your problem. How do you know that this job is going to work out? And if it doesn't where does that leave you?'

'It will work out because I shall make sure it does.'

All the same Laura felt the chill of fear. Aunt Peggy was saying what could happen. She would do her best but what if her best wasn't good enough? What if she didn't prove satisfactory, or another thought: Mr Cunningham was still a young man, an attractive widower, and he could remarry. Would his wife want her or would she be told to go? These were dangerous thoughts and she couldn't afford them.

Laura got up and forced a smile to her face. 'You'll have to excuse me but I've masses of work to do.' She waited for an offer of help but none came. Instead, as though to hasten her departure, Aunt Peggy collected Laura's coat from the sofa and helped her on with it.

Laura had been to Braehead on two occasions. On the first she had met Annie who was on her knees scrubbing the kitchen floor though it was really Jean Fairley's job. She didn't get to her feet but looked up when Mrs Mathewson introduced Laura. Her hands holding the wet cloth were red and swollen.

'A bairn to look after a bairn, that is what it looks like to me. What is the man thinking of taking on a bonny lass like that?'

'Miss Morrison is very capable as well as being bonny.'

'That may well be but she'll be snapped up by some young lad and married before that wee soul gets to know her.'

'No, Annie, no chance of that,' Laura said firmly as the woman smiled, displaying wide gaps between her badly stained teeth. Laura thought she would be much improved if the teeth were pulled and she got a mouthful of false ones. 'I do have one young man in my life, he's eleven and he is my brother.'

'That's different,' she said quietly. 'Left to look after him, were you?'

'Yes.'

'You'll be all right here, it is a fine place to work.'

'Ronnie won't get into anyone's way. He is quiet and studious.'

She smiled. 'It'll be real fine to have a wee laddie about the place.'

'He'll keep to his own room.'

'The bairn will need to eat?'

'Well, yes, I suppose he'll come to the kitchen for meals.'

'What about school? Will he take a piece?'

'Yes, he'll have to but I'll see to that.'

'Don't dare, lass. That's Mrs Barclay's territory. She'll make up the laddie's piece and I'll grant you he won't go hungry.'

'He most certainly won't,' Mrs Mathewson added.

They left Annie and walked away.

'What I have seen of the house is lovely.'

'It is a fine house and the late Mrs Cunningham should get the credit for that. She had excellent taste though some would say that there was a lot of extravagance. Why not, I say? Just so long as there is the wherewithal to carry it out.'

Laura nodded. She would go along with that.

'Very little has changed since she died. Mr Cunningham, like a lot of men, has simple tastes. Comfort comes before appearances but that said he does like everything looking nice.' She stopped. 'Here we are. This is the dining-room,' she said, opening the door. It was a large room, oblong in shape, and the long, beautiful mahogany table and the eight high-backed chairs looked well in it. A water-colour of a lake surrounded by trees that were reflected in the water hung above the mantelpiece. The heavy brocade curtains at the window were floor-length.

'Does Mr Cunningham do much entertaining?'

'Not since his wife died. He does have friends in occasionally for a drink but when he feels it is his turn to offer hospitality he books a table at the hotel. You'll see her often enough so I had better mention that Mr Cunningham has a lady friend, a Miss Davina Dorward – did Laura imagine it or was that a slight sniff of disapproval – 'and she is a frequent visitor. I'm not a gossip and it isn't my place to say this but the lady in question has hopes of becoming the next Mrs Cunningham.'

Laura felt a cold hand wrap round her heart. She was barely in the door and the uncertainties were back. The smile she gave was strained.

'Is she likely to succeed?'

'If she doesn't it won't be for the want of trying. Mind you, you can't blame the woman altogether. When Mr Cunningham is invited to some function or other and needs a partner he takes her along. They make a good-looking couple and they appear to get on well. You've seen all you want here?'

'Yes, thank you.'

The older woman led the way up the wide stairway with its thick carpeting held in place by brass rods that shone brightly.

'This is the wee lass's room. Miss Yeaman is looking after her.'

'Is Miss Yeaman a friend?'

'A very good friend. You'll like her. Betsy Yeaman is a lovely woman. In her forties I would put her but never had a life of her own. Her mother was an invalid and for many years Betsy devoted her life to looking after her. Sadly she departed this earth a few years ago, five years after her husband, leaving a daughter who had no friends of her own age.'

'Always the daughter, isn't it?'

'Yes, she is always the one to lose out. Not with Betsy though. She was the quiet retiring type and she didn't consider it a hardship to care for her widowed mother.'

'Is she very lonely?'

'She will have come to terms with her loneliness by this time. Of course it makes life a lot easier when you have no financial worries and I imagine Betsy was well provided for. Needless to say a few gentlemen have made advances but didn't get far. Betsy is no beauty as she would be the first to admit but neither is she a fool.'

'Sent them packing, good for her,' Laura said, laughing.

'On your day off Betsy will take charge of Sylvia. She adores children and is so good with them.'

'Would have made a good mother?'

'Not necessarily,' Mrs Mathewson said wisely, 'it is much easier to be patient when you don't have endless questions to answer day in and day out. Betsy only has it for a specified time, remember.'

'You have a point, I'm sure.'

'Does Miss Yeaman live alone?'

'All but. She has an old housekeeper who is as deaf as a door post and they rattle around in that big house.'

'What do you think of it? A pretty room for a pretty little girl.'

'It's lovely,' Laura said softly. The walls were papered in a light shade with figures from nursery rhymes. On the bed with its pretty pink cover and pillowcase to match was a teddy bear with a torn ear and an assortment of fluffy animals beside it.

'The teddy was her daddy's.'

'I thought it was second-hand by the state it is in.'

'Funny how it is always the teddy they cuddle for comfort.'

Laura's eyes had gone to the top of the wardrobe where there was an array of dolls.

'Aren't they just gorgeous?' she enthused.

'Brought back from different countries and too valuable to be played with. Strangely enough the child seems to accept that.'

'By the look of it she has plenty to play with without them.'

'What she wants she gets and when she doesn't get her own way she can be a little madam. You'll have to be firm and mean no when you say it. Her daddy can't say no to her and he has her ruined.'

'Are your own arrangements going well?' Laura asked.

'Not much arranging to do and I can safely leave what there is to the end. Since you're pushed for time we'll leave the drawing-room and the rest for now. You'll want to see where the boy is to sleep.'

'I would, please.' She paused. 'Once I see it I'll know what to bring in the way of furniture.'

'Plenty of spare furniture in the attics. You don't have to bring anything, unless that is you want to.'

'I would, Mrs Mathewson.'

'Then you do that. The lad will settle better with his own belongings around him.'

'Yes.'

'What do you think of this for your brother?'

Laura was looking at a fairly large room with a window that let in plenty of light.

'This is just perfect, Mrs Mathewson. It is much bigger than Ronnie's bedroom at home. He is going to be thrilled with this and so he should be.'

'Annie and Jean between them cleared it out and I gave them a hand.

The painter is coming for the woodwork and to put on a plain wallpaper. Boys of that age don't want anything fancy.'

'Ronnie likes everything plain.'

'Mr Cunningham had a look at the room and he suggested getting the joiner to fix up shelves on one wall since the lad is keen on books.'

'Did he? How very kind. Ronnie has a bookcase and that will be coming with us but he has more than enough books to fill it.'

'Bring the laddie along and let him see where he is to be living. I'd like fine to make his acquaintance before I go.'

'Ronnie is anxious to come,' Laura lied.

She knew that he wasn't looking forward to the move one little bit and when she had suggested he come with her every possible objection was put forward.

'I'll go when I have to. I see no point in going before.'

As the removal date drew near they were both hiding their feelings from each other.

For Ronnie it was all getting too much. Fairfield Street had always been home and he didn't want to leave it. Why couldn't he be like David with a mum and a dad and a house? It wasn't fair. Everything was going wrong. This was home and how could that other place be home when it belonged to someone else? It was hard to know what his sister was thinking. He was angry with her and he couldn't think why. She didn't laugh very much and sometimes she would snap at him for nothing. Only Mrs Turnbull understood him and knew how he felt. She was easy to talk to and she seemed to know what was wrong with Laura. She would be missing Michael, she said, and that was why she wasn't her usual self. Ronnie could understand that, he missed Michael too. Wonder why he didn't send Laura a letter from Manchester? Maybe they had had a row before he went away and hadn't had time to make it up.

'No, Ronnie, I am not making excuses for you.'

'Why does he want to see me? You said I didn't have to see anyone unless I wanted to,' he said angrily.

'Neither you do once we are living there but this is just an introduction. It is good manners.'

'Why do I have to go this very day?'

'Because you have been asked,' Laura said sharply. She was getting angry. 'You were so keen to come with me, terrified I would leave you, and here you are being shown all this kindness and you haven't the good manners—'

'All right! All right! Don't go on and on. If I have to go I have to.'

A very reluctant boy accompanied Laura to Braehead. Apart from a glum face he was looking very smart in his new suit and his unruly hair had been brushed into some order. The furniture from her father's bedroom and the front room hadn't fetched as much as she had hoped but enough to get Ronnie new clothes and a pair of shoes.

Mrs Mathewson came to the door. She welcomed Ronnie but didn't make a fuss and for that she went up in his estimation.

'You can show your brother his room, it's all ready, but wait a while. Mr Cunningham has an appointment so the lad had better see him now.'

They followed her to the sitting-room where Laura had had her interview. Sylvia was playing with building bricks on the floor and Mr Cunningham dropped the paper he had been reading when they entered. He got to his feet and so did his small daughter.

Ronnie was nervous. He didn't know what to do with his hands and his new shoes were hurting his heel. It was all too posh for him and it was terrible not knowing what was expected of him. Laura had been precious little help. 'Be polite and answer when you are spoken to.' As for that little girl, did she have to stare at him like that? Staring without blinking. Come to think of it that must be difficult to do. He must try it when he got home.

'So this is your brother, Miss Morrison?'

Laura murmured an introduction and Ronnie's hand was firmly shaken.

'Pleased to meet you, sir.'

'What is your name?' the child lisped but Ronnie hadn't quite heard.

'Pardon?'

'What is your name?'

'Ronald Morrison.'

They were all laughing and for the life of him Ronnie couldn't see what was funny. He shot his sister an anguished look.

'That is his full name, Sylvia,' Laura said, 'but he's called Ronnie.'

'Can I call him that?'

'You must ask the young gentleman, not Miss Morrison,' her daddy smiled.

'Suppose so,' Ronnie muttered. 'I mean yes you can,' he corrected himself when he saw Laura's raised eyebrows.

They were all seated by this time and the man was asking him sensible questions that he didn't mind answering. Not silly talk like asking what you are going to be when you are a big boy. A big boy. He never bothered to answer. After all eleven was nearly grown-up.

'Made any decisions regarding your future, Ronnie?'

'No, sir, I haven't quite made up my mind.'

'Well, eleven is a bit early and I take it you are not in a hurry to leave school?'

'No.'

The little girl had climbed on to his knee and made to speak.

'No, dear, you mustn't interrupt, you'll get your turn later.'

She pouted but obeyed and Ronnie was glad that she had to keep quiet, he wanted to hear what the man was going to say.

'You remind me a little of myself at that age.'

'Do I?'

'Yes, I used to like my own company and slip up to my bedroom to read. My brother was the opposite. He had no time for books, never sat still long enough to read one, but he was a wizard at sport and very popular. He made me sick. You see, Ronnie, I was jealous.'

Ronnie burst out laughing. 'That's just the way it is for me. I get called a swot and I'm not. My dad,' he faltered, 'thinks it is important to be good at sport. He would have liked me better if I had been.'

The man nodded thoughtfully. 'Very often we come off better in the end and that is something you should bear in mind.'

'Because it means getting a better job with more money?'

'The money part aside and that is seldom the most important, Ronnie, no matter what is said to the contrary. What is important is doing a job well whether that job be in a trade or profession.'

'May I ask you something, sir?' Ronnie said eagerly and Mrs Mathewson exchanged a smile with Laura. Sylvia was sucking her thumb and her eyes were closing.

'Of course you may.'

'Did you get to do what you wanted when you left school?'

'That is difficult to answer and I have to think about it.' He paused.

'I made a decision which I haven't regretted but I may well have had equal satisfaction in some other profession.'

'But you must have wanted to do what you are doing?'

'Ronnie!' Laura said warningly.

'No, Miss Morrison, I started this and the question shall be answered to the best of my ability. As a wee laddie, Ronnie, I wanted to be an engine driver, no doubt you went through that stage too?'

Ronnie nodded. He hadn't but he wanted this man to think he had so it made them more alike.

'An uncle of mine was extremely good to me. He was a man of the cloth—'

'Is that a minister?'

'A minister of religion, yes. I wanted to please him and for a time, a very short time I have to add, I wanted to follow him. That, however, is a special calling and I think the family were in general agreement that I was not cut out for the ministry. In the end I followed the path intended for me and after university I joined the family law firm.' He looked at his watch. 'Sadly I must end this very interesting conversation, Ronnie, but no doubt we can continue it at a future date.'

'Shall I?' Laura said, making to take the sleeping child from him.

'No, I'll put her on the sofa, she's quite a weight.'

They were outside. 'He's all right, Laura.'

'I told you that and you wouldn't believe me.'

'It's still rotten having to leave home but it won't be as bad as I thought.'

'You must be pleased with your bedroom?'

'I am, it's great, and the shelves will hold my school books, jotters and things.'

Laura smiled at his enthusiasm. She could stop worrying about her brother. His own little world had been shaken but was settling again. Life for him wouldn't be all that different. He could disappear to his own room whenever he pleased. Changing schools would have been an ordeal but thankfully that hadn't proved necessary.

The items on Laura's list were being ticked off. She cancelled the newspapers and paid Mrs Grieve, the woman assistant who had been behind the counter for as long as Laura could remember.

'Sorry to see you going, Laura, but needs must, I take it?'

'Yes, I'm afraid so,' Laura smiled. She wondered about the stories going around and just how far wide of the mark they were. It didn't matter. Her departure would be a nine days' wonder and then there would be something else to gossip about.

'Good luck to you and Ronnie but seeing as you aren't leaving Miltonsands we'll maybe see something of you.'

'Sure to.'

'Mrs Brand going too, I hear.'

'Yes, nothing but changes, Mrs Grieve.' She put the change in her purse. 'Goodbye, Mrs Grieve.'

'I'm just saying cheerio and good luck.'

Laura's next call was to the dairy. She paid her bill and the owner, a dour man who seldom smiled, managed one for her.

It was all over and Laura marvelled at how smoothly it had gone.

An empty house looked so cold and cheerless but the one she was leaving had escaped the worst with the flooring and curtains remaining. The linoleum was very worn in parts and perhaps she wouldn't be thanked for leaving it since if the new tenants wanted new wax-cloth they would have the trouble of lifting the old. The curtains were in good condition so maybe that would make up for the shabby flooring.

Aunt Peggy had thought it ridiculous to leave the curtains and Mrs Brand had been surprised.

'What was to hinder you taking them down?' Aunt Peggy wanted to know.

'What would I have done with them? Where could I have put them?'

'In one of the cases,' she pointed out.

Her father had taken the best cases and what was left had broken catches and had to be held together with string. Once Laura had emptied them they would be flung out.

Time for the final goodbyes. Ronnie was next door with his old chum. Both boys seemed happy to be together and Alan was inviting Ronnie through to Montrose for the holidays.

'Ronnie can come, can't he, Mum?'

'Yes, Ronnie, you'll be made very welcome.'

Laura was alone and going from one room to the other for a last look. Her eyes went to the faded wallpaper shown up by the removal of the furniture and to the wall where too boisterous play had caused a tear in the paper and her mother, after a good deal of scolding, had repaired it as best she could, but it still showed. It was so sad saying goodbye to a house that had always been home and Laura was having difficulty in holding back the tears. It wasn't so much the house that she would miss but rather remembering her mother in it. In the kitchen humming a tune while she prepared the meals. Coming upstairs to say goodnight and when she was very young to hear her say her prayers. Laura didn't pray much these days and when she did it was only when she wanted something. Perhaps it was time she gave thanks to Him for showing her a way out of her difficulties.

She was silly to imagine a house had feelings and that it would miss them. What she and Ronnie were leaving was an empty shell and another family would make it into a home again. Was this what life was all about? The pain of partings. Was change inevitable? Was life mapped out and what we did made little difference? Or were we in charge of our destiny? So many questions and no real answers.

Her mother dead. Her father gone and Michael had found someone else to love. She had dreamed of a future with him and maybe, just maybe, that dream could still come true. Michael had been deeply hurt, they had both said things she regretted anyway, but time was a great healer and if he really loved her . . . She sighed. All she was doing was making matters worse for herself. Nothing had changed, she wasn't free and wouldn't be for a very long time.

She began to wonder about her own feelings. She had felt betrayed when she had met Michael and his new love. Betrayed because she had believed their love to be very special and that it would all work out. It hadn't and she must face that fact. Those first weeks after seeing them together had been filled with despair but she had hidden her unhappiness. There was so much to do that she had gone to bed and slept the deep sleep of exhaustion. During the day Michael was now just a dull ache.

Time to go. Time to leave her old home but the sadness was lifting. Her memories wouldn't remain here, they would go with her. She shut the door for the last time and with a smile on her face went into the house next door. Soon they would be leaving too and in Mrs Brand's own words, the house was in a pickle, but they would sit down and have a meal together. There would be talk and laughter, then she and Ronnie would take their leave and set out to start a new life.

Chapter Fifteen

George Morrison was only a shadow of his former self. He was sitting up in bed with the pillows at his back and watching the activity below. Nurses in their white, stiffly starched uniforms were crossing from one part of the hospital to the other. George was hardly aware of them, his eyes were searching for the one person he wanted to see and when she came into sight his eyes brightened.

Connie knew the window, knew that he would be watching and waiting, and she waved. The bandages weren't so bad now, he did have some movement but not enough to raise his arm and wave back. His was a small ward, only two beds in it. The other was empty, the patient gone home to recuperate there. Soon another case would be brought in. This ward was kept for serious car accidents, automobile accidents as they called them here. A nurse was in constant attendance except at visiting times when she was mostly in the corridor directing visitors to the larger wards and making sure her own patients were not over-tired by well-meaning but too talkative visitors. Connie was never that, she could read the signs and when she saw her husband's distress would take his bandaged hand and hold it gently in hers and stay quietly by his side. A sensible woman, the nurse thought, and wished there were more like her.

How dreadful that it should have turned out this way, Connie thought as she went through the wide entrance and followed others up the stairway. The only view of New York that George had seen so far had been from a hospital bed. Connie hated the smell of hospital, it brought back her own stay in it. Conscious but traumatised, she remembered the ambulance screaming its way through the traffic with George unconscious and the driver of the cab who had been declared dead on arrival at the hospital. Her own injuries had been severe bruising to the body, a broken left arm and a nasty gash to her forehead. She had been very, very lucky.

Poor George had been less fortunate. He had been sitting behind the driver when the cab had skidded and gone into the back of a lorry and lodged itself there. The police and the fire service had been quick on the scene and had got her free but it had taken longer to get the other two from the tangled mess.

For four days George had lain in a coma, his life hanging in the balance. He had taken a very severe knock to the head which had everybody worried. Broken bones would mend, bruises would eventually disappear, but there could be severe and permanent brain damage that could leave George little better than a vegetable. Fortunately George began to show signs of improvement and the doctors were much more hopeful that there would be no lasting damage. Even so he would require to be kept under observation for some time yet.

When George did come out of the coma he remembered nothing of the accident or of his life before it. The doctors told Connie, when she was well enough to be wheeled to her husband's bedside, that amnesia in cases like his were not uncommon. Memory could return quickly and completely or it could be a slow process. Nobody said that it might never return but they were all aware of the possibility.

George had terrible headaches which were easing now. Sometimes in confusion he would have flashes of memory when he would shout for Ellen and want to know about Laura and Ronnie. Then he would know by the silence that something was wrong since it was an embarrassed silence. This woman sitting beside the bed was a stranger but a stranger who seemed familiar. There would follow a foggy recollection when he would struggle with a memory that Ellen was dead and Laura and Ronnie had disappeared.

Throughout it all Connie had been wonderful and he remembered when he'd called her Connie and she had bent over to kiss him and he had tasted the salt of her tears.

'Welcome back, darling,' she had said.

The door opened and she breezed in. No tiptoeing now, not today anyway. The other bed was empty and George no longer suffered the agonising pains in his head when every small noise was like a hammer blow and every footfall a crash of cymbals.

'Darling, here I am,' she said, pressing her lips to his.

He smelt her perfume and with it came the familiar longing. He wanted her near him always.

'You look wonderful.'

'Do I?' she smiled.

He nodded. The navy costume with its large white lapels was very smart and stylish. She wore a hat but it didn't hide the beauty of her blue-black hair.

'The mark on your forehead is almost gone.'

'Camouflaged with make-up. We women do have the advantage there,' she smiled. 'Thank goodness you still have your handsome looks.'

'Had I been badly marked would you have still loved me?'

She crossed one elegant silk-stockinged leg over the other. 'What a question to ask and I suppose you want a truthful answer?'

He didn't reply just watched her face.

'I never lie just because it is easier to do so,' she said in her husky voice.

'I know that.'

'Your looks were the attraction to begin with. Love followed and a badly marked face wouldn't have altered that or at least I hope it wouldn't. Happily I won't be put to the test because I still have my good-looking husband.'

He smiled. The answer had satisfied him.

'I don't seem to have asked the most important question. How are you?'

'Well enough to go home, that is if we have one to go to. I don't want to land on your sister and your brother-in-law. Bad enough that he is paying to keep me here. How in God's name am I going to pay that back?' He sounded angry and frustrated.

'Sh-sh,' she said, putting her finger against his mouth. 'Getting into a state will only hold back your recovery. Dr Steele, I had a word with him, is very well pleased with your progress but you need a few more weeks.'

'I've had enough of this place, I want out of here,' he said sulkily.

'Darling, I couldn't possibly give you the attention you get here.'

'I'd be too much trouble, is that it?'

'Don't be childish and difficult or I won't give you my news.'

'What news?'

'You promise to behave?'

'Yes! Yes!' he said irritably.

'I've found an apartment for us and I'm sure you'll approve.'

'Since you are paying for it—'

'Oh, for heaven's sake, George, if it wasn't for your bandages I'd give you a good shake. Harry will not be looking for repayment for the hospital bill. He feels terrible about what happened and considers he was partly to blame.'

'That is nonsense.'

'No, not entirely. Harry is a decent sort. He was coming to meet us, remember, but there was an emergency, something to do with business, and he arranged for a cab instead. Had that not happened there would have been no accident.'

'I don't hold him responsible.'

'Neither do I but I can understand how he feels. For him this is an easy way out of his guilt, he'll hardly miss the money. Satisfied?'

'Relieved anyway.'

'Good. I hadn't finished but I can see that I am tiring you and the rest will keep until the next time.'

'I am not tired and how often do I bloody well have to tell people that, including you.'

'Language, dearest, it's a good thing that sweet little nurse isn't here or she would be scandalised.'

'Just tell me if there has been a letter from Laura.'

'No, dear, and I waited for the post before I left Lottie's.'

'You did write? You are sure you put on the correct address?'

'George,' she said quietly, 'I wrote quite a long letter to your daughter explaining everything. I checked the address carefully and posted the letter myself.'

'Then why hasn't she replied?'

'Maybe she and this Michael decided to get married and have moved away from Miltonsands.'

'It would have been re-addressed. Mrs Brand, our next-door neighbour, would have known Laura's address.'

'Perhaps you have to face it that Laura has decided not to reply.'

'She wouldn't do that.' He was looking distressed and she said sharply, 'In London you weren't all that concerned about your family.

According to you Laura took after her mother and would be well able to look after herself and her brother.'

'Maybe I wasn't concerned enough. Lying here day in day out I have had plenty of time for thinking. Connie, I've treated Laura badly, I see that now. I can't blame her if she doesn't want anything more to do with me.' He paused for a rest. 'She got a place in college and she and Ellen were in seventh heaven about it.'

'And you thought education was wasted on a girl?'

'I still think so. All right for a plain girl but Laura is pretty and she'll never be short of admirers. No chance of her being left on the shelf.'

'I know reasonably nice-looking women who didn't want marriage but we'll leave that aside. You have done some soul-searching and you are feeling guilty?'

'Yes, a bit anyway. I just want to satisfy myself that they are both all right.' He looked at her pleadingly. 'If I could only use my hands, if I could only hold a pen.'

'It'll come.'

'Write to Laura again, please.'

'What good will that do? Far better to write a short letter to one of your sisters and presumably they will know what has become of your son and daughter.'

'No, Laura would hate that. They don't get on all that well.'

'It was just a suggestion,' she said mildly.

'I know,' he said excitedly. 'I know exactly what to do. Write a letter to Laura, please Connie, and enclose it with another. My boss in my old office is very obliging and if he doesn't know where Laura is he'll make it his business to find out.'

'How would he do that?'

'One of the other clerks has a lad in Ronnie's class at school and if Ronnie has moved to another school it will be perfectly possible to trace him.'

'Do you remember the office address?'

'As well as I remember my own name.'

'Very well,' Connie said resignedly, 'I'll get the letters off as quickly as possible.'

'Have you a piece of paper to write down the office address?'

'Yes, I have in my bag.'

'Do it as soon as you can.'

'Yes, yes and yes again.'

'What was the other thing you wanted to tell me?' She heard the weariness in his voice.

'That can wait. My time is up and I don't want the nurse to think I am taking advantage. She has been extremely good about bending the rules for her favourite patient.'

His eyes were closed as Connie let herself out of the ward. Pity she had to keep the rest of her news for the next visit. She thought he would be pleased but it wasn't always easy to know with George. Much as she loved him he was difficult to understand.

On the next visiting day Connie looked attractive in a coat dress in lime green.

'The Lamberts were here,' George said.

'Lottie and Harry? How nice?'

'Take a look in the locker: you'll find it stuffed with candies. Better put some in your bag.'

'Give them to the nurse.'

'Don't you want any?'

'Can't afford to eat anything sweet. I must try and keep my figure since I am at an age when it is very easy to put on weight but not so easy to take it off.'

'You did write?'

'Of course I did and spent most of the evening doing it. You must remember it isn't easy to write to strangers.'

'I'm sorry, I do ask a lot of you.'

'George, you must at times wish that you had never set eyes on me. You could be in London or back in Miltonsands instead of coming through all that pain and suffering.'

'Wrong, my darling, you couldn't be more wrong. This has been sheer hell, I won't deny that, but until I met you I didn't know what love was. Ellen and I were happy together and when she died it was dreadful but if I ever lost you I wouldn't want to go on living.'

'Somehow one gets the strength to go on. I know because I so nearly lost you.'

They were both silent – both remembering.

'George, am I ever going to tell you my news?'

'I'm listening.'

'I'll keep my voice down, I didn't notice that there was someone in the other bed.'

'Poor devil was brought in this morning. Haven't discovered who he is.'

'Poor soul, is he badly hurt?'

'Don't know, seems to be sleeping most of the time.'

She nodded. 'You know how keen I was to get a job in the fashion world?'

'Is that it? You've got yourself a job.'

'A bit more to it than that and it could involve you.'

'Beggars can't be choosers.'

'I cannot stand people who dismiss something before they even hear it.'

'I stand corrected or in my case sit.'

She smiled at his attempt to joke. 'Lottie and I got talking about the fashions in New York. They concentrate almost exclusively on the young woman. Those in their forties and older are ignored. Such short-sightedness since these are the people with money and a great desire to look smart and attractive.'

'So?'

'So we aim to show them real style. Create fashions just for them. So many New Yorkers go too much for fripperies and that is a big mistake. Simplicity is the keynote here and I mean to educate them that this is the look for the older woman.'

George was trying to show an interest he didn't feel.

'Who is going to finance it?'

'Harry is —'

'Harry again! Good old Harry.'

'Yes, Harry and Harry again,' she said sharply, then looked in consternation over to the hump in the other bed but it hadn't moved. The nurse came in, smiled at Connie, looked at the form in the other bed and went out.

'This is to be a partnership. Lottie is bored, she hasn't enough to do. The house runs efficiently and the kids are taken care of.'

'Comes of having money.'

'Yes, it does. Lottie is keen that we should undertake this venture together. Harry is to look for suitable premises in a good district and put up the money to get us started. He is all for Lottie having an interest outside the home and he is financing his wife, remember. Once we get started and begin to make a profit I'll repay Harry.'

'If it is a success?'

'I am as confident as I can be that we have found a niche in the market. Women love to be cosseted and told by someone knowledgeable what they should wear and the look they should strive for.'

'Sounds all right but where do I come in?'

'On the financial side. We need someone who understands the other kind of figures,' she smiled.

'I'm not an accountant.'

'No.'

'Maybe you need a trained accountant or maybe again you don't,' he said thoughtfully.

'You could be interested?'

'Perhaps.'

'Not for a while, not until you are fully recovered. I'm no wizard with figures but I'll manage until you are ready to take over.'

'We'll be in business together.'

'I like the sound of that, don't you?'

George did. The job that was to be his would now be filled. He wondered if there had been a job or was one to be made for him?

Chapter Sixteen

Laura wasn't long in settling into life at Braehead. In that first week she had met Betsy Yeaman, the friend of the family who lived nearby and who would be looking after Sylvia on Laura's day off. Fergus Cunningham had introduced them and in those first moments both knew that they had made a friend. Betsy Yeaman was of average height and thin rather than slim. She had slightly sloping shoulders that made what she wore hang awkwardly. She had no interest in clothes for herself, just happy to wear what was comfortable, and the number of layers were added to or taken away according to the vagaries of the weather. She did, however, admire fashionable clothes on others and would give her carefully considered opinion on an outfit if asked to do so. Fergus was one of the very few who knew her age. She was ten years his senior and he was thirty-one.

Betsy had been a plain but much-loved child of parents who had been denied children until both had reached the age of forty. She in turn had adored her parents and returned that love by nursing them until they were both taken from her. She was quite alone apart from an elderly and deaf housekeeper and those days spent at Braehead with little Sylvia Cunningham were the highlight of her week.

Davina Dorward, whom Laura had also met in her first week, was a very different person. Betsy was plain and Davina was beautiful but Davina's was a cold beauty. She was quite tall with a good, curvacious figure and chestnut-brown hair which she wore in the short, cropped style that was becoming fashionable. Her features were perfect, her complexion clear, and she had an air of sophistication that Laura couldn't help but admire and envy. She also dressed beautifully.

Discovering that there was someone in the hall, Laura had been about to turn back but Fergus Cunningham had seen her and spoken. 'Don't run away, Laura, come and meet Miss Dorward.'

Laura went forward, a smile on her face.

'Davina, this is Miss Morrison who has come to take charge of Sylvia.'

Davina Dorward looked startled for a moment, then drawled a disinterested 'How do you do' before turning away. There had been no attempt made to shake hands but in Miss Dorward's eyes Laura would be a servant and not someone to whom she would give her hand. She would have forgiven her for that but not for the insolent way her eyes had looked her up and down before taking Mr Cunningham's arm and all but leading him away.

Laura flushed at the slight and knew that it had been deliberate. Clever too since it had happened in the moments when Fergus Cunningham's attention was elsewhere.

In Betsy Yeaman, Laura had found a good friend. Had she also made an enemy? Time would tell and this was the woman who could be the next Mrs Cunningham. She wouldn't think about it. She would forget Davina Dorward.

Davina Dorward couldn't dismiss Laura so easily. For a start there was Fergus making free with the girl's Christian name and her appearance had been like alarm bells. She had expected Mrs Mathewson's successor to be someone similar to Mrs Mathewson but a few years younger. Not a girl with the bloom of youth and one who was quite lovely. There was a grace and dignity about her too that only added to her disquiet. What was a girl like that doing in such a job?

Davina was thoughtful as she got into the car. They were on their way to spend the evening with mutual friends. Davina liked it to be taken for granted that they were a couple. Fergus and Davina. Davina and Fergus. She looked at his profile, the firm chin, the grave attention he gave to the road. He drove fast but not too fast and was always in control. Davina sighed inwardly and wondered if she was wasting her time. Fergus was proving more difficult than she would have believed. She had always been in love with the attractive, quietly spoken lawyer and believed that if she hadn't been so stupid as to play hard to get he would never have married Mavis. How she had hated that woman. She had done no mourning. Indeed she had just bided her time thinking her day would come and that after a decent interval Fergus would turn to her. He had but just as a friend and so far it had remained just that. Was he blind? Couldn't he see what an asset she would be? She had looks that other men admired and a figure that other women envied. Over and above she had the social graces and would make an excellent hostess. In short she was the right wife for a successful lawyer. Mavis had been a vivacious and scatterbrained creature who had died in tragic circumstances. Fergus never spoke of the tragedy, neither at the time nor since, For weeks he had gone about grey-faced and with a haunted look. The newspapers had made a lot of it – TRAGIC DEATH OF PROMINENT LAWYER'S WIFE. There had been an inquest and the verdict, as expected, was accidental death. Not everyone was satisfied.

The rumours did not concern Davina but the death left the way clear for her. She had always wanted Fergus Cunningham and he had been the reason for turning down offers of marriage. Then he had gone and married Mavis and she had been devastated. A man in her life was necessary, always had been and always would be. She had tried to hang on to the more presentable but when they finally tumbled to the fact that there was no future in it for them they dropped the lovely Davina to look elsewhere.

Time was not on her side. She would be thirty this year and the only one of her set as yet unmarried. Her looks wouldn't last forever and the day was fast approaching when she would look in the mirror and see the first faint lines. It was a depressing thought and Davina shivered. Why was Fergus so slow? What was he waiting for? Not the period of mourning that was long over. Folk expected him to take a wife, particularly when there was a child. Davina had little time for children, she didn't understand them and didn't want to. As to that spoilt little brat, Sylvia, she could see her far enough. Davina had seethed to see how willingly the child went to everyone but her. No manners either since she had to be prompted to say thank you for the presents Davina brought.

There was almost a desperation in the jagged thoughts going through her head but there was also a steely determination. How should she go about it? Mustn't scare him off. Perhaps just half-jokingly bring the matter to his attention. Tell him that the others were asking her when they were going to name the day. Yes, that would be a good approach, and if she played her cards right Fergus would see no honourable way out of it. He was the perfect gentleman and would ask the question she was eager to answer.

That all but settled in her mind, she would think about the changes she would make at Braehead. Ideally, of course, they would sell the family house and buy something bigger and better. Davina didn't expect to win there. Fergus loved the old house. The next best would be a facelift for Braehead. The existing furniture and furnishings would have to go and she would get in the professionals to discuss and advise. New staff would replace those already there and first out the door would be that Laura girl. Her lips curled. Fergus might be a good lawyer but he hadn't a clue about organising his own home. A middle-aged woman would be engaged for the child, a strict disciplinarian who would stand no nonsense and prepare Sylvia for boarding school.

'You are very quiet, Davina. Penny for them.'

'Sorry, dear, I was deep in thought.'

'What about or shouldn't I ask?' She saw his smile. Fergus wasn't interested but good manners made him ask since he would know that she wanted to tell him. He was right.

'Sylvia was in my thoughts. Darling, what on earth possessed you to engage a young, inexperienced girl and entrust her with caring for your precious little daughter?'

Fergus shot her a surprised look before returning his attention to the road.

'I have to agree that she is very young but she is also very capable and dependable.' He smiled as he remembered the interview with Laura. 'She pointed out to me that the child needed someone young, someone with the energy to run about and play with her. She mentioned the park and feeding the ducks.'

'How very rude and forward of her.'

'She was neither rude nor forward.'

'She must have been and hadn't you always found Mrs Mathewson satisfactory?'

'Yes, I had no complaints but I do see that the child is too much with older people. In the park she will be able to play with other children.'

'A man doesn't notice things that a woman does and I have to confess to feeling very unhappy. Not only unhappy but worried too.'

'Why should you be worried?'

'You ask that? I'm worried, Fergus, because I care for Sylvia and I don't want any harm to come to her.'

'What possible harm could come to her?' he said sharply, then regretted the sharpness of his voice. Davina was after all only voicing what had been his own first impression. He had thought Laura too young for the responsibility.

Davina was getting more frustrated by the minute but she couldn't let it go there. Perhaps she could still make him see sense.

'Girls of her age have boys on their mind, that was what I meant. She isn't unattractive and her young charge may not get her whole attention.' She smiled. 'Had you given a thought to boys?'

'It crossed my mind,' he said, amused. 'She is a very lovely girl.'

Davina swallowed hard. 'You don't see difficulties?'

'I always see difficulties, Davina, it is part of my training but I deal with them if and when they arise. I don't meet them half-way if I can help it.'

Only with difficulty was she managing to hold back her anger. 'You surprise me, you really do, Fergus. I hadn't expected you to be quite so offhand about something that should concern you very much.'

'Of course it concerns me, Davina, and if I hadn't thought Laura suitable she would not have been engaged. I pride myself on being a good judge of character.'

'Nobody is infallible.'

'I hope I didn't suggest I was, but I believe the girl to be level-headed. Her life in the last year or two has not been easy.'

'Fobbing you off with a hard-luck story, you are too—'

'I'm not one to be fobbed off with any hard-luck story,' he interrupted.

'Then tell me why a young girl should answer an advertisement clearly intended for a mature woman with child-caring experience?'

'Probably caught her eye since it offered a home and she felt herself qualified to apply.'

'Homeless as well as everything else, dear me.' She couldn't keep the sarcasm out of her voice.

'No, not homeless but the very real possibility of that sometime in the future. Had she had only herself to consider Laura could have coped but she has the responsibility for her schoolboy brother.'

'You are having this boy to live at Braehead?'

'It was the only way to get Laura.'

'Part of the bargain?' The words were out before she could stop them.

'You could call it that,' Fergus said frostily.

Davina took a deep breath. 'I sincerely hope that you don't come to regret it.' She turned her head to look out at the darkness and to hide her anger.

Fergus said nothing, there was just the tightening of his lips.

As they approached their destination and to avoid further conversation, Fergus gave more concentration than was needed to parking the car.

Davina adjusted her cape and wondered unhappily if she had gone too far and perhaps damaged her own chances. Then she brushed that thought aside. For this evening she had taken special care over her appearance and was confident of the many admiring glances that would come her way. Fergus couldn't fail to notice and she would be at her wittiest and sparkling best.

Fergus Cunningham was becoming increasingly uneasy. Just of late Davina had turned very possessive, acting as though there was an understanding between them when nothing was further from his mind. He did have a twinge of conscience. Perhaps he had made use of Davina but only because she had shown such willingness to partner him. Surely to God he hadn't given her the wrong idea? There was the way she kept addressing him as darling and that he found irritating but he made allowances since the endearment was so widely used and so meaningless in their circle.

Another uneasy thought came to mind. The invitations that had come since his wife died had said Fergus and partner but now as often as not they said Fergus and Davina. Which was to say that they were now accepted as a couple by a few of his friends and all of hers. A few, he now recalled, had gone as far as hint that it was time he remarried.

They could be right and Sylvia did need a mother, he mused. Braehead required a mistress for the smooth running of the house, although there was nothing terribly wrong with the way it was run at present.

Poor Davina, she was only trying to help and he had been quite nippy. He really must put matters right and be especially attentive this evening.

Marriage! Was he having serious thoughts about it? He and Davina had known each other for many years and they got along well. He had seen and been amused by the envy he had seen in other men's eyes, so what was holding him back? He didn't even pretend to himself that he

198

loved her but there was liking and she could be very charming. His thoughts shifted. Why did she stick with him? Surely she wasn't in love with him? If so, was she waiting with growing impatience for him to propose?

There was one very big obstacle. His daughter hadn't taken to Davina and poor Davina made the mistake of trying too hard. One couldn't win over a child by showering gifts on it.

Laura had made a conquest in the first few minutes. Fergus sighed. His trouble was, and he recognised it, that he wanted the best of both worlds. He didn't want marriage to Davina but then again he would miss having her around. Fergus thought back ruefully to those dinner parties he had been obliged to attend. The way the seating had been carefully arranged so that he had a single or widowed woman beside him. Sometimes as they searched for a common interest he was sure their embarrassment was as great as his. The one thing they then had in common was a longing for the evening to end.

He went to open the car door for Davina. 'I'm sorry,' he whispered, 'blame overwork for my boorishness.'

Davina smiled brilliantly. She had been about to apologise and had been searching for the right words. 'My fault just as much as yours,' she said, linking her arm in his.

The evening turned out to be like so many others. The food was excellent and beautifully served and drink was plentiful. The women were fashionably dressed but none outshone Davina. Fergus joined in the laughter but he kept thinking of home, Sylvia rosy from her bath and cuddled into Laura for her bedtime story. They had been seated on the sofa and for a little while he had been with them. A happy family scene and he had been reluctant to leave.

Chapter Seventeen

Mrs Mathewson had fully intended showing Laura over the whole house but something always got in the way. As the days went by the usually calm housekeeper was becoming more and more flustered and apprehensive. It had been lovely to think of retirement when it wasn't quite on her but now that her final day at Braehead was fast approaching she was less sure. Would it turn out as she hoped? For so long she had thought of the peaceful days ahead but she hadn't considered the loneliness when she could find herself with too much of her own company.

Laura didn't remind Mrs Mathewson, time enough to see over the house when she took up her duties. It wasn't as though she were taking over from the older woman in the true sense. Mrs Mathewson had been a housekeeper but Laura's position in the house was more difficult to define. Her main task, the one for which she had been engaged, was to look after Sylvia and that would take up a large part of the day. But not all of it and Laura felt that she should do more since Ronnie was to be living at Braehead. She was to be in charge of the household accounts and the paying of the wages to the kitchen staff as well as the gardener and his assistant. The house, apparently, ran itself. She would just have to wait and see.

The child was beyond the toddler stage and should be getting more freedom. Constant supervision was bad, it was stifling. She needed space to express herself, find her own amusements and not have everything handed to her. Laura was thinking of her own childhood. Her mother had always been there in the background, keeping an eye on her, but giving ample freedom to an eager, enquiring child who wanted to explore on her own.

For the first few days Laura was grateful to Annie for her guidance and help.

'Anything you're not sure of be sure and ask. You can't be expected to step into Mrs Mathewson's shoes and carry on as she did without some help.'

'I'm not really stepping into her shoes, Annie. I wasn't engaged as a housekeeper.'

'Maybe not, but it is what you are.' She smiled. 'Here I am calling you Laura when I should be addressing you as Miss Morrison.'

'I'm more comfortable with Laura.' She gave a nervous laugh. 'I can't see me giving orders.'

'You'll learn to do that but there is little need at the moment. We all do what is required of us and in return we get a fair wage. I won't be stepping out of line and that goes for Mrs Barclay and Jean Fairley. You won't get a rough ride from any of us. For one thing we wouldn't want to risk losing our job and these are difficult times.'

'Thanks, Annie, you make me feel better already.'

Sylvia was a handful but Laura was well able to control the child when she became too boisterous. Jumping up and down on the sofa as well as being harmful to the springs was not acceptable behaviour. The child would have to understand that.

'Sylvia, if you must jump do so on the floor and not on the sofa.'

She continued to jump on the sofa but with sly glances in Laura's direction.

'No means no, Sylvia,' Laura said severely as she lifted the child down.

'Daddy—' she began indignantly.

'Daddy would not allow that. He wants to come home to a nicely behaved little girl and not to a silly little baby who jumps up and down on the furniture.'

'I'm not a silly little baby.' Sylvia looked on the verge of tears.

'Most of the time you are a very good little girl.'

The child sat down and looked at Laura through half-veiled eyes. 'I've nothing to do,' she complained in a babyish whine.

'We could go out. Would you like that?'

'It's raining.'

'I like being out in the rain.'

'And get all wet?'

202

'We won't get wet if we put on a raincoat and have something to cover our hair.'

Sylvia seemed interested but uncertain.

Laura got up. 'Come along, Sylvia, we'll put on wellingtons and walk through all the puddles. That'll be fun, won't it?'

Sylvia giggled. 'I'm going to splash you.'

'And if you do, Sylvia Cunningham, I'll splash you back. Where are your wellingtons kept, do you know?'

'I'll show you.' Eager now to be outside, Sylvia took Laura's hand and pulled her towards the cupboard next to the kitchen, and sure enough the place was filled with an assortment of rainwear and two pairs of shiny red wellingtons. Both pairs looked new and Laura lifted them to see the size. She chose the larger size.

'I'll get socks.'

'Why?'

'It's better to have two pairs to keep your feet cosy.'

When they were dressed and ready for outdoors Sylvia looked like Little Red Riding Hood in her red raincoat, matching souwester and red wellingtons. Laura wore her old navy raincoat, a beret to cover her head and a pair of wellworn black wellington boots.

The rain had become a constant drizzle as hand-in-hand Laura and her little charge went out the back door, through the garden and into the lane. Traffic used the lane and mindful of this Laura kept well to the side. There were plenty of puddles on the uneven road and soon Sylvia was happily splashing herself and when she got more daring began to splash Laura. Laura gently returned the splashing to Sylvia's delight and her squeals of excitement could be heard all around.

They were so engrossed that neither heard the car and were only aware of it when the vehicle slowed and stopped.

Laura looked at the driver and flushed to the roots of her hair. At the same moment Sylvia became aware that it was her daddy and rushed over to him.

'Daddy, I splashed Laura and she splashed me and I'm having lots and lots of fun.'

'So I see.'

Fergus Cunningham had opened the car door and to her relief he was smiling broadly.

'She won't come to any harm, Mr Cunningham,' Laura said anxiously.

'My dear girl, this is what the child needs. You only have to see her face to see how much she is enjoying herself.'

'Daddy, you come out and play too.'

'Can't do that, poppet, Daddy has to work to make the pennies.' He smiled at Laura. 'I left some papers at home and needless to say they had to be those I require for the case I am working on.' He closed the car door, gave a wave of his hand then drove on.

He was smiling to himself. At first he hadn't realised that it was Laura and his small daughter. What a delightful picture they made and he found himself wishing that he'd had a camera to capture that happy scene. It would have been nice to send a snapshot to his parents and reassure them that their grand-daughter was well and happy.

By the time Laura and Sylvia returned to Braehead the child was healthily tired and went to bed for her rest without a murmur. Almost at once the eyelashes fluttered, then the eyes closed and the regular breathing showed she was asleep. Laura left the door slightly ajar. Household noises wouldn't disturb the child, only unusual ones did that. After an hour she would go up, it was long enough for an afternoon nap, any longer and it would put her off going to bed at her usual time.

This was a good time to see those rooms of the house that she had not as yet inspected. She started with the drawing-room with its big bay window fronting the garden that at present looked bleak and uninteresting. By spring and summer, she was told, the gardens would be a blaze of colour and the view from the window quite spectacular. Laura stepped into the room and was impressed with its grandeur but a little uncomfortable too. It was too lavish and spoke of money. Laura much preferred the sitting-room with its hint of shabbiness that made it so homely and inviting. The sitting-room had character. The drawing-room was a showpiece.

There was the breakfast room where the master ate his meals, all but dinner which was set for him in the dining-room. Laura thought it a shame and rather sad that it shouldn't be used more often. Fancy having a good cook like Mrs Barclay, a lovely dining-room and taking his friends to a hotel! Maybe this was an area where she could help. It shouldn't be beyond her to organise a dinner party, a small dinner party for eight or ten people. Once she was more confident she would suggest it to her employer.

Laura was surprised to find that Sylvia had all her meals in the kitchen. She saw no harm in having breakfast there, at least until the child was of school age, but other meals should be taken in the breakfast room where she would be taught proper table manners in readiness for the big move to the dining-room.

Cook liked nothing better than spoiling children. Sylvia ate what she wanted and left what she didn't. It was bad for the child and wasteful. It would have to stop but Laura would have to go about it carefully.

Ronnie got his plate heaped up with whatever he fancied and the 'piece' he took to school for his lunch made him the envy of the other boys. They were all going to be killed with kindness.

Expecting to be teaching young children, Laura had done a lot of reading. Some of it dealt with the pre-school child and what to notice. No two children were the same and each child required a totally different approach. It emphasised that point. There were chapters about the children who had imaginary friends and speaking to them as though they were real people. In the short term it was safer to ignore. More than likely when the child had other interests it would stop. Sylvia had her soft toys with her in bed and there was no harm in that. Teddy was her favourite and at the table he had his own plate. Mrs Barclay put food on each plate and Sylvia spooned some to Teddy. Laura wanted that to stop.

'Leave Teddy on the bed and come and have breakfast.'

The child shook her head vigorously. 'Teddy hungry.'

'No, Sylvia, Teddy isn't hungry.'

'Yes, he is and if he eats a lot he gets sick.'

'That is because he doesn't want to eat. He just wants to stay on your bed with the rest of your soft toys.'

She had the teddy bear in her hands but after a struggle with herself she put it down on the bed.

'Good girl.'

Only children were often lonely children and clung to their Teddy for comfort. Sylvia had seen too many changes in her short life. How could one tell how much a child remembered? There was the closeness of the mother and baby in the womb followed by the nursing of the infant. That was a special bond, and did something of it remain with Sylvia? No one could tell. Only her daddy was a constant figure and he was with her for only short spells. Poor little Sylvia.

Fergus Cunningham had finished his meal and his coffee cup was empty. It was half past six and early for him. This could be an opportunity to have a talk with Laura and iron out any problems. He hardly dared admit it to himself that it was no more than an excuse to have her company.

Laura had come in quietly. 'Would you like more coffee, Mr Cunningham?'

'No, thank you.'

'Then I'll take this away,' she said, putting the coffee things on a tray.

'Do that, then come back here if you will. Incidentally where is the little minx? I seldom get my coffee in peace.'

'Shall I get Sylvia?'

'No, I just wondered where she was.'

'I hope you don't mind but she's followed Ronnie to our sitting-room,' Laura said half-apologetically.

He laughed. 'Is she being a nuisance?'

'No, not at all. Ronnie would rather die than admit it but I think he is tickled pink to have Sylvia follow him around.'

'Most certainly he wouldn't admit to that, I wouldn't have at Ronnie's age.'

She smiled. 'Your daughter's education has begun. Ronnie is teaching her to count and according to my brother she isn't bad which is praise indeed.'

'I'm sure it is.'

'One to five with ease, six to ten with some difficulty.'

'Very good. You get rid of that tray and come back.'

Laura returned very smartly.

'Sit down, Miss Morrison.'

Laura sat down in the chair he indicated, her hands in her lap, and waited.

'Since the child addresses you as Laura, you won't mind me using your Christian name?'

'Not at all. I'm not used to being called Miss.'

'Had you become a teacher it is how you would have been addressed.'

'Yes.'

He seemed to have forgotten what he was going to say and Laura, uncomfortable in the silence, said hastily, 'Was there something you wanted to see me about, Mr Cunningham?'

'Only to ask if you are settling in and if there are any problems you wish to discuss.'

'I'm settling in happily and so is Ronnie. Everyone is so kind and helpful.'

'I'm glad.' He looked pleased.

'If you have the time there are one or two—'

'Problems?'

'No, not problems, I just need guidance.'

'Then now is a good time to hear them. I am in no particular hurry.' He gave her an encouraging look and settled more comfortably in his chair.

Laura, without being aware of it, did the same.

'As you may know, Sylvia has her meals in the kitchen and although that is fine for breakfast meantime, I do think she should have her other meals in the breakfast room.'

'To be honest with you I wasn't aware of the arrangements. I agree the kitchen is not the place for Sylvia although breakfast there is probably acceptable. I'm glad you brought this matter to my attention. Where do you take your meals?'

'In the kitchen or sometimes I have a tray in my own room.'

'In future please have your meals in the breakfast room and supervise Sylvia. I have no idea what her table manners are like – probably awful.'

'Oh, no, please don't misunderstand,' she said hastily. She didn't want Mrs Mathewson or Mrs Barclay blamed. 'Sylvia eats her food very nicely.' It was taking a liberty with the truth. The child banged her spoon on the table for attention and fingers were much in evidence when eating with them proved to be easier.

'Nevertheless I would like you to correct any bad habits she has acquired. She may, as you say, eat nicely but I am sure there is room for improvement.'

Laura smiled. 'Yes, some room I think.'

'What about your young brother?'

'He is being killed with kindness, Mr Cunningham, and having his meals in the kitchen suits Ronnie.'

'I'm sure it does but even so you don't want Ronnie's table manners to suffer. Have Ronnie eat in the breakfast room when he can be persuaded. Anything else?'

'I wondered about Christmas.'

'Christmas! Yes, I suppose it will be soon upon us.'

'What are the usual arrangements, Mr Cunningham?'

Laura wanted to laugh, he looked so mystified.

At last he shrugged. 'I can't recall much about the previous Christmas. Presumably cook will produce the traditional Christmas fare. The staff get something extra in their pay packets and that's about it.'

'I didn't mean that. What about Sylvia?'

'The child gets a great many gifts and if you have any suggestions as to what she would like, or what you would like her to have, please let me know.'

'I really meant about a Christmas tree and decorations,' Laura said desperately. 'Children love those and if you have no objections to holly and a few decorations in here—'

'My dear girl, you have a free hand. Do what you wish and buy what you need.'

'I promise not to go too rash and overdo it.'

'Just make it a happy Christmas for the child, Laura, and for Ronnie. I think we should have Christmas lunch in the dining-room and it might be rather nice to invite Betsy Yeaman. She isn't likely to be doing anything and she may enjoy the company.'

Laura showed her delight. 'Betsy is a lovely person and she is marvellous with Sylvia.'

'She is a good soul.' He paused. 'We've settled that point and I calculate we shall be five for lunch.'

Laura wondered how he arrived at five and then thought with a sinking heart that Miss Dorward, as Mr Cunningham's lady friend, would be invited. Ronnie would have his in the kitchen but she, herself, would be present to attend to Sylvia.

'Betsy, Sylvia, yourself and Ronnie, and myself as host.'

Laura felt a wave of relief that there was no mention of Davina Dorward. Ronnie would prefer his in the kitchen and she tried to say so.

'Certainly not, Laura, Ronnie will dine with us.'

In the time left before Christmas Laura promised herself that table manners would come high in her priorities. She wanted her employer to be pleased with his daughter, and Ronnie's manners could do with a bit of polishing.

She made to get up but he waved her back. 'No, not just yet. There was one other thing I wanted to say regarding the haphazard domestic arrangements in this house. You see, Laura, when my wife was alive she supervised the staff and there was, I distinctly recall, a young girl who served at table. Perhaps she left and Mrs Mathewson didn't see the necessity to replace her or perhaps again she brought it to my notice and it had slipped my memory. No matter, we do need a maid to serve the meals and I want you to see about engaging a suitable person right away. May I leave that with you?'

'Yes, I'll see to it.'

He got up and opened the door for her. What a delightful girl she was and so lovely. Her face was smooth with the warm glow of youth and as she thanked him her mouth curved tenderly when she smiled. As he sat down again with his newspaper, Fergus Cunningham was smiling. What a stroke of luck it had been that the girl had applied for the vacancy and thank goodness he'd had the good sense to employ her. The nagging worry that the child wasn't getting the attention she needed was gone. Laura had breathed new life into Braehead and made a little girl very happy. He amended that to include the child's father. Ronnie was a nice, quiet, sensible lad, a bit like a big brother to Sylvia. Such thoughts must be kept from Davina, she would be quite horrified. To her Laura was a paid help and should be kept in her place. To him she was an intelligent and brave girl. The work she was doing was so far removed from what she had expected but she had accepted it for her brother's sake. Fate had not been kind to Laura Morrison and her brother. Fergus found himself wondering about a father who could desert his own children. Most fathers would be very proud to have such a lovely daughter and clever son.

Mrs Barclay was beaming. 'Christmas lunch for five in the dining-room, it's a start anyway and maybe we'll be doing some entertaining before long,' she said as she waddled to the oven. There was a rush of heat as she checked the meat sizzling in the tin. Deciding it could do with a few more minutes, she shut the door smartly and continued with what she was saying. 'There was a young lass, no' bad at her job either, but she didn't stay long.'

'I'll have to advertise.'

'Maybe I could save you that bother.' Alice Barclay was a small, stout woman with a rosy complexion and small buttons of eyes that disappeared when she laughed. Her sleeves were rolled up and she wore a white apron tied at the back. There were a few brown stains on it. 'Would you look at that?' she said, fingering the stains, 'I hate a mucky pinny, that was me stirring too vigorously. Now where was I? Oh, I mind now, I was to bring Jinny Ingram to your notice.'

'Who is Jinny Ingram?'

'Tell you in a minute. That tea in the pot should be drinkable. Be a good lass and pour me a cup and one for yourself.'

Laura got two cups and saucers and poured the tea. With Ronnie it had been coloured water, this was black as tar, the way the cook liked it. Laura added hot water to hers while Mrs Barclay brought over the biscuit tin. On it was a picture of Queen Victoria and some lettering but over the years it had faded and little of it could be made out. Mrs Barclay, like so many stout people, sat down with her feet well apart.

'You were going to tell me—'

'About Jinny. She's a lass that might do you. Honest and reliable I would say. Her granny brought her up.'

'Is she looking for a job?'

'That I wouldn't know but she might be. She was training to be a tablemaid when her old granny took ill and she had to give it up and look after her.'

'I take it the old lady has recovered?'

'She's as well as she's ever likely to be but she doesn't need Jinny with her all the time. You wouldn't be wanting her full-time?'

'To be truthful I hadn't thought that far but no, it doesn't need to be full-time.'

'You can work out the hours between you, that shouldn't be diffi- cult, and she could come in at other times if wanted.'

'That sounds ideal but I would have to see her for myself.'

'I can arrange that for you.'

Two days later Jinny was in the kitchen talking to Mrs Barclay when Laura went in.

'Here she is, Miss Morrison. This is Jinny Ingram.'

'Hello, Jinny,' Laura smiled.

Jinny smiled shyly and got up.

'We'll have our talk in the breakfast room.' Laura opened the door, noticing as she did the encouraging smile the cook gave to Jinny.

The girl wore a brown tweed coat with a belt and was hatless. She carried an old-fashioned clip bag that Laura guessed must have belonged to her grandmother. There was little difference in the age of the two girls but Laura felt much older.

'Mrs Barclay mentioned your previous employment,' Laura said once they were both seated.

'I was training to be a tablemaid, Miss Morrison, and I was sorry when I had to leave.' She swallowed nervously. 'I couldn't do nothing else 'cos there wasn't anyone to look after my gran.'

'I do understand,' Laura said sympathetically.

'Everyone was pleased with me and they were going to keep the job open only they didn't 'cos I was away too long.'

Laura nodded. 'Can your grandmother be left alone?'

'Yes. She can get about with a stick and a next-door neighbour would keep an eye on her.'

'Working a few hours daily would suit you?'

'Yes, nothing would suit me better, Miss Morrison, and I can come in at other times if I was needed.'

'From time to time that could be necessary and I am thinking about Christmas Day.'

'I could work all day if you wanted,' she said eagerly. Her face lit up. 'It would be more fun than just sitting with my grandmother. She nods off for much of the time.'

'Old people tend to do that.' She explained the hours, her duties and the wage. 'Would you consider that satisfactory?'

The girl's eyes opened wide. To be asked if it was satisfactory, no one had said that to her before.

'Oh, yes, Miss Morrison, very satisfactory,' she breathed.

'You'll start on Monday and I shall look forward to seeing you then.'

'Thank you.' The girl stood up clutching the bag to her chest. 'I'll be ever so careful. I never had no breakages in my last place.'

'What did you think of Jinny?'

'I liked her and I think she'll prove very satisfactory, Mrs Barclay.'

'She'll need a uniform, a maid's outfit. It's come to my mind that there are two or three frilly aprons in the linen cupboard. The mistress ordered them and a lacy thing for the head.'

'Will they do for Jinny?'

'Do for anyone but she'll need a black dress.'

'Is that part of the uniform?'

'It is. The last lassie would have left hers behind and with a bit of alteration it should do.'

Jean had come in to wash the floor and heard some of the conversation.

'A good bit of alteration I would say. Yon was a hefty lass and there isn't much of this one.'

'Well, it shouldn't be beyond Jinny to shorten it and a belt will do the rest,' she said as if that was the end of the matter.

Laura laughed. 'I'm sure Mr Cunningham won't mind the girl getting two new dresses. He will want her to look smart.'

Already the shops in Miltonsands were displaying their Christmas goods. Children pressed their noses to the window and screamed to each other what they wanted. Mothers grumbled that Christmas got earlier every year. Some declared that the Christmas clubs were to blame but most took advantage of them. It was a way of spreading the expense over the year. Housewives, factory workers and shop assistants paid a regular sum each week from their wages or housekeeping and were able to reserve the goods of their fancy.

Laura's mother had subscribed to none of the clubs. She had been strong willed enough to put aside her own money without fear of dipping into it.

At home the same decorations had gone up year after year with the occasional replacement when one was too tattered and torn to be stuck together with glue. Laura wondered if there were boxes of decorations and perhaps crackers hidden away somewhere at Braehead. Annie would be the most likely to know.

'No, there are none about the house.' Annie shook her head vigorously.

'Surely they weren't thrown out?'

'None to throw out. Never did much at Christmas, not after the old folk left. The young mistress didn't bother with Christmas decorations.'

'Didn't she celebrate Christmas?'

'Of course she did, but she and the master always spent Christmas with friends and we didn't object, it made for an easy time for us.'

'Annie, what was the young Mrs Cunningham like?'

'In appearance? Bonny and fair-haired. The wee lass takes after her.'

'You must have known her?' Laura thought it was like pulling teeth to get any information on the young Mrs Cunningham.

'How could I have known her? I would see her about the house but orders came through Mrs Mathewson and I doubt if I ever got the time of day.'

'I see,' Laura said resignedly.

'Tell you this much. She was a restless creature always needing to be on the go. Not enough to occupy her. The bairn had a nursemaid—'

'Didn't she look after Sylvia at all?'

'Oh, at the start the baby was a great attraction and shown off to everybody, then when she got tired of that she looked elsewhere for amusement.'

'Not an easy person to live with?'

'No, and he must have been real fond of her to put up with all he did, but then don't they say that love is blind?'

Laura thought he must have loved his wife very much. Occasionally he must have longed for a quiet night in his own home instead of having to dress and take his wife to the theatre or wherever they went.

She had discovered a little more, but not all.

Chapter Eighteen

The days went by. Mostly they flew and Laura wondered where the hours had gone. There was no discord, everyone was quietly content. Jinny had settled in and always arrived early to begin her duties. For her work in the kitchen she wore an overall on top of her own clothes. Her uniform was kept strictly for serving at table. Two black dresses had been ordered from a shop in Dundee that specialised in servants' wear. They were plain but well cut, had a slightly flared skirt and a neat white collar that was detachable for easy laundering. Everybody agreed that Jinny looked a treat in her black dress, stiffly starched apron and the piece of lacy nonsense settled on her hair which was how Annie described it.

Jinny was thrilled and happy. No one had ever taken such an interest in her before except her gran and she didn't count. What really had her singing with happiness was the master taking the trouble to compliment her on her appearance and saying how well she served at table. Fergus Cunningham had spoken to Laura too.

'That girl is extremely good. You chose well.'

'Yes, Jinny is very good but I can't take the credit. I didn't need to advertise. You see, Mrs Barclay suggested Jinny since she lives within walking distance and had some experience.'

'Excellent. Do sit down, please.'

'Thank you.'

'Christmas preparations going well?'

'Yes. I've ordered a tree and I'm reasonably well organised. May Sylvia borrow one of your longer socks or better still kilt stocking to hang up?' she said with an impish smile.

'You think of everything.'

'I try to.'

'Reminds me of when we were very young,' he said softly. 'My brother and I used to hang up our stocking and one year Roger decided that his wasn't big enough for all he hoped to get. Somehow he managed to get hold of a pillowcase and hung it at the foot of his bed.'

'Did he get it filled?'

'He did not. My stocking was filled with the usual – you know, an apple, an orange and a new penny and a few more interesting gifts on top. Roger got nothing, just a note pinned to the pillowcase which had words to the effect that greedy boys got nothing and that was what he was getting.'

'Rather hard, wasn't it?'

'Just my father's way of teaching him a lesson. Roger received his gifts later in the day but he had a long, anxious wait.'

'There was something *I* meant to ask you, Mr Cunningham—'

'And what was that?'

'I wondered – I know you sometimes entertain your friends at the hotel—'

'That is true.'

'It seems so unnecessary.'

'I felt it saved a lot of work for Mrs Mathewson who would have had to arrange it.'

'Things are different now. We have Jinny to do the serving and I would be happy to arrange a small dinner party.' She paused and then went on. 'Mrs Barclay and I could go over the menu together and then you could see if you wanted to make any changes.'

His face brightened. 'Why not, Laura? We have an excellent cook, an efficient tablemaid and I have every confidence in you as the organiser.'

'You are serious?'

'I am. We'll get Christmas and the New Year over and then settle on a date. I'm grateful to you for the suggestion.'

'I feel it is the least I can do. You are very good about Ronnie.'

Laura left with her spirits high. Arranging a dinner party would be a new experience and she wanted to make it a huge success so that it could be repeated and there would be no necessity to return to the hotel.

She kept reminding herself that it would be a mistake to let herself be lulled into a false sense of security. Circumstances could change so quickly and she must remember that Fergus Cunningham was an attractive man and Davina Dorward must have high hopes of becoming his wife. Saving was important and most of her wage was found money. The time might come when she would need to find accommodation for herself and Ronnie. She would have to approach the landlord for a two-roomed house and find herself another job. Not easy but she would get a good reference. Sadly there weren't many employers like Mr Cunningham and she couldn't expect to be taken on at the post office. Each day she prayed that nothing would change at Braehead but her prayers were not always answered.

She was young and felt she could be forgiven for wanting to look nice for Christmas. Surely she could treat herself to a new dress? Why it should be so important to look her best Laura couldn't have said. Her employer wouldn't notice what she wore, there was no reason why he should. He would, however, be interested in what his small daughter was wearing.

'Buy Sylvia the prettiest dress you can find, Laura.'

'Yes, I'll have a good look round but honestly, Mr Cunningham, Sylvia has some lovely dresses hanging in her wardrobe, a few haven't even been on.'

'Blame her grandmother,' he smiled.

Laura knew about the parcels, usually dress-boxes, that arrived from the child's grandmother in Devon. Inside were lovely little dresses and frilly underwear packed in masses of tissue paper. They came direct from an exclusive children's outfitter.

'No, I wouldn't do that but it is a pity when they don't fit.'

'My mother keeps on asking me to send on the child's measurements but how on earth should I know? She knows Sylvia's age and I would have thought that enough.'

'I'm afraid it isn't, Mr Cunningham. There are fat children and skinny children and those in between who share the same year of birth but not the same measurements.'

He smiled. 'I stand corrected. I have asked Mother to stop sending so many parcels but her trouble is that she has only to see one of her friend's grand-daughters in something she admires and she is ordering one of them for her own grandchild.'

'That is lovely and very natural. It would be a shame to spoil her pleasure and if you don't mind I'll keep you supplied with Sylvia's measurements allowing a little for growth.'

'In case she shoots up?'

'Yes.' She paused. 'Any particular colour of dress you would like me to get for Sylvia?'

'No! No! No! You deal with it.'

It was laughable but everyone seemed to congregate in the kitchen. Mrs Barclay moaned about it, asking how she could be expected to get through the work when she was never left in peace. The truth was, and they all knew it, that she liked nothing better. This was her castle and she was the queen.

At the moment she was giving all her attention to carving the meat, a big piece of tender beef.

'We'll have it hot today for everybody then cold for ourselves tomorrow and what's left after that I'll mince. I hate waste and no one could accuse me of it nor of being extravagant.' She looked up.

Laura, Jinny and Annie gave the appropriate answers and she continued.

'There's a good lot of beef dripping and that will do for stovies. Young Ronnie is partial to a plate of stovies when he gets in from school.'

'You spoil him,' Laura said as she made some calculations on a scrap of paper.

'Away with you and I like to see food enjoyed. Ronnie is a mannerly lad and he never rises from that table without saying thank you.'

Laura was pleased to hear it.

'Mind you, it isn't the same without that wee bairn and I'm missing her.' The cook pursed her lips. 'Tell me truthfully, Laura, how the lass is taking to having her meals' – she sniffed – 'in the breakfast room?'

'To begin with there were tantrums but not now. It had to come, Mrs Barclay, you knew that. Mr Cunningham will be expecting Sylvia to dine with him when she is a bit older.'

'That won't be for a while yet.' She sighed. 'I'm not blaming you, lass, like the rest of us you have to do as you're told.'

The postman arrived at Braehead about eight o'clock and in time for Fergus Cunningham to see his mail before leaving for the office. He went through the bundle, most were for him, one was for Mrs Barclay and one for Miss Laura Morrison. She had just come into the hall.

'Letter for you, Laura.'

'Is there?' she said, sounding surprised. It couldn't be from Montrose because it was only a week since she had replied to Mrs Brand's letter. Who could be writing to her? It would have to wait until she had more time. Laura put it into the pocket of her skirt and went to see to her charge. Sylvia would be awake. The child had a bath before going to bed so a wash was all that was necessary in the morning.

Dressing took a bit of time since Laura insisted that Sylvia dress herself. After that she would brush the child's hair, put a ribbon in it, then together they would go for breakfast. Laura made do with a cup of tea and a biscuit and she and Sylvia had their breakfast together.

She didn't wonder too much about the letter since it had a local post-mark. When she was free she went along to the sitting-room and took the letter from her pocket. She didn't recognise the writing and slipping her finger into the flap she opened it and drew out a page of writing together with a folded letter. When she saw that the letter had an American stamp her heart began to thump alarmingly. Her hand was shaking as she began to read the page of writing.

Dear Laura,

The enclosed letter came to me together with
a request that I make enquiries as to your whereabouts,
and if successful to have the letter forwarded to
you. No one in Fairfield Street appeared to be
acquainted with your new address.
Success did come through a member of my staff
who has a son at the same school as your brother.
I do hope to hear that the letter has reached you
and that the news in it is good.

Yours sincerely,

It was signed William Hart.

How very good of Mr Hart and she would certainly write to thank him. She fingered the letter and wondered at her reluctance to open it. Hadn't she longed for some word and it didn't have to be bad news?

What worried Laura was that it wasn't in her father's writing. At last
she opened it and smoothed out the pages. Laura began to read the
neat, slightly backhand writing.

Dear Laura,

My other letter must have gone astray or otherwise I'm sure we
would have heard from you.

Your father and I had only just arrived in New York when the car
in which we were travelling went out of control and got entangled
with another vehicle. Your father was very badly hurt but let me
hasten to say before I go into further details, that he is making slow
but steady progress. For a time it was touch and go as to whether he
would live. George was in a coma for some days and when he came
out of it he could remember nothing of the accident or of his life
before it. We were dreadfully worried but I'm happy to say that his
memory has returned and the terrible headaches have largely gone.
The broken bones are mending but the right arm and hand are
taking longer. George is very frustrated that he cannot as yet hold a
pen and has to depend on me.

He was greatly concerned about you and your brother but
consoled himself by remembering how capable you are.

To return to the accident the driver was dead when the ambulance
reached hospital. I had to be cut clear too and spent some time in
hospital but I was incredibly lucky, suffering no more than a few
broken bones, cuts and bruises and a very ugly gash to my forehead.

When no reply came to my letter to you I suggested to George
that I send a short letter to his sister but he didn't seem to think that
was a good idea. Mr Hart, I understand, is a former employer and
your father has every confidence that this letter will eventually
reach you.

Do please write at your earliest and put your father's mind at rest.
The address given is our apartment and that is where to send your
letter. At the time of writing George is still in hospital but not for
much longer.

My best wishes to you both

Connie

* * *

Laura was crying, the tears pouring down her cheeks.

'Oh, Dad, I'm so sorry, so very, very sorry for thinking the awful things I did. You didn't forget us after all.' Her whole body was shaking and when she got up her legs almost gave way. Tea, sweet tea, would help, it was supposed to be good for shock. She would make herself a cup then she would be able to carry on. She couldn't bear to answer questions just yet but she would tell Mr Cunningham at night. She wanted him to know the reason for her father's long silence. Ronnie would see the letter just as soon as he got in from school.

Her mind kept wandering and she would start something and forget to finish it. If it was noticed no one remarked on it. It had been a long, long day but at last it was four-thirty and Ronnie would be home from school at any minute.

'Jinny,' Laura called and the girl turned.

'Yes, Miss Morrison.' She always addressed Laura that way and Laura thought it better that she did.

'Find Ronnie, please, and tell him to go up to my sitting-room, will you?'

'Yes.'

'And keep an eye on Sylvia for me. She's happy with her crayons at present.'

'Don't worry about her, I'll keep her occupied but I'll get Ronnie first.'

'What's the matter? What's all the panic?' he said, coming in.

'A letter from America, Ronnie.'

'From Dad?' he almost screeched.

'Connie has written it but read it for yourself. Start with the letter from Mr Hart.'

Ronnie looked up after reading it. 'If Mrs Brand had still been here—'

'Yes, she would have known but we didn't tell anyone else. Didn't seem any need for it. And Ronnie, before you read Connie's letter Dad is recovering.'

'Recovering from what?'

'Read it for yourself and sit down.'

She watched the changing expressions crossing his face. Shock, horror, concern, and was that shame?

221

'I feel so rotten.' His eyes filled with tears and he wiped them away with an impatient jerk of his hand.

'I do too,' Laura said quietly.

'Dad could have died, Laura, that other man was killed. Do you remember what I said to you?'

She shook her head.

'You must. When we didn't hear I said that he should be shot.'

'You didn't mean it. We all say things we don't mean when we are hurt and angry.'

'I still said it though and maybe I did mean it at the time.'

'No, you didn't. Poor Dad. Mum used to say he was a terrible patient, that he was worse than a child.'

'That was for a bad cold or something like that. I bet he was brave when this happened.'

'Yes, I'm sure he was.'

'You'll have to let Aunt Peggy know.'

'I will once I get Sylvia to bed. I'll go over then. Do you want to come?'

'Only if you especially want me to.'

'No, it's all right, I'll go myself.'

'I want to write to Dad.'

'Of course you must.'

'Connie isn't bad is she?'

'No, I think she must be a truly nice person. I'll write to them both.'

'You'll have to tell Dad about giving up the house.'

'I know but I have a feeling that having come through so much he won't bother himself about that.'

Fergus Cunningham insisted that Laura be seated. He saw how pale she was and told Jinny to bring another cup so that they could have coffee together.

'Laura, just let me say how pleased I am to know that you have heard from America. I felt all along that there would be some explanation because no father would willingly abandon such a delightful son and daughter.'

'He could have been killed,' she said unsteadily, 'in fact it was a miracle he wasn't.' She bit her lip. 'I feel so ashamed that I didn't give

Dad the benefit of the doubt, but instead I just blamed him for everything that went wrong.'

He shook his head. 'Don't blame yourself, Laura. From what I gathered you were left with rather too many problems and too much responsibility before your father even left for America.'

'I should have coped better.'

'No,' he said firmly. 'You did your best in very difficult circumstances.' He smiled gently. 'And leaving your dreams in ruins.'

'My lost dreams,' Laura said with a tired smile. 'If I have learned anything from all this it is not to build up one's hopes too high or to make judgments. I was so wrong about my stepmother, she comes over in her letter as a very nice, caring person.'

'Not a wicked stepmother after all?' he smiled.

Jinny came in with an extra cup and fresh coffee and they waited until she had gone before continuing with their conversation.

'Far from being a wicked stepmother she is probably just what my father needs. My mother was managing but in the nicest possible way and Connie could well be the same.'

'There you are then, Laura. Everything is beginning to work out far better than you would have believed.'

'Yes, Dad is recovering, but slowly and it is going to be a very long time before he is able to work. Poor Dad.'

Fergus Cunningham poured coffee into Laura's cup and filled his own. Until he put the cup before her Laura didn't seem to notice, then she came to with a start.

'I'm so sorry, forgive me, I'd quite forgotten.'

'My dear girl, I am quite capable of pouring out a cup of coffee.'

'I know, but I should have done it for all that.' She gulped down some of the coffee. 'You have been so kind and understanding all along and I want you to know how grateful I am.'

She looked up at him with a hint of tears in her deep blue eyes and Fergus had an almost overwhelming desire to take her in his arms, to hold her close, but he had to fight it. Laura was so young and when she fell in love it would be with some charming young man and not a widower with a young child.

'I do have a favour to ask,' she said hesitantly.

'Then let me hear it.'

'Once I have Sylvia in bed would you mind if I took the bus over to see my aunt? She is going to be in a dreadful state when she hears about the accident but greatly relieved that there is word about her brother. They were very close.'

'My dear girl, someone else can see to Sylvia.'

'No, she is used to me and she goes down without any trouble. I know I'm free after that but I like to be nearby until she is sound asleep.'

'You are very conscientious. You do as you wish, then when you are ready I'll run you over to your aunt's house.'

'No, please, you mustn't go to all that trouble.'

'No trouble, I assure you. I'll have the car waiting at the front.'

Laura watched the capable hands on the wheel and thought what a gem of a man she had for an employer. He was far too good for Davina Dorward and Laura hoped that when he did take another wife it would be to someone worthy of him. Perhaps he wouldn't remarry – some men who had loved deeply were quite unable to think of another marriage. They had hardly spoken in the car but it was a comfortable silence.

'You had better direct me from here, Laura.'

'Yes.' Her mind had been wandering. 'Turn first left and then it is quite a bit along or you could drop me here.'

'Certainly not, I complete what I set out to do.'

He drove to the door of the house and as Laura got out she saw the curtains twitch.

'Thank you very much, Mr Cunningham.'

'My pleasure.' He drove away and Laura went to ring the bell.

The door opened smartly. 'Well, well! Laura, this is a surprise.'

'And a pleasant one,' Uncle Archie added as she went into the sitting-room. There was a good fire burning. Uncle Archie had been reading the newspaper and judging by the work basket Aunt Peggy had been mending socks. It was a cosy, domestic scene.

'Heard a car stopping and thought it was you getting out.'

'My employer gave me a lift over.'

'Well in, aren't you?'

'Let the lass get her coat off before you bombard her with questions.'

Aunt Peggy took her coat and Uncle Archie brought a chair closer to the fire. 'Sit yourself down, Laura, and how is the world treating you?'

'All right, I think.'

'What brought you, it must be something?'

'I've had a letter from America,'

'From George?' she said eagerly.

'No, from Connie, from his wife.'

'Why should—'

'Wheesht, woman, you'll hear more if you hold your tongue.'

'Dad was in an accident, a serious accident—' Laura filled in all the details and saw the deep concern on her aunt's face.

'Dreadful! Dreadful! We might have lost him and none of his dearest beside him.'

'He has Connie, Aunt Peggy,' Laura said gently.

Her aunt shrugged as though Connie didn't count. 'You didn't bring the letter?'

'I didn't think to, but that is more or less word for word. I had it off by heart.' Laura would have given the letter to her aunt to read but then remembered in time the reference to her aunts and her dad's wish that the letter should be sent to Mr Hart rather than to his sister.

'You did bring the address?'

'Yes, I've written it down,' Laura said, taking two folded pieces of paper and giving them to Aunt Peggy. 'One for Aunt Vera and that is the address of their apartment.'

'Thanks, lass, I'll write to George tomorrow once I've seen Vera and now I'll get that kettle on.'

'No, please, Aunt Peggy, don't make tea for me. I want to get back and I want to write a letter. So does Ronnie, so Dad is going to get a bumper mail.'

'You put that kettle on, Peggy, we'll have a quick cup and I'll see Laura to the bus.'

'No, really, Uncle Archie, don't leave the warm fireside.'

'You got a lift here and I'll see you safely on the bus.'

Chapter Nineteen

With Christmas only a week away Sylvia could talk of nothing but Santa Claus. Jack Deuchars, the gardener, had filled a box with sand and when the Christmas tree arrived he and Tim White, his young assistant, planted it firmly in the sand.

'That's a fine place for it, Miss Morrison, I couldn't have chosen better. Very wise it is to keep bairns a distance from the fire.'

Laura smiled. She was getting caught up in the excitement herself.

'Once I tie the ornaments on and drape some tinsel over it the tree is going to look lovely.'

'You'll be needing a bright star for the top.'

'No, Jack, it was to have been a star but Sylvia wants a fairy. So a fairy it is.'

'Somebody is a very lucky lass.'

Sylvia tugged at his sleeve. 'Santa Claus is coming.'

'Never!'

'He is! He is!' she squealed.

Jack shook his head. 'Now I wouldn't be so sure of that. Santa Claus only comes to good little boys and girls.'

Sylvia's face fell and she looked worried. 'I'm a good girl.'

'Is she, Miss Morrison?'

'Most of the time,' Laura smiled. Jack was a family man and had a nice way with children.

'Most of the time, you say?' He seemed to be pondering, then began to nod his head slowly. 'Yes, lass, I have a feeling you would qualify.'

Sylvia looked to Laura for enlightenment. 'Yes, Sylvia, Santa Claus is sure to come.'

Her little face brightened and she turned to Jack again.

'I'm going to hang up my stocking.'

'No, dear, your stocking is too small and you are going to hang up one of Daddy's,' Laura corrected her.

'You aren't the only one,' Jack said, 'I'm hanging up mine too.'

'What are you getting in yours, Jack?' Laura asked, though she thought she knew the answer.

'Same as always, my foot.'

The child looked mystified and ran away to find other amusement. A few minutes later she was back.

'When Santa comes down the chimney will he get all black and sooty?' she wanted to know.

'Oh, no, that would never do,' Laura said. 'Once you are in bed and fast asleep a good fairy comes and sweeps the chimney until it is all clean.'

'You'll be giving me the name of that good fairy, Miss Morrison. My good lady declares her sweep leaves as much soot behind as he takes away with him. And now I must stop blethering and get back to work. Come on, Tim,' he said to the thin-faced boy who had been standing saying nothing but taking it all in.

'You won't forget the holly, Jack?' Laura reminded him.

'No, you send that wee lass, Jinny, round and I'll have some ready for her. Tim here will be more than happy to give her a help with the carrying.'

Tim went bright red and his eyes fell to studying the toes of his heavy boots. Laura shot Jack a reproving look but she couldn't keep the smile off her face. Tim was painfully shy and Jinny nearly as bad, but it was obvious to all that the two young people were attracted to one another. Laura was for letting love develop in its own time but others, like Jack and Mrs Barclay, were all for giving it a helping hand.

By the time Ronnie was back from school the tree was decorated. There was holly on top of the pictures and Laura had paper chains ready to criss-cross the room. She hoped she wasn't overdoing it.

'B'oons,' Sylvia said. 'I want b'oons.'

'Balloons, dear. Ronnie, that is a job for you. You can blow up some and we'll tie them together and fix them to the ceiling.'

'With what?'

'I don't know. A drawing-pin or something. Use your imagination.'

'Is this the only room getting decorated?'

'That is enough don't you think?'

'What about our own room?'

'Anything left over you can put up, and come to think about it I want more holly.'

'To put where?'

'In the hall. A big vase of it would be sort of welcoming. Go and ask Jinny to get me more.'

'I could get it.'

'No, leave it to Jinny.'

'Is that because she is sweet on Tim?' he grinned.

'Nothing much misses you, does it?'

'Heard it in the kitchen.'

Laura spent her day off in Dundee. She had prepared a list of what she wanted and was looking forward to a browse before buying. Miltonsands prided itself on its good shops but when it came to clothes for special occasions the choice was limited. Top priority was finding a dress for Sylvia. There was such a wonderful selection that choosing was difficult. Had price been a consideration it would have been easier but it wasn't. Only the best was good enough for Mr Cunningham's daughter. The buttercup yellow very nearly won but in the end she settled for pink. Not a sweetie pink but a lovely soft shade that should be perfect with Sylvia's colouring. It was a party dress to appeal to a child as well as to adults. Laura loved the tiny rosebuds on the net covering the skirt.

The assistant, young and obliging, was waiting for Laura to make the final decision.

'Thank you for being so patient. I'm sure you won't want too many customers like me.'

'Don't you believe it, this is a pleasure,' she said when Laura handed her the pink dress. 'Some people come in and want to see everything in the shop. They know and we know there will be no sale but there is nothing we can do about it.'

'Except a frosty look and a few sighs,' Laura smiled.

'Wouldn't put that lot up nor down.'

'No, I suppose not.'

'This is for my employer's child. I do hope I have chosen well.'

'If it helps any I was hoping you would choose that one.'

'Were you?'

'My favourite when it came in. The buttercup yellow is gorgeous but it isn't a Christmas colour.'

'No, it isn't, I thought that too.'

'Shall I have it sent?'

Laura was undecided. 'I don't know, perhaps I should take it with me.'

'A bit awkward if you have other shopping and then getting on a bus.'

'I know, and it might be standing room only. Could you promise—'

'My word on it you'll have the dress by midday tomorrow.'

'Thank you.'

The assistant smiled. Serving was a pleasure when you got someone nice.

'I'll go right away and get this packed in a box and marked urgent for tomorrow morning.'

Laura was in high spirits when she left the shop. Plenty of time to look around for something for herself. She began browsing in the less expensive stores and one dress caught her eye. It was on the stand and she went over for a closer look. An assistant was hovering nearby.

'Beautiful shade, isn't it? Midnight blue it's called.'

'Very nice.'

'Like to try it on? Should be your size.'

Laura already knew that it was. She loved the colour, the simplicity of the style, and the sweetheart neckline was a favourite of hers.

'I'm not pushing for a sale but you should try it on.'

'It's the price I'm worried about and if I can't afford it there is no use trying it on.'

The price ticket had been pushed inside. 'Not as expensive as you thought, is it?' she said, showing Laura the price.

It was more than she wanted to give but not by so very much. 'All right, I'll try it on.'

The woman took it from the stand and they went along to the cubicle where Laura slipped out of her skirt and jumper and the assistant helped her into the dress.

Laura looked at herself in the mirror. 'It's just what I wanted but I really shouldn't.'

'Why not?'

'I won't have many occasions to wear it and I did put a ceiling on what I was to spend on myself.'

'Could be your lucky dress and you'll meet your Prince Charming.'

'Not a hope but that's a new line in patter,' she laughed.

'I have a persuasive tongue but I would never tell someone a garment suited them unless it did.'

'No, I don't think you would.'

'Others aren't so fussy, anything for a sale. Now I would say if you went home without this dress you'll regret it.'

'That's what I'm afraid of. You win,' Laura said, 'I'll take it.'

'Want it sent? Wouldn't advise it myself. Better to be on the safe side and take it with you.'

'Yes, I'll do that and thank you so much for your help.'

Next stop was a restaurant or small café. She'd had nothing to eat or drink since breakfast and she could do with something now. The restaurants were full and people were standing waiting for a table. No use joining them, she would find a small café. She did and sank down gratefully on the wooden chair. Tea and a buttered scone would do her until she got back to Braehead.

Refreshed and ready to do the rest of her shopping, Laura visited a bookseller's and chose a picture book for Sylvia. Ronnie was always delighted with books providing he had the selecting of them himself. She would give him money but wanted a surprise for Christmas morning. Clothes were out of the question. That wasn't a gift since he had to get them. Almost despairing of finding something to please him, she eventually settled on book-ends in polished wood. She wished she could afford a fountain pen or a watch for her brother.

Satisfied that her shopping expedition had been a success, Laura walked from the bus stop to the house. She went in the back door and up to her own room to deposit her shopping. After taking off her coat Laura put the gifts at the bottom of her wardrobe. When she had the time she would wrap them in Christmas paper. Last of all she took the dress from its box, shook it clear of tissue paper and hung it up. It looked lovely but accusing. A better use could have been had for that money but it was too late for regrets. As to her Prince Charming that was laughable.

There was no Prince Charming for Laura Morrison. Once upon a time it had been Michael but that was all in the past and only very occasionally did she give him a thought. Why had she bought a new dress? Was it to impress her employer, make him notice her? Of course not, that was ridiculous. Any attraction she felt for Fergus Cunningham had better be hidden, she mustn't make the mistake of confusing kindness with something more. How awful if he were to suspect that she thought of him in any other way but an employer. The Christmas excitement was going to her head. Davina Dorward would one day be mistress of Braehead and the only question was when. They were ideally suited coming from a similar background and knowing many of the same people. Together with that Davina had poise, beauty, elegance and sophistication. Other women didn't much like her but she wouldn't let that trouble her. Men did, she appealed to them, and many must wonder why Fergus Cunningham was taking so long to pop the question.

Laura had enjoyed her day in Dundee but now for some unaccountable reason she felt depressed. The dress had been a spur-of-the-moment buy, a stupid purchase since one of the dresses in her wardrobe would have done very well.

'Daddy! Daddy! Come and see,' Sylvia was trying to pull her father.

'Can't it wait?'

'No, I want you to see it now,' she said, pulling him into the sitting-room where Laura was tidying the floor of toys.

Fergus looked at the decorations. The curtains were drawn and the light glinted on the tiny ornaments hanging on the tree. There was holly on the mirror and pictures and paper chains criss-crossing the room.

'I do apologise, it is terribly overdone.'

'Nothing of the kind, I find it quite charming and you are to be congratulated. Without you here, Laura, it would have been a very dull Christmas for Sylvia. Mrs Mathewson was too old to bother and I must confess I didn't take much interest.'

'The fairy, Daddy?' She pointed.

'Where did she come from?'

'Laura found her.'

'Would you like to see the dress I got for Sylvia? It will be here by tomorrow.'

'No, I'll see it on the child on Christmas Day.' He paused. 'I have a small favour to ask.'

Laura looked at him.

'Don't get me wrong but there are occasions when Sylvia forgets to say please and thank you.'

'That surprises me very much, Mr Cunningham, I think she is very mannerly for her age.'

'I would agree with that but for some unknown reason the child always has to be prompted to say thank you to Miss Dorward. Embarrassing too since Davina is so good to the child.'

'I'm sorry, I'll have a word with Sylvia and make sure that Miss Dorward is thanked in future.'

'Thank you, I'm sure I can depend on you.'

'Sylvia, you do know that you must always, and I mean always, say thank you when you get a present?'

She nodded.

'Daddy says you don't always remember to say thank you to Miss Dorward.'

'She wants me to call her aunt and I don't want to,' she pouted.

'Maybe Daddy would like you to?'

'She isn't my real aunt and I don't like her, so there.'

'Sylvia, you are being naughty. Miss Dorward is very kind to you.'

'She isn't, she just wants Daddy to like her.'

Children even as young as Sylvia were surprising. They noticed a lot more than one imagined. 'Daddy does like her, that is why he wants you to like her as well.'

Her lower lip trembled. 'Are you angry with me, Laura?'

'Of course I'm not.'

'Why have I got to like *her*?'

'You have to be polite and you want to please Daddy, don't you?'

'I love Daddy and I love you too.'

Laura gave her a hug. 'I love you too and you are going to promise me, aren't you, that you will be nice to Miss Dorward and if she gives you a gift you'll remember to say thank you?'

'Yes,' she said and turned away. Laura busied herself and the child turned to her again. 'You love me best and Daddy second best.'

The door had been off the catch. How long had he been standing there? A moment or two, long enough to hear what the child had said. He had, she could tell he had by his smile. Not a trace of embarrassment whereas she didn't know where to look.

'Another moment and I might have heard the answer to that but alas I'll never know. I came to see if I'd left my pipe here.'

'Over on the coffee table,' she managed to get out.

'So it is. I'll take myself off to the study and make a start on work that should have been done last week. A lawyer's job is not always a happy one as I tell young Ronnie but it doesn't seem to put him off.'

'Has he hopes of becoming one? I didn't know.'

'Then I am more in his confidence than you.'

'So it would seem.' She smiled. 'It's early days, he is only beginning senior school and there is no guarantee that he'll get to university.'

'He has the ability and I was privileged to see his school record card. My parents would have been over the moon if I or my brother had gone home with results like that.'

'You must have made the grade?'

'Yes, but I had to work hard in my final two years at school and burn the midnight oil. I wished then that I'd read books to improve the mind rather than adventure stories that had me biting my nails.'

'What about your brother?'

'Roger did as little as he could and he hasn't changed much. He didn't make university but then it was never expected that he would. That said, he isn't stupid, not by any means, but quite unable to put his mind to something for very long. Roger is in India,' he added. 'No rest for the wicked,' he said as he left the room.

'Ronnie, you didn't tell me, but you must be having talks with Mr Cunningham.'

'What is wrong with that?'

'Nothing. He just mentioned to me that he had seen your school record card.'

'I wasn't showing off if that is what you are thinking.'

'I wasn't.'

'We just got talking and it sort of came up,' he said awkwardly. 'I like him, Laura. I know I said I wouldn't like living here but I do. In my letter to Dad I told him that we are living in a great place.'

Laura was worried and thought it better to warn him.

'Ronnie, don't get carried away, this might not last, you know.'

He looked at her strangely. 'Why not? I thought you liked it here.'

'I do.'

'For a wee kid Sylvia isn't bad. I thought she might be a pest but most of the time she isn't.'

'Sylvia is no problem, she is a sweet little girl.'

'I was going to tell you I bought her something for Christmas out of my money,' he said proudly.

'That was very nice of you. A book, I suppose?'

'You suppose wrong. Everybody doesn't like books.'

'What did you buy?'

'I'm not telling and you're not getting told what you're getting.'

'I don't want to know. I want to be surprised on Christmas morning.'

She saw the worried frown. 'What did you mean about not getting carried away?'

'If I tell you you keep it to yourself.'

'All right.'

'There is always the possibility, Ronnie, that Mr Cunningham will get married and it is unlikely that his wife would want us.'

'You mean that Dorward female, don't you?'

'Ronnie!' she said, shocked. 'I will not have you talking like that and I don't know what Mr Cunningham would have to say if he heard you.'

'Well, he won't, will he? That is what they call her in the kitchen. She is just his lady friend but I'll shut up about it.'

She should leave it there but she couldn't. Laura was curious to know what was being said in the kitchen. There was never any gossip when she was around.

'What are they saying in the kitchen about Miss Dorward?'

'Only that if he was interested in marrying her he would have done it before now. Is that what you are worried about?'

'I'm not worried,' she lied, 'but it would be a mistake to think that this could go on for ever.'

'When will Dad write do you think?'

'Connie said his right hand was badly hurt and trying to write with it would be too much of a strain.'

'Does he just dictate to Connie like she was his secretary?'

Laura smiled. 'I doubt if Connie would agree with that.'

'Sometimes she makes me laugh, what she says in the letter.'

'She has a sense of humour.'

'Dad didn't, not much of one.'

'He's changed, Ronnie. It's said you know that a brush with death can change a person.'

'Do you know what I hoped?'

'No. What did you hope?'

'That Dad would get a good job in New York, make more money than he got here and send us some.'

'I'm sure he would like to do that,' she said gently, 'but just now he is dependent on Connie and that could go on for a long while yet.'

'When one door closes another opens.'

Laura laughed and looked amazed. 'Where did you hear that?'

'David's mum. It was a long time ago but I remembered because it was about you. She meant leaving the post office and coming here.'

'That's true.'

'You won't be mad if I say something?'

'I might, it depends. Come on out with it, you've got me curious.'

'Mr Cunningham likes you.'

'How do you know?'

'I just do and it would be great if he married you. We could stay here for ever then.'

'Ronnie, for a clever lad you do talk a lot of rubbish.'

'Bet it could happen.'

'It isn't going to.'

'No harm in me hoping, is there?' he grinned.

He went away and left her smiling. Ronnie was a changed boy. He had so much more confidence and was a bit too cheeky at times. But that was better then before when he had been tongue-tied. Poor lad, like the rest of us he was entitled to his dreams. For a moment she allowed herself to think what life would be like were she to become the next Mrs Cunningham. No more financial worries. She would have a beautiful home and Ronnie too would live in Braehead for as long as he wished. He could stay on at school and hopefully go on to university. Sylvia was a dear little girl and she saw no problems there. She blushed when her thoughts strayed to Fergus Cunningham. She imagined being in his arms, of being loved, and she felt a tremor of longing. Was it love? She couldn't be sure of her own feelings. What she was sure about was Fergus Cunningham. He was a man who would be totally dependable. Laura sighed and then got on with her work.

Chapter Twenty

It was Christmas Eve and there was an air of expectancy at Braehead. Upstairs an exhausted child was sound asleep in her bed, a faint smile curving her lips. Laura smiled down at her and tucked the clothes around the hot little body. Every child felt it, this special magic about Christmas that had nothing to do with gifts. Fergus Cunningham's small daughter could have any toy that money would buy yet no little one could be more excited. The highlight of her day had been helping to find one of Daddy's stockings, the kind he wore with his kilt. Then, her eyes huge, she watched Laura hang it at the end of her bed.

Gifts for the child had been arriving in all shapes and sizes. One was from Devon. Sylvia's grandmother, much to that lady's relief, was now in possession of the child's measurements. Marked clearly were the instructions that the box was to be opened on arrival.

'You had better open it, Laura,' Fergus Cunningham said, handing her the box.

'You want me to open it?'

'Yes, it is probably something to wear.'

'I love opening parcels,' Laura said as she undid the string. When she opened the box she gasped.

'Look! Isn't it beautiful, absolutely gorgeous?' Laura said, taking it out of its fold and holding it up for his inspection.

He nodded. 'I take it the size is right?' he said lazily as he reached for his paper.

'Perfect.' Her hand touched the smooth velvet and she simply adored the shade, a deep cherry-red. The dress had a small white lace collar and pearl buttons to the waist. 'I shouldn't have got that other one, Mr Cunningham, Sylvia should wear this on Christmas Day. I'm sure her grandmother would like that.'

'Very probably. Let her wear both – not at the same time, I hasten to add,' he smiled across at her from above his paper.

'One in the morning and the other after lunch?' Laura suggested.

'If the child can be bothered to change, that is?'

'Little girls love to dress up.'

'Problem solved then.'

Fergus thought how pleasant and relaxing it was with Laura in the room with him. She was quiet, never intruding, and he was impressed with the way she handled Sylvia. When firmness was called for she was in control and made sure that the child behaved. Unlike Mrs Mathewson she didn't give in to tears and sulks. It worked too, he thought admiringly. Sylvia wanted to be in Laura's good books and very soon she would say sorry, get a hug, and all would be forgiven. He owed the girl a great deal.

'May I say how pleased I am at the way you handle Sylvia? She was getting horribly spoiled but she isn't that now.'

'Thank you. She is a lovely little girl and I've grown fond of her.'

'Are you happy here, Laura?'

'Very happy,' she said quietly, 'how could I not be? You have been very kind and I'll always be grateful to you for what you have done for Ronnie.'

'He seems happy enough.'

'He is.'

'Poor little chap, none of us likes the upheaval of being removed from the house we knew as home to the uncertainty of strange surroundings.'

'Given the choice, he would be reluctant to return.'

His eyebrows shot up. 'I'm so glad.' He folded his newspaper and deposited it on the floor.

'I'm sorry, I'm keeping you from reading your newspaper.'

'Not at all. After two or three attempts I've given up. The concentration has gone. Could be I'm getting into the Christmas spirit. No, don't run away, this is an opportunity to finalise the arrangements for tomorrow. Miss Yeaman, or Betsy as she prefers to be called, is coming over about ten. I thought Sylvia could open her gifts then. What do you think?'

'A good idea. Betsy would love to be there for the opening of the presents and Sylvia will be perfectly happy playing with what she gets in her stocking, or yours to be more correct.'

'Mine?'

Laura dimpled. 'Someone found a pair and I borrowed one. Perhaps you would like to fill it?' she said, greatly daring.

'What do I put in?'

'That is all taken care of.'

'Then come along and we'll get on with this very important job,' he said, getting up.

They went in and looked down at the sleeping child.

'Such innocence, not a worry at that age,' he whispered.

'Do you really believe that?' she whispered back, 'about no worries I mean.'

'Don't you?'

'Children worry. I did when I was small. Silly little worries but none the less very real.'

'I can't remember, I go back a bit further.'

'Not by all that much,' she said before she could stop herself.

'Very kind of you and much appreciated I'm sure but by my calculation a good ten or eleven years separate us. Let me cheer myself up by saying it isn't such a huge gap.'

Laura was embarrassed and kept her face averted.

'Did you check for holes in the stocking?' he joked.

'I did and there aren't any.'

'What goes in first?'

Laura handed him an orange then an apple.

'Where is the new penny?'

'Couldn't find one.'

'Never mind,' he said, putting his hand in his pocket and drawing out a number of coins. 'No pennies but a half crown should do.'

Laura took it from him and wrapped it in tissue paper before placing it beside the fruit.

Fergus looked at the neat pile waiting to be put into the stocking.

'You've gone to an enormous amount of trouble.' There was a packet of coloured crayons and one of coloured pencils along with picture cards and puzzles. There was also a china doll dressed in pink and a fluffy rabbit with a tartan collar round its neck. All items to bring joy to any little girl.

'Ronnie gave me a lot of help.'

'Then I am grateful to him too.'

The pink shaded lamp gave a soft light to the room and they had both been on hands and knees dealing with the filling of the stocking. With the task completed they chose the same moment to get up and their heads bumped together. He was full of concern.

'I am sorry, Laura, how clumsy of me.' His arm went to steady her and for a moment he held her close. Standing there with his arm encircling her, Laura felt a sort of breathlessness seize her and she moved away.

'It's all right,' she said shakily, 'no harm done. I have a thick enough head.' The child stirred, and fearful of disturbing her they both remained still. 'She's over again, probably just dreaming.'

On tiptoe they slipped from the bedroom. Fergus had been more shaken than he would have believed. Another moment and he would have crushed her to him. No use hiding from himself his interest in this lovely girl but he would do well to hide it. The very last thing he wanted to do was frighten her away. Laura, and Ronnie too, had breathed new life into Braehead and he found himself looking forward to returning home whereas before there was no pull other than his child, and by the time he got home Mrs Mathewson had the child in bed. Mostly it was just weekends he and his daughter were together.

Life was very different now. Ronnie no longer hid himself away though that could have been Laura telling him to keep to their own apartment. The boy seemed to enjoy it when they could talk man to man. Poor lad, he was very confused by that father of his. And was it any wonder? The man had behaved disgracefully, putting his own happiness first. Fate had decided to step in and deal him a cruel blow. A close brush with death had changed the man, or that was what he had gathered from Laura. He was taking a belated but nevertheless welcome interest in his family.

Earlier in the week there had been a few flurries of snow and hopes rose that this might he a white Christmas. It wasn't to be. The snow melted as soon as it touched the ground and Christmas morning dawned crisp and bright.

Screams of excitement brought a smiling Fergus to his daughter's bedroom. He was casually dressed and his usually sleeked-back hair was in disorder, giving him a boyish look. Laura had managed to get

Sylvia into her dressing-gown and slippers on her feet before she fell on the stocking bulging with little packages.

Laura's reward for all her work was the sheer delight mixed with wonder on the child's face.

'Santa Claus came and he must have come right into my bedroom,' she said almost fearfully.

'He must have, Sylvia,' Laura smiled, 'and aren't you a lucky little girl?'

'Did he bring you anything, Daddy?'

'No,' he said, pretending disappointment.

'Is there not a Santa Claus for big people?'

'No, dear,' Laura said gently, 'but big people exchange gifts and that is nice too.' She paused and looked at her employer. 'May I thank you for mine? It was very generous.'

'You have more than earned it.' He looked at his watch.

'Daddy, you're not going out?' his daughter wailed.

'No, I'm not, but I am going into the study for the next hour.'

'I'll see you are not disturbed,' Laura said.

'Would you? No matter how one tries to get ahead the unexpected always happens and has to be dealt with.'

'Daddy, I've got a present for you.'

'Have you, pet? That's nice but I'll wait until Aunt Betsy comes.'

'Laura helped me choose.'

Laura looked at her employer and shook her head vigorously. 'Don't blame me,' she whispered.

'Bad as that?' he grinned.

Laura raised her eyes to the ceiling.

Everybody at Braehead was happy and good-humoured and with reason. The extra in their pay packet had been generous and they were to have their own party after the lunch was served and the clearing-up done. They would enjoy the same traditional meal with the accompaniments. Two bottles of wine and a bottle of port were hidden away in case someone was tempted to a tipple before the time. Jack and Tim, the gardeners, could have had the day off but both chose to come in for half a day rather than miss out on the slap-up meal served in the kitchen.

Jinny was flushed and happy. She hadn't expected a Christmas bonus since she had only just started work. But there they were, two half crowns, and that was a great deal of money to Jinny.

Tim was racking his brains for a way to hand his gift to Jinny without anyone seeing him. Jack had taken pity on him but wished the lad had a bit more gumption. He didn't remember being so bashful when he was that age. Still, better that than being too forward like some he could mention.

'You bide here, Tim, and I'll get that lass down here. Use the shed, better than standing out in the cold.' He winked.

'That would be great, Mr Deuchars.'

'Well, I didn't see you going up to the kitchen.'

Tim's eyes widened in horror. 'I could never do that, Mr Deuchars.'

Jack shook his head and strolled away. Some time later Jinny arrived with her coat flying open. She had come over in a hurry and was pink with excitement.

'Happy Christmas, Tim,' she said breathlessly.

'Same to you, Jinny,' he said gruffly and held out a package. A nicely wrapped packet with a bow to finish it off. 'That's for you.'

'Thank you very much and that's for you,' she said, giving him a very small packet. It did have Christmas paper round it but it wasn't as neat as she would have liked.

'You shouldn't have done that,' he said, looking pleased and surprised.

'It isn't much,' she said apologetically.

'We can open them in the shed, that is if you want to?'

'Better than standing out here. I don't think anyone would be watching but you never know.' She giggled nervously, stepped in and he followed.

'Go on, open yours first, Jinny.'

'Better both do it together.'

'No, I want to see your face.'

She touched the package lovingly. 'It's so pretty, it's a shame to open it.'

'That's daft. You have to open it to see what is inside.'

'I know,' she laughed.

She undid the bow carefully, then slowly removed the paper thinking she would keep it for next year. The box had a cellophane top and

Jinny's eyes widened. The pale pink handkerchiefs had been made up to form a perfect rose.

'Tim, it's like real, and the best, the prettiest present I've ever had. You know this, I'm never, ever going to use them.'

'That would be stupid 'cos when all's said and done them are only hankies to blow your nose.'

'I've got plenty of old ones for that, these are special. Did you get the woman in the shop to wrap it up for you?'

'It was a girl and she offered, I didn't have to ask.' He was smiling.

Jinny felt a faint disquiet. The girl must have taken a fancy to him when she offered. Not many did that or made such a good job of it. Still, Tim had bought the hankies for her and maybe that meant he wanted her to be his steady girlfriend. Her heart gave a queer little jump. Tim couldn't help being nice looking and when they started going out together there were some she could name who would be envious. She hugged the thought.

'Open yours, Tim.' Jinny wished now that she hadn't let the assistant talk her into buying a tie-pin. She had believed it when the woman said they were all the rage with young gents but she should have known better. It was a very silly gift and Jinny was almost apologising for it.

Tim didn't know what it was, that was plain enough by the look on his face. She wouldn't have either if she hadn't been told.

'It's a tie-pin, Tim,' she said quietly.

'Knew that, I just couldn't mind the name for the moment. Like you I'm going to keep it in a safe place. Awful if it fell out of my tie, not that I wear one very often' – now why had he said that – 'only on special occasions—' He floundered to a stop.

'Are you pleased with it?' she asked uncertainly. Why was she asking? She couldn't exchange it.

'Of course I am. Couldn't have given me anything I fancied more.'

'You're not just saying that?'

'No, I'm not. Like I said, you couldn't have chosen anything better.'

Jinny thought he was overdoing it, but it just showed he was a nice lad with a kind heart.

'I'll have to go, Tim, there's all that work to get through.'

'Not too much for you?'

'No, I manage. There's the dining-room table to be set and there are crackers at each place. It'll be ever so bonny when it is all ready.' She smiled. 'Wish you could see it.'

'Yes – well—'

'You'll be along later?'

'You can bet on it.' They had been sitting on opposite corners of the bench and both got up.

'Must go.'

'Seeing as it's Christmas,' Tim said, putting his hands on her shoulders and bringing his face level with hers. Startled, she moved slightly and their very first kiss landed on her nose. It didn't matter, it was a beginning, a move in the right direction and two young people were very, very happy.

Betsy arrived a few minutes before ten and Jinny took her cloak, a warm garment in a dark blue and green tartan, and showed her into the sitting-room. Not one to display affection, Laura was surprised to get a kiss on the cheek and Sylvia a warm hug.

'I can't tell you how much I've been looking forward to this,' she smiled as she looked around her at the decorations and then the tree.

'Aunt Betsy, I've got two party dresses,' Sylvia piped in.

'Aren't you a lucky girl? Stand up tall, dear, and let me look at you.'

The child obeyed willingly and like all little girls she liked to be told how pretty she looked.

Laura had dressed her in the pink dress and she would keep it on until the Christmas luncheon was over. A spot on it would be easier to remove than from the velvet, where it always left a mark.

'This one is from Daddy, Aunt Betsy, and my other one is from my nana.'

'You look good enough to eat in that one.' She turned. 'Did you choose it, Laura?'

'Yes, you should have been with me to help me choose. I almost came away with the buttercup yellow.'

'A spring colour, cool and fresh. Pinks and reds are Christmas colours, warm and bright.'

'Wait until you see the red velvet.'

Betsy smiled and the smile lit up her whole face. For a moment she was almost beautiful. She had taken care over her appearance and

Laura thought the dress had been bought specially for the occasion. It was in very fine wool and in a lovely shade of lavender.

'You suit that colour, Betsy, and you look very, very nice.'

'Thank you, Laura. I thought the occasion worthy of a bit of effort.'

Sylvia tugged at Betsy's sleeve. 'That's Laura's party dress and you haven't said it is pretty.'

'I know, dear, I'm searching for the right words. Lovely, delightful, they all come to mind. Let me just say that you are a very beautiful young woman and the dress is quite perfect.'

'Thank you. Not too dressy, is it?'

'How could it be that?'

'A bit too dressed up for a housekeeper?'

She shook her head. 'I think of you as my young friend and I hope that I may be included among yours?'

'You are. When I started I was nervous and you helped me a great deal by putting me at ease.'

'We all need friends. Fergus has been a good one to me. He is a fine man and believe me he hasn't had his sorrows to seek, but those are better forgotten.'

'Mr Cunningham is in his study but he promised to be with us by ten o'clock.' They were both seated and Sylvia was engrossed with her picture cards and spreading them over the floor.

'When was a lawyer ever on time for an appointment?' Betsy said as Fergus came in.

'We would be if clients turned up when they should.' He kissed her on both cheeks. 'Happy Christmas, Betsy.'

'Thanks to you it looks like being just that.'

Laura noticed that her employer had changed into a dark suit that was both formal and smart.

'You look nice, Betsy, very nice indeed.'

'More of a compliment if there was less surprise in your voice,' she said tartly.

Fergus threw back his head and laughed. 'Don't mind us, Laura, Betsy and I are good at trading insults, that comes of being the best of friends.'

'As I told Laura, I made the effort. I didn't want to arrive looking like something that had fallen off the back of a lorry. You do remember my dear, departed papa used to say that?'

'I do, but never to describe his daughter.' He looked at Laura. 'Betsy's father was a wonderful old gentleman and as a boy I used to be enthralled with his story-telling.'

Betsy saw the admiration in Fergus's eyes when they rested on Laura and she smiled to herself.

Sylvia felt she had been ignored long enough. 'I want to open my presents.'

'So you shall, dear, but we are one short. Where is Ronnie?'

'Shall I get him, he'll be in his room?'

'Let me! Let me! I'll go.'

'No, Sylvia,' Laura said gently but firmly, 'you pick up all those cards off the floor and I'll get Ronnie.'

Ronnie shut his book with a show of reluctance. 'I don't need to put a jacket on. What's wrong with the way I am?'

'I would rather you were properly dressed.'

'Let me go like this and I'll promise to take off my pullover and put on my jacket before we sit down to eat.'

She swithered.

'I would be uncomfortable and another thing, Laura—'

'What?'

'After we've eaten I'm coming back here to read.'

'That's all right, just remember to excuse yourself.'

Ronnie smiled with relief. 'That's not bad, the thing you are wearing.'

'Thanks,' she said drily, 'now come on, Sylvia has been very patient.'

He did look smart in his short grey trousers and a grey V-necked pullover over a white shirt. Ronnie had spells of shyness and this was one. He grunted 'Happy Christmas' and sat down.

Fergus went over to the tree and the pile of gifts. 'You can open that one, Sylvia,' and glanced at Laura.

She nodded. 'I'll take note—'

'A splendid idea,' Betsy said, 'that way there is no confusion as to whom one should thank.'

'Give that to Laura. It's from you.'

The child put the package on Laura's knees.

'Thank you very much, Sylvia.' Laura opened it and saw that it was a small bottle of very expensive perfume. 'I'll keep this for special occasions,' she said, her voice shaking. Fergus must have bought it and she smiled over at him.

'Good thing I didn't give you scent this year,' Ronnie said.

'May I ask what Ronnie gave you?' Betsy said.

'A lovely chiffon scarf.'

'I can't get this paper off,' Sylvia said, her face red with anger and effort. 'It won't come.'

'Leave it for the minute. You hand these over. One for Laura, one for Aunt Betsy and three for Ronnie.'

'For me?' Ronnie said in a voice of total disbelief. He recognised the writing on one gift tag as Laura's and opened it first. 'Great, Laura, thanks,' he said, looking as pleased as punch as he saw the book-ends. 'You gave me money and I didn't expect anything else. Thanks.'

Sylvia was interested in Ronnie's gifts. 'I want to see yours, then you can see mine.'

'Did you ever,' Fergus said in mock disgust, 'she is more interested in Ronnie's than her own.'

'She had her stocking filled by Santa Claus and there is just so much excitement in one day.' Laura smiled.

Betsy had given Ronnie a card with a ten-shilling note.

'Thank you very much, Miss Yeaman.'

'Thought you would prefer to buy something yourself.'

'Yes, it'll get more books.'

When he opened the long, narrow package he seemed to have lost the power of speech. When he recovered he stammered out his thanks.

'Thank you, sir, I've never had anything like this. Look, Laura, it's a fountain pen.'

'That was far too much, Mr Cunningham.' He saw that she really did look upset.

'It was a fountain pen or a tie.'

Ronnie looked alarmed. 'This is much, much better than a tie, sir.'

'Save dipping into the inkpot at school.'

'This isn't going to school. No fear. I'll use it for my homework.'

'Daddy, from Laura,' Sylvia said, showing him the book.

'Did you thank Laura?'

'Yes, she did, Mr Cunningham.'

'A lovely book,' he smiled as a small Swiss-dressed doll was thrust almost into his face. 'From Aunt Betsy. That's lovely too,' he laughed.

Laura got embroidered handkerchiefs from Betsy and Ronnie handed an untidily wrapped package to Sylvia.

'For you,' he said gruffly.

She plonked herself on the floor and in no time had the paper off. Laura looked to see what it was and was pleased to see that it was a jigsaw puzzle, the pieces were in wood and suitable for a pre-school child.

'Do you like Sylvia's dress?' Laura said quietly.

Fergus looked quickly over at his daughter. 'Yes, very pretty.'

'Laura, he didn't even notice.'

'Sorry, too many other things on my mind,' he said apologetically, 'but let me say again, very pretty, and now after that exhausting hour I think a sherry is called for.'

Ronnie was feeling that he should do something after all the kindness shown to him. This was going to be a wizard Christmas.

'Look for a corner piece,' he said, going down on the floor beside her.

'Like that?'

'That's not a corner.'

'Is that?'

'Yes. Put it there.'

'Like that?'

'Yes. Now find the pieces with smooth edges.'

'I can't see any.'

'You will if you look a bit harder.'

The three adults, glass in hand, were watching with amusement.

'That's all the outside done, now look at the picture on the box.' He pointed. 'Find a piece that colour.'

'That's red. My new dress from Nana is red.'

'That doesn't matter. You look for a piece with red on it.'

She sighed, then pounced on the only piece with red.

'Found it.'

'Fit it in.'

'It won't go.'

'Yes, it will. Press harder but turn it a little bit. There, that's it finished now.'

'I did it all by himself,' she said proudly.

'Just about,' Ronnie said generously.

'Well done, Ronnie, I think you need a refreshment after all that.'

'I'll go and get it,' Laura said, making to rise.

'No, you are on holiday. Ring through to the kitchen and that little girl Jinny can bring it.'

Sylvia was examining Laura's bracelet. 'Pretty,' she said.

'That's the one you got from Michael last Christmas, isn't it?'

'Yes.'

Ronnie was getting talkative. 'Laura's old boyfriend, he's in Manchester now.'

The dining-room was comfortably warm and festive-looking. The seating arrangements had worried Laura. Fergus Cunningham would be at the head of the table but what about the other end? Should Betsy sit there, on the other hand would Betsy want to? Laura dismissed that thought. The place belonged to the mistress of the house and since there was no mistress the place would be left vacant. The chair would be removed since it served to focus attention on the fact that there was no Mrs Cunningham. As for herself she would sit next to Sylvia to assist her with the food should that be necessary. Laura was rather proud of her small charge who was becoming increasingly independent. Betsy and Ronnie would sit together on the opposite side.

Just before leaving the sitting-room Laura noticed a small Christmas-wrapped package half down the side of the chair and found it to be Sylvia's gift to her daddy. As they were about to take their seats for the luncheon Laura whispered something to Sylvia and gave her the package.

'Is it too late?' she said and was on the point of bursting into tears.

'No, this is a lovely time. Go and give it to Daddy now.'

'For you, Daddy?'

'For me?'

'Yes, open it. It's the bestest present you've got,' she said, dancing about with excitement.

Fergus pretended to be having great difficulty in getting inside the package but at last he held up a tie for all to see. Betsy spluttered into her handkerchief and Ronnie was grinning.

'You like it, don't you?'

'Poppet, I've never had one like it,' he said in all honesty and caught Laura's eye. 'Did you help to choose it, Laura?'

'No, I chose it all by myself. Laura wanted me to take a different one but I wouldn't.'

'It is nice and bright, sir,' Ronnie said and Sylvia beamed.

The tie had pink and purple stripes and was as far removed from Fergus's quiet taste as could be. He was having difficulty in keeping his face straight.

'Will you wear it to your office, Daddy?'

'Could be good for business,' Betsy said wickedly.

'Much too good for the office, Sylvia, dear, this is going to be kept for very special occasions.'

Sylvia's interest had turned to her cracker when Ronnie spoke.

'One of my pals at school told us that when his dad got a tie or scarf or something he didn't like his mum sent it to someone the next Christmas.'

'How awful,' Betsy laughed.

'You are giving me ideas, young man.' He checked that his daughter was paying no attention and added, 'You could find it in your stocking next year.'

It was a happy and relaxed meal with cook excelling herself and Jinny being quick and efficient. Fergus was enjoying himself and wished that he hadn't been going out in the evening. The Galbraiths were very good friends and congenial company, and no doubt it would be a very pleasant evening, but he wished that he had been staying at Braehead. The evening ahead made him think of Davina. He would have to bring her over to the house first since she wanted to hand over her gift to Sylvia. He hoped the child wouldn't be too tired or over-excited and forget her manners.

Laura was delighted to see Ronnie so happy. It was a lovely atmosphere with everybody laughing and talking as the crackers were pulled and paper hats put on.

Mindful that the kitchen staff hadn't eaten and would be hungry since Laura knew that Mrs Barclay would frown on nibbling since it would put them off their meal, she was glad to see Mr Cunningham put down his napkin and make a move.

'Jinny, have the coffee and mince pies taken to the sitting-room, please. I'll serve it and don't worry about the clearing-up here, it can be done later.'

Jinny was surprised and pleased. She had expected to do the clearing-up before having theirs in the kitchen.

'I'll speak to Mrs Barclay myself, Jinny, but do tell her that it was a splendid meal and you did extremely well yourself.'

Jinny blushed. 'Thank you, sir,' she said breathlessly.

Chapter Twenty-One

Around six o'clock Fergus went upstairs to dress for the evening ahead, showing a marked reluctance to do so, Laura thought. It had been such a happy day so far. Ronnie hadn't disappeared to his room as he had said he would. Neither had he gone up for his jacket.

'Do I have to?' he had asked and earning himself a sharp look. Mr Cunningham had come to his rescue.

'I see nothing wrong with Ronnie's appearance.'

'He should be properly dressed to go into the dining-room,' Laura said stubbornly, 'everybody else is.'

'Laura, Ronnie looks very smart and more important he looks comfortable,' Betsy put in, 'so do stop fussing and leave the boy alone.'

Ronnie turned to her in gratitude and had he not known that she was a lady he would have said the movement of her eye was a definite wink.

'I seem to be outnumbered,' Laura said, giving in with good grace. She did want Ronnie to be comfortable but the jacket had been bought especially for the occasion and she could have saved herself some money. It had been chosen for its good fit and not for growth as was the usual.

When Fergus Cunningham came in looking very handsome in his dinner suit, Laura's heart skipped a beat. Then came the thought of her employer with the lovely Davina and Laura felt a stab of loneliness and some of the brightness had gone from the day.

'Daddy, why have you got to go out?' Sylvia pouted.

'I have to, darling, these arrangements were made a long time ago.'

'Did you forget that it was Christmas Day?'

'I'm afraid I must have.'

The child looked a picture in her cherry-red velvet dress but her face had grown pale, a sign that she was tired. Laura made no objections when she climbed on her knee and snuggled up. The thumb went into her mouth, a habit she had largely outgrown, but Laura chose to ignore it.

'Your lovely dress, I'll take her,' Betsy offered, but Laura shook her head. 'Poor little lamb, she's dead beat.'

'Yes, she is. My fault, I should have insisted she had her rest.'

'She wouldn't have gone down and where's the harm? There are no rules on Christmas Day.'

'True. I'm not bothered for myself but Miss Dorward is apparently coming with a gift for Sylvia.'

'Rather late in the day. What was to hinder her handing in whatever it was on Christmas Eve?'

'I don't know but Mr Cunningham made special mention that Sylvia is to say thank you to Miss Dorward without any prompting.'

'She won't need prompting, the child is well-mannered.'

'Usually she is but for some unknown reason she isn't at her best with Miss Dorward.'

'Which must tell us all something. I have met the lady in question on several occasions and I will just say she is not one of my favourite people.'

Sylvia's eyes were open and Laura was turning the pages of a picture book. Ronnie was sitting in a corner deep in a book. Only Laura couldn't relax until Davina had been and gone. At last she heard the door then voices.

They came in. Fergus was smiling and Laura smiled back nervously. Davina Dorward's presence seemed to fill the room. She wore an evening gown in a silvery grey and over it a fur cape. There was a sparkle of jewels at her throat and diamond studs in her ears.

'Good evening, Davina,' Betsy said. Her paper hat was still on and set at a rakish angle and Laura felt a giggle coming on.

'Good evening, Miss Yeaman, I trust you are well?'

'Never felt better.'

'Sylvia, dear, come over here, I have something for you.'

The thumb had gone back in her mouth and Davina looked very disapproving.

'That can't be Sylvia sucking her thumb like a baby and sitting on the housekeeper's lap? Fergus, love, what are you thinking about?'

Fergus gave a deep frown and Laura could only think the frown was for her.

She got the child gently to her feet.

'You have to make allowances, Davina,' Betsy said sharply, 'the child is tired after all the excitement.'

'I'm sorry, I do apologise, Miss Dorward, Sylvia is more tired than usual since she missed her afternoon rest.'

'And why was that?' Davina smiled but the smile didn't reach her eyes.

'Davina, is it so long since you were a child that you have forgotten the excitement? Laura is extremely good with the child but even she can't do the impossible.' Fergus had been out of the room during this exchange but was back.

'Haven't you handed it over yet? We are going to be very late.'

'Just about to.' She gave her sweetest smile. 'Come and see what Aunt Davina has for you.'

Laura gave her a gentle push. The large cardboard box very obviously held a doll. The lid was kept on with a large pink bow.

'You take one end of the ribbon and I'll take the other, then pull.'

The child obeyed, then looked up at her daddy and he smiled encouragingly.

'A dolly, I knew it was going to be that.'

'That was clever of you. This is a very special one that can open and shut its eyes.'

'I've got one that goes to sleep.'

'She's pretty, isn't she?'

'Yes.' There was a pause then at last it came. 'Thank you very much.'

Laura breathed a sigh of relief and Betsy nodded smilingly.

'Dolly hasn't got a name and you must think of one.'

'I'm going to call her Laura.'

Laura marvelled. The child had suddenly come to life.

'No, we want a pretty name. I thought of Carol since it is Christmas.'

Sylvia's fair hair swung as she shook her head. 'No, I want it to be Laura.'

'Accept it, Davina, she gets her stubbornness from me, remember.'

'I think it is time we were on our way.'

Fergus held the door open, smiled to those in the room, then closed it gently. Betsy gave them time to be out of the house then she burst into laughter.

'Sylvia, you did us proud, you little monkey.' The child didn't hear, she had curled herself on the sofa and was sound to the world.

Laura decided to let her sleep where she was. 'Ronnie?'

'What?'

'Go along to Sylvia's bedroom, would you, and take the top cover from her bed.'

Ronnie returned with it. 'I nearly brought the pillow.'

'The cushion will do.' Laura tucked the cover round the sleeping child.

'I would have preferred if I'd got her velvet dress off.'

'I wouldn't worry, not worth disturbing her and the creases will come out of velvet I imagine.'

'I hope so.'

'I'm sorry to keep going on about it, Fergus, but I cannot help but be concerned,' Davina said as the car moved off. 'Did you notice that for the whole time I was in your house that boy never as much as lifted his head from his book? Such deplorable manners, but he, I imagine, is your housekeeper's brother?'

'Yes, that is Ronnie,' Fergus said in a clipped voice that should have warned her.

'I thought so. The boy probably knows no better. You cannot let this go on, Fergus, leaving little Sylvia, your own daughter, in the care of someone who doesn't know the meaning of good manners.'

Perhaps she would have stopped sooner if she had seen the anger in Fergus's eyes and his stiffened jaw.

'Davina, I think I said on one previous occasion that I was well satisfied with Laura and as for her brother I cannot let that pass. Ronnie was at the far end of the room and for much of the day he has entertained Sylvia. Not many boys of his age would have been so good-humoured about it. He did ask my permission to read which I readily gave. The boy was prepared to go up to his own room but I suggested he take himself to a quiet corner where he could get peace to read. And another thing, I can remember myself at that age being so enthralled in a book that I was totally unaware of what was going on around me.'

Davina realised that she had gone too far. 'I've angered you.'

'Not at all, but I would prefer it if Laura's name wasn't mentioned in future.'

'I wouldn't have believed it possible.'

'Believed what possible?'

'That the young woman has made such an impression on you.'

'Let me just say this, Davina, it was a lucky day for me and my daughter when Laura came to Braehead. Only now am I realising that Mrs Mathewson, caring soul though she was, was too old and set in her ways to be able to look after an active and demanding child.'

'I thought Mrs Mathewson very good, I much preferred her, but there we must agree to differ.' She paused and softened her voice. 'You do know that I am only thinking of the child's good?'

'I never doubted it for a moment.'

'Fergus, my love, you are much too kind-hearted.'

'A lawyer kind-hearted? Try telling that to some of my clients.'

'Your clients, I happen to know, hold you in high esteem.'

For the rest of the journey they were silent but both were busy with their own thoughts.

Fergus was wishing himself back in Braehead. It was a long time since he had enjoyed a Christmas so much. It had been like a real family day with Sylvia so happy and everyone laughing and in good spirits. He found himself smiling. Laura had looked lovely in her blue dress but then she would look lovely in anything. She had a natural beauty with an inner goodness that shone through.

No use fooling himself, he was in love with the girl. Probably had been from the first moment he saw her. Such a brave girl and proud too. Her brother was a credit to her, a fine boy. The thought of proposing marriage was with him all the time and he was just waiting for the right moment. Once or twice the way she had looked at him gave him hope but then again that could be no more than wishful thinking. It could be a way out of her predicament, a roof over her head and security for the future. Added to that, Ronnie would be able to go on to university. He would willingly do that for the boy.

It wasn't the best foundation for a marriage with love only on one side but it could work. He would have her affection and respect and perhaps in time that would turn to love.

Davina was distinctly alarmed as well she might be. She had handled the evening very badly and it had been a mistake to let her dislike of the girl show. Obviously she had wormed herself in and to make matters worse she had most of the advantages. She was there every day pampering to that tiresome child and trying to show herself as being indispensable. Couldn't the stupid man see that she was only interested in getting a home for herself and that brother of hers?

Her face hardened. She wouldn't succeed. It must never happen and she would see that it didn't. There had to be a way, there always was if one just exercised patience. Not too long a wait though. Time was running out for her. She shivered and it had nothing to do with the cold.

There was another worry. With Fergus out of her life the good times would come to an end. Davina loved nothing better than the cut and thrust of good conversation with intelligent people of wide interests and she could hold her own with the best. All that would stop. Invitations would cease to come her way. She wouldn't be welcome on her own. Few single women were and most certainly not one who could claim beauty. A lovely woman was a threat to wives. Her lips curled and she felt a delicious little thrill. If she chose to use it, she had the power to attract any man who sat around the table. A certain look from her and they would come running. It was a heady feeling but Davina sighed. She didn't want an affair with a married man, she wanted Fergus and marriage. Her own age group were all married or spoken for and she could be left. It angered her to think that she may have missed her chance by concentrating all her charm on Fergus Cunningham.

'You are very quiet, Davina.'

'So are you.'

'Are you looking forward to the evening?'

'Of course, aren't you?'

'Yes, but I'm afraid I've already over-indulged in food. Mrs Barclay surpassed herself.' He smiled, remembering the meal.

'That was thoughtless, darling, you should have known better. Anna will have gone to great lengths to produce something extra special.'

'I'll try and do justice to it and hope I won't have to suffer too much afterwards.'

'Darling, pay attention and slow down, we are almost at the gate.'

'Sorry,' he said, braking suddenly.

'That wasn't at all like you,' she said as she picked up her evening purse.

Silently he agreed with that. It hadn't been like him but he kept picturing the scene at Braehead. Sylvia would be asleep, worn out after all the excitement. How sweet she had looked in both dresses. He must remember to write and tell his mother how lovely her grand-daughter had looked in her red velvet dress. She was a happy child, not a poor motherless little child, and for that and so much more he had Laura to thank. She was so loving and generous and he couldn't bear the thought of her leaving them one day.

As they entered the Galbraiths' house he promised himself no more thoughts of Laura. He owed it to his host and hostess to look as though he were enjoying himself. That shouldn't be such an effort. All those present were friends and stimulating company, and Davina would be in her element. She had a sharp but wicked intellect but unfortunately she was uncaring if her words caused hurt and embarrassment. Laura would never be guilty of that. She was all too familiar with hurt, anguish and near despair. If only Laura could be here with him instead of Davina. They were both beautiful, intelligent women. They would sparkle in any company but the difference was that other women would like Laura whereas a number of them heartily disliked Davina. Hadn't he promised himself not to think of Laura? But he couldn't stop himself.

He must break completely with Davina and soon. It would be far from easy and he certainly wasn't looking forward to it. If he was truthful he was dreading it because he did feel some guilt. He had allowed himself to drift into this relationship without a thought to where it was leading. Or was that quite true? Had it not been for Laura coming on the scene it was just possible that he and Davina would have made a match of it. What had held him back was Davina's lack of interest in children. She did her best with Sylvia but the child hadn't taken to her. Children instinctively knew what was genuine and what was sham.

The New Year was over before the snow arrived but it was a good fall that delighted the children if not their elders. Ronnie had invited David over and the two boys were supposed to be making a snowman for Sylvia. They were all in the garden at Braehead, warmly clad and with wellington boots for the deep snow. Ronnie and David were engaged in horseplay, each trying to ram a handful of snow down the other's neck. Sylvia was squealing and dancing around them.

'Enough of that, you two. You are supposed to be making a snowman.'

'It's nearly finished.'

'You call that nearly finished? I've never seen such a pathetic effort in my life.' Laura shook her head at the pair of them. 'I'll show you how to make a real snowman but don't think for a moment that I am doing all the donkey work.' She pointed. 'Is that supposed to be the head?'

They looked sheepish. 'Not big enough?' David said.

'Not nearly big enough. Go and roll it in the snow until it is three times that size.'

'Then it will be bigger than the body,' Ronnie grinned.

'No, it won't because you are going to make the body a lot bigger. Sylvia and I will help.'

The final result wouldn't have taken a prize, it was lopsided but it delighted Sylvia.

'Ronnie, ask Mrs Barclay for a carrot.'

'For the nose?'

'Yes.' She smiled as he and David disappeared to the kitchen. No doubt they would scrounge something to eat. 'Come on, Sylvia,' she said, taking the child's hand, 'we'll look for two black pebbles for the eyes. We could use currants but the birds might eat them.'

'He looks like a real snowman now.'

'Yes, David, but he needs a pipe.'

'I'll get one of Daddy's, I know where he keeps them.' Sylvia made to dash away but Laura held her back. She didn't want the child taking one of Mr Cunningham's favourite pipes.

'No, dear, when Daddy comes home you can ask him for an old one.'

'I know what will do meantime,' Ronnie said, running inside.

Ronnie returned. 'Wasn't sure if it had been thrown out. Laura is awful good at throwing away things that she thinks I'm finished with.'

'Just like my mum,' David said gloomily.

'My daddy's pipe is better than that,' Sylvia said scornfully.

'I know that, this is just for blowing bubbles with but it will do, won't it, Laura?'

'Just the job, Ronnie,' she said, pushing the pipe into the snowman's mouth.

'I'm going to keep him for ever.'

'He'll melt.'

Laura frowned and both boys dissolved in laughter. Sylvia didn't know what they were laughing at but she joined in.

Fergus was just getting out of the car after collecting his briefcase when he saw the tall young man at his neighbour's house. He watched him come out of the gate then hesitate.

'May I help? Are you looking for someone?'

'Yes, I am.' The boy had a nice friendly face, Fergus thought. 'I'm looking for a house, Braeside or Braehead—'

'This is Braehead.'

'Would Laura Morrison work there?'

'Yes, she does, Miss Morrison is my housekeeper.'

'That's a stroke of luck.'

A very confident young man and not much older than Laura, he thought.

'You must be a friend of Miss Morrison's?'

'A bit more than that, at least we were until I went off to Manchester.'

Fergus's heart dropped like a stone. By what the boy had said they had been sweethearts until he had gone off to work in Manchester. Probably had a silly quarrel and this was him hoping to patch it up.

'You had better come in.'

'Thanks very much.'

Fergus led the way to the sitting-room where a fire blazed and all signs of a child's play things had been removed.

'Do be seated and I'll get someone to find Miss Morrison for you.'

Michael smiled disarmingly. 'We've a lot of catching up to do and I'm hoping very much that she'll be able to get a bit of time off.'

'I don't see that a problem.'

'Great!'

Fergus left the young man and seeing Jinny told her to find Laura. Laura appeared at that moment.

'There you are. You have a visitor, Laura.'

'I do? I'm not expecting anyone.'

'Then presumably this is a surprise visit.' He opened the sitting-room door and she stared in amazement at the very last person she had expected to see.

'Michael, what on earth are you doing here?'

'Came to see you and I can tell you this, you weren't easy to find.'

Laura was about to introduce Michael to her employer but she didn't get the chance.

'I'll leave you,' Fergus said quietly and went out, closing the door behind him. This then was the Michael Ronnie had spoken of, the young man who had given her a bracelet for Christmas. Feeling depressed, he went into his study, sat behind his desk and gazed at the opposite wall.

'What brings you, Michael? Why are you here?'

'Do I have to have a reason?' The smile was still there but it had slipped a little. He was less sure than he had been.

'I would have thought so.'

'You're mad about that time I brought Alice to Miltonsands.'

'I wasn't in the least mad.'

'You were hurt though. You tried to hide it but I knew.'

'How very perceptive of you,' Laura said sarcastically.

'Meaning you were?'

'If I was it was for a very short time.'

'You have to try and understand, Laura, I was lonely in a strange city and Alice was company. It was never serious, you can take my word for that.'

'Serious enough to bring her here to meet your parents.'

'It wasn't like that. Alice had never been to Scotland and pestered me until I agreed she could come.'

'If you say so. How do you like Manchester and the job?'

'The job is good and I'm getting plenty of experience and as to Manchester it's all right but, I do get homesick at times.'

'Yes, I suppose you must.'

He was looking around him. 'You doing all right here?'

'Yes.'

'Funny job for you though. What happened to the post office?'

'Nothing. Circumstances changed, that's all.'

'Heard your old man got himself married.'

Laura was getting annoyed. 'My father remarried and is very happy,' she said coldly. 'They now live in New York.'

'New York? I didn't know that. In a few years that is where I hope to be.'

'Dad had a very serious accident, Michael.'

'Did he? I'm sorry to hear that. He's recovering though?'

'Yes, but slowly.'

'Give him my best regards when next you write.'

She nodded though she didn't see herself doing it.

'How about the two of us going for a meal? You haven't eaten, have you?'

'No, I haven't.'

'Seems a decent sort your employer, said you were free to go out.'

'It happens to be my day off,' she smiled.

'Then you'll come?'

'There is nothing to talk about, Michael.'

'Don't be like that, Laura. We are all allowed one mistake surely.' He paused and looked at her pleadingly. 'We can remain friends, can't we?'

'Of course I'll always look on you as a friend, Michael.'

'I'd hoped for more but I suppose that'll have to do. How about the Royal then the cinema to finish off the evening? I'm just here on a quick visit and I go back tomorrow.'

A night out would be rather nice and where was the harm? She had made it clear where she stood.

'Give me time to get changed.'

'Don't rush. Is that today's paper?'

'It will be.' There was a good fire burning and Michael would be quite happy with the newspaper until she joined him. First, however, she must tell Mr Cunningham though it wasn't necessary. Then she thought guiltily that he should be in the sitting-room until his meal was served. He would have gone to his study. She went along and knocked.

'Come in. It's you, Laura.' He raised his eyes from the papers on his desk.

'The young man – that's Michael, an old friend of mine, and he has asked me to go for a meal.'

'You don't need my permission. What you do in your free time is your own concern.'

It was like a slap in the face. Surely there had been no necessity for that. 'I'm aware of that but I thought I would just let you know since you invited Michael into your home,' she said coldly.

'Then I have to say thank you. I hope you have a pleasant evening.' His head went down and she was dismissed.

When she had gone and the door closed, Fergus Cunningham shut his eyes. Why had he spoken like that to Laura of all people? In part he could blame the day, a hard day made more difficult by having to come down heavily on a clerk whose carelessness had almost lost them a valuable client. To think that he had all but decided to propose marriage to his housekeeper, but then he'd had no inkling that she would go off with a young man who very likely had the same thought in mind.

Since they were to be dining at the Royal, Laura changed into the blue dress she had worn last on Christmas Day. She finished dressing then went to join Michael.

'That's me ready,' she smiled.

Michael folded the newspaper and put it back on the chair. She saw that under his coat he wore a dark business suit, white shirt and self-coloured blue tie.

It was a cold, starry evening as they walked the half-mile to the hotel and she made no objection when he tucked her arm in his. To do so would have been churlish since his nearness no longer affected her as it once had.

'Must get a car when funds allow.'

'That would be nice for you.'

'Probably won't though until I'm over in the States.' He pressed her arm. 'Can't get over your dad being in New York. Strange if one day we should meet.'

Laura laughed. 'With a huge city like New York I find that highly improbable.'

'Even so, stranger things have happened.'

'Not all that often, you have to admit.'

'To go back to that night, we had our disagreement—'

'No point in that.'

'Yes, there is. Had I been more patient and you more understanding—'

'In the end it wouldn't have made the slightest difference.'

'I don't agree.'

'Michael, Ronnie was the problem and he hasn't gone away,' she smiled.

'Not yet.'

'What do you mean?' Laura said sharply.

They had been walking but now they stopped and faced each other.

'Don't you see? Another year or thereabout and we, you and I, could be in New York.'

'What have you done with my young brother?' She sounded amused.

'He is in New York too,' Michael said impatiently. 'You aren't following me.'

'That's true.'

'Let me make it clearer. Your dad is happily married and living in New York. Right?'

'Right.'

'As I said before, but it is worth repeating, Ronnie is your father's responsibility and he could make his home with his dad and his stepmother.'

She shook her head.

'If you are thinking about education there are plenty of opportunities in America.' He took her arm again and they began walking. 'Laura, we would all be in the same city but we would start our married life together which is as it should be.'

'Michael, it's too late,' she said softly.

'You don't forgive easily, do you?' he said angrily. 'One small fling that meant nothing and you're going to throw it back in my face.'

'I am doing nothing of the kind and stop looking so furious. This has got nothing at all to do with Alice.'

'Then what?'

'I don't love you, Michael.'

'I don't believe that.'

'It's true.'

'You did once,' he said sulkily.

'I thought I loved you and perhaps I did. Or perhaps, Michael, we both imagined that what we shared was love.'

'You've met someone else?'

'There is no one else,' Laura said quietly. For a little while she had imagined that Fergus Cunningham was attracted to her but she knew

267

now that it wasn't the case. In future she would do well to remember her place and she would. Her face burned as she remembered his cold indifference to her going out this evening.

'I have a feeling there is but you are not prepared to say. You've changed, Laura.'

'We both have.'

'You more than me.'

'Perhaps.'

Suddenly he grinned and she saw no pain. He wasn't heart-broken, that was clear. 'We can look back on some wonderful times together and I wouldn't want to forget those,' he said.

'Nor me.'

'We'll part the best of friends so let's enjoy the evening for old times' sake.'

She nodded and felt a lump in her throat. Partings were usually sad and she and Michael had so many happy memories.

'An evening to remember, we'll make it that,' Laura said a little unsteadily.

'And where better than the Royal? Remember how we used to wish that we could afford to go there?'

'Still, those evenings in the Pavilion were pretty good.'

'I wish – no, never mind.' He steered her into the hotel.

'Have you a reservation, sir?'

'No, I just hoped there would be a table.'

'I believe there is, sir. May I take your coats?' They were taken and handed to another waiter. 'This way, please.' They were shown to their table and a menu handed to each of them. The wine list was left on the table.

'Who are they trying to kid?' Michael whispered. 'I knew they wouldn't be busy.'

Laura smiled as she looked around the dining-room. Apart from theirs only two other tables were occupied. They studied the menu, made their choice and Michael chose the wine.

She giggled.

'What's so funny?'

'This is a long way from fish and chips in a newspaper.'

'Might not be any tastier but the surroundings are a bit of all right.'

'Very posh.' She smiled to him across the table. 'We should be more adventurous with our choice of dish and it is a good menu.'

'I don't know. A little of what you fancy does you good.'

The waiter arrived, pad in hand. 'Have you decided?'

'I think so. Laura?'

'Fresh fillet of haddock and French fries, please.'

'No starter?' he asked with an air of disapproval.

'No, not for me, thank you.'

'I'll have the same - haddock and French fries.'

'Do you wish wine with your meal, sir. I could recommend—'

Michael wasn't interested in what the waiter could recommend. He had a fair bit of money in his pocket but he didn't want to make himself too short and with wine one never knew how much they would charge.

'Two glasses of house white wine.' The waiter departed.

'I don't know much about wine, to be honest,' Michael said apologetically.

'I don't care for it all that much. You can finish it for me.'

'Not done in the best of circles.' He put his hand over hers. 'We don't have to pretend, we know each other too well for that. Pity we weren't making a go of it,' he said wistfully.

'It wouldn't work, Michael.'

'No putting the clock back?'

'No putting the clock back, Michael.'

'Do you remember when we used to go to Tony's, especially when it was raining, and sit and sit —'

'And people waiting and glaring—'

'And then Tony himself asking if we were stuck to the seats.'

'Cheeky monkey.'

Laura sighed. They had been happy times and maybe she was making a big mistake. She could be throwing away a chance of happiness and Ronnie was a different boy now. Connie wasn't keen or so it would appear but if her dad insisted she would have to go along with it. Ronnie could make his home with them and perhaps Michael could arrange it that they didn't live too far apart. Would she like life in New York? A difficult question to answer. She would like to see it as a tourist but as to making her home in America she wasn't so sure.

Chapter Twenty-Two

In the early afternoon Laura got herself ready and set out for Jane's home. To have caught a bus would have been a big help but there was no direct service and it was quicker to walk than go to the High Street and wait for transport. Few people were abroad since only those who had to would venture out on such a day. There were rain puddles everywhere and a thin wet mist hung about and clung to the skin like cobwebs. To avoid them Laura dipped her face further into the collar of her coat.

Jane had been at the window and seeing the hurrying figure had the door open.

'Lovely to see you, Laura, I hardly dared expect you to come out on such a day,' she said, closing the door behind her and giving a shiver.

'I very nearly had second thoughts,' Laura smiled as she stepped into the narrow hall. The layout of Jane's house, like Aunt Peggy's, was very similar to the house in Fairfield Street but she had done some modernising. The old fireplace in the living-room had been removed and one with a tiled surround installed. The wallpaper had faint stripes on a cream background and with no heavy furniture the room looked larger than it was.

'I'm glad you didn't have second thoughts. Give me your coat and your other things, they'll dry in the kitchen.'

'Thanks,' Laura said, handing them over.

'That's right, get yourself near to the fire. The kettle's on the boil and I'll have everything through in a jiffy.' She pulled forward a small table. 'No ceremony, we'll have our cuppie at the fire.'

'Lovely.' Laura picked up a seed catalogue and glanced over it until Jane came in with the tray and placed it on the table between the two comfortable chairs. Then she returned for the teapot and began to pour the tea. 'Is this you planning for the spring, Jane?'

'Yes, I find it cheers me up. Don't know about you but February is my least favourite month. Thank goodness it is the shortest.'

Laura nodded. 'I do love flowers but as you know I didn't make much of a success of the garden at Fairfield Street.'

'Oh, I wouldn't say that, I thought you kept it tidy.'

'Nothing much to look at though. I don't have green fingers like you and sadly I don't have the patience for gardening. What I am looking forward to, Jane, is seeing the spring show at Braehead. It is spectacular, so Mrs Barclay says and Jack, bless his heart, has promised to keep me supplied with flowers for the house.'

'Lucky you.' Jane paused to offer her home-baking.

'Thanks, I will,' Laura said, putting a sponge cake on her plate. 'You've been busy.'

'My day for filling the tins. This Jack you mention, he'll be the gardener?'

'Yes.'

'Think you could talk nicely to him and get me some cuttings or small plants? Spring is the best time and I'd be grateful for anything. I'm having a clean-out of all the old plants and making a fresh start.'

'A bit drastic I would have thought.'

'I know but I just feel like it. I'm sending for a flowering cherry, made up my mind. It'll go in that dull patch just as you come in the back door.'

'That should be nice. I do love that delicate shade of pink cherry blossom,' Laura said, then drank some of her tea.

Jane put down her cup. 'That takes care of the gardening, now I need to be brought up to date with your news.'

Laura smiled. 'Would you believe it, Jane, Michael found out my whereabouts and called at Braehead to see me.'

'Did he now?' Jane's eyes widened. 'Is this him back for good?'

'No, just a short visit to his parents.'

'You must have been surprised?'

'Understatement of the year,' Laura laughed.

'You were out with him?'

'Yes.'

'This is like pulling teeth. Where did he take you?'

'The Royal.'

'Dinner at the Royal?'

'Yes.'

'Very, very nice. That is where we went for my birthday treat.'

'After that the second house of the cinema. I had seen it but I didn't let on.'

'Back seats?'

'No, Jane,' Laura laughed, 'nothing like that.'

'Pity. I was hoping you were going to say the romance was on again.'

'No romance.'

'Could have been, but you said no. Am I right?'

'Yes, but that said I don't think Michael was terribly upset.'

'Hid it from you?'

'No, he couldn't, I know him too well.'

'Just good friends,' Jane said with a deep sigh.

'We'll always be that,' Laura said quietly, 'I'll think of him with affection and in time that is the way he'll think of me.'

'I'm being very inquisitive and I make no apologies. Is there someone else?'

'No one else, Jane, absolutely not,' Laura said firmly, then felt her cheeks go rosy.

Jane seemed on the point of saying something but stopped herself and Laura, to hide her embarrassment, rushed in with the first thing that came to mind.

'You know, Jane, when I told Mr Cunningham that I was going out with Michael he was quite curt and it was so unlike him. He's always been so courteous. 'Still, maybe he'd had a rotten day or something.'

'Maybe you going out was inconvenient.'

'No, not at all. It was my day off. I wasn't asking a favour.'

'Did they happen to meet, your employer and Michael?'

'Yes.' Laura told her how it had come about.

'Want to know what I think?'

'Yes, I would.'

'First, though, tell me is he still offhand with you?'

'No, Mr Cunningham is just as he has always been.'

'Laura, you are young and very attractive and this employer of yours is still a young man. He could be in love with you and if so he wouldn't be exactly overjoyed to see you going off with an old boyfriend and a good-looking one at that.'

'Jane, your imagination is running away with you. Mr

Cunningham,' her voice softened though she wasn't aware of it, 'is a perfect gentleman and so kind. He is marvellous with Ronnie, you must see a difference.'

'Yes, he has a lot more confidence.'

'Thanks to Mr Cunningham.'

'So that's it,' she said softly.

'What is?'

'My dear girl, you are no longer interested in Michael because you have fallen for your employer. It's true, I can see it in your face.'

'No, you are wrong. I like and respect him but that is all and as for Mr Cunningham he has a lady friend. I look after his child and his house and that is all there is to it.'

'He must have a first name, this very interesting man?'

'Fergus, but of course I don't use it.'

'Does he use yours?'

'Not to begin with he didn't, but since his daughter calls me Laura and she objected to him addressing me as Miss Morrison—'

'I get it.'

'This lady friend, have you met her?'

'Yes.'

'Do you like her?'

'Not much. Not at all if I'm to be honest and—'

'Are they engaged?' she interrupted.

'They may have an understanding but there is nothing official.'

'Taking his time then, isn't he?'

'I don't suppose he is in any hurry.'

'She may be if she is getting on a bit. Looks don't last that long and if she is passed the first flush of youth—'

'She is, but her kind of looks will last. Jane, she is very beautiful and sophisticated and wears marvellous clothes.'

'How does she get on with the wee lass?'

'She does try but Sylvia doesn't like her.'

'There you are then, nothing will ever come of it, you can be sure. Your Fergus won't marry someone his daughter doesn't like. Stands to reason.'

'Miss Dorward brings lovely gifts and tries her best to gain the child's affection.'

'That doesn't work.'

'I don't think Fergus will ever marry.'

'Why not?'

'From what I gather he was very much in love with his wife and was devastated when he lost her.'

'I expect he was and maybe as you say he can't bring himself to take another wife.'

Laura nodded.

Jane was silent. The girl deserved some happiness and she just hoped that Laura hadn't made a mistake by sending Michael away. She decided to change the subject.

'I wonder about the boys, Laura, do you think they will stay friends?'

'Why shouldn't they?'

'Ronnie will be staying on at school, won't he?'

'I hope so.'

'Then in all likelihood going on to university?'

'Jane, I don't think that far ahead.'

'It's what you hope?'

'Yes.' She paused. 'It is what I would like for Ronnie and what he wants for himself but I still don't understand what you mean.'

'David will be leaving school when he is fourteen. I wanted to give him another year but his dad says no. Very determined about it too. He sees it as a waste with David gaining nothing.' She paused. 'He is good with his hands—'

'Very good, I know that.'

'If he leaves at fourteen the joiner down the road from us is willing to take him on as an apprentice and he could serve his time.'

'What does David have to say about it?'

'He wants to leave and get a job.'

'Seems you'll have to let him, Jane.'

'I know that, I accept it, but I could be forgiven for wishing that he was more academically inclined. I wanted David to be a white-collar worker,' she said wistfully.

Laura knew her friend's hopes and sympathised. 'Let's face it, Jane, we'd all change bits of ourselves if we could.'

Jane gave her usual cheerful smile. 'I suppose so. We mothers won't admit it but we are selfish. We want what we think is best for our children because it is what suits us. David's dad shares my disappointment, he had his dreams too, but he has the good sense to

accept things as they are. David will make a good joiner and take a
pride in his work.'

'One day he may have his own joinery business.'

'Now there's a thought, Laura,' Jane laughed. 'My son with his own
business. Yes, I could live with that. I like it.'

'What is to stop the boys remaining friends?'

'What do you think, Laura?'

'Honestly?'

'Yes, be completely honest.'

'Then I think they will both make new friends. It is inevitable since
they will be seeing a lot less of each other.'

'Their interests will be so different.'

'Yes, but that need not stand in the way of friendship.'

'I hope not. They have been good for each other.'

Jane smiled. 'Ronnie didn't manage to make a scholar of David but
he kept him from slipping too far behind.'

'We met through them, Jane, and I hope you are not going to walk
out on me.'

'No fear. I'll always be here for you.'

The mist had largely cleared when Laura began her walk back to
Braehead. She had enjoyed her visit to Jane and when she got back she
would write to her father and stepmother.

She wrote three pages and then added a final paragraph. Laura had
intended mentioning it before.

Dad, Connie, could I ask you to address your next letter to Ronnie
instead of to me? He would so love it if the envelope with the American
stamp had his name on it. You have been very good about writing,
Connie, and believe me it is very much appreciated. We love hearing
about the business you are setting up with your sister. Most of all we
like to hear about New York and you have the magic touch of bringing
the city to life. Sorry, Dad, your letters, delightful though they were,
never managed to bring London to us in Miltonsands.

George Morrison had been out of hospital for some time and was
pleased with the apartment that Connie had managed to acquire. It had
one large L-shaped room and two others of reasonable size. One now
held a double bed, wardrobe and dressing-table while the other could
become a spare bedroom. At the moment it served as a store-room. It

was in a particularly pleasant area and the apartment looked out on to mature trees and green grass. Nearby were appealing walks that didn't overtax George's strength. Loneliness troubled him at times but he made no mention of it to Connie. She was the breadwinner as he kept constantly reminding himself. His greatest distress was the damage to his right hand and his inability to use a pen.

'Darling, you must have patience,' Connie had said on more than one occasion. 'Your hand will come all right. You really should be thankful that you have reached the stage you now are.'

'All right you saying that but it shouldn't be taking this long. I'm completely useless if I can't use a pen,' he said gloomily.

Connie looked at his face, the greyness hadn't quite gone and became worse when he was overtired. She felt a wave of pity and underneath that the guilt that wouldn't go away. Indirectly she was responsible for his condition. Not the accident, she didn't accept any responsibility for that. Her guilt came from the fact that George was in New York.

'You are not useless,' she said sharply, 'but you are becoming a trial to me.'

'There you are, you are admitting it.'

'I am doing nothing of the sort. Just let me repeat myself. Your hand is improving, the exercises are doing that, and if the experts say it is only a question of time then believe them. They know what they are talking about.'

'I expect they do,' George said but without conviction in his voice. 'But I want to be able to earn my own living.'

'Don't be silly,' Connie said briskly, 'you more than earn your keep. When it comes to the financial side of the business I need your advice and guidance. Talking problems over with you helps to straighten them out.' She smiled. 'Believe me, George Morrison, I am living for the day when I can chuck invoices, accounts and all the rest of it over to you.'

She saw his face brighten and knew that she had said the right thing. The poor lamb hated the thought of living off her.

'When that day comes there won't be a happier man.'

Connie kissed him lightly and patted him on the shoulder. 'Be a dear and see if the postman has left anything.'

George got up and went down to the hallway where one wall was given over to post-boxes. His was marked G. MORRISON. Turning the key he opened it and drew out the solitary letter.

'Just one,' he called when he got inside the apartment, 'from Laura.'

'No bills, we can breathe again,' she joked. 'Did you say it was from Laura?'

'Yes.'

'Good! You know, dear, I've surprised myself.'

'In what way?' he asked as he handed her the letter.

Before answering she slit the envelope open and drew out the pages. Then she handed them to him. 'I've become rather fond of my stepdaughter and stepson. I wish now that we'd made the effort to see them before leaving London.'

'If you recall there wasn't the time.'

'There is always time, George. One makes it for what one considers important. In a way it is very like – you know the expression – if you want something done ask a busy person.'

'I don't see the connection.'

'Don't you? Never mind. You read your letter then give it to me.'

Connie kept silent and busied herself doing a quick tidy. It was all the apartment ever got. Business came first, it had to, their future depended on it.

'Here you are, the pair of them seem to be getting along fine. Mind you, Connie, I don't like the thought of Laura being a housekeeper or childminder or whatever she calls herself. She was better off in the post office, at least it kept her brain working.'

'The girl had no choice. She wrote and told you her financial position, even going so far as to supply the figures. The plain truth was Laura couldn't afford to carry on as they were, especially when that wretched landlord of hers put the rent up.'

'It wasn't my fault. You know yourself I was to arrange for an allowance to be sent and it would have if—'

'Of course you weren't to blame but try putting yourself in Laura's shoes. She knew nothing about the accident and it was extremely careless of you not to send her Lottie's address.'

'I thought I had but obviously I hadn't. You're blaming me.'

'Of course I am blaming you for that. Who else was responsible if you weren't?'

'She could have asked Peggy for a loan to tide her over.'

'Would your sister have helped? Was she in a position to do so?'

'How should I know?'

278

'George, much as I love you there are times, like now, when you exasperate me, you really do. Has it escaped your mind completely that Ronnie is your responsibility and not Laura's? Had she not had her brother to look after she might well be married by now. There was that boy you spoke of—'

'Michael.'

'You said they seemed serious about each other but not many young men would want to be saddled with a schoolboy.' She was showing him up, exposing his guilt and at the same time her own.

'You've changed your tune,' he said angrily.

'Calm down and please remember I wasn't in possession of the facts.' His face was tight. 'Very well, Connie, you tell me truthfully—'

'I am always truthful,' she said coldly.

'All right, tell me, would there have been a home for Ronnie with us?'

Connie was silent for a long time then she gave a deep sigh. 'There I have to say I don't know.'

'I do. There would have been no marriage.'

'Very possibly not,' she said quietly.

'So things are better as they are?'

'For us, certainly.'

'That storm over?' George smiled. They did have occasional flare-ups but they never lasted long.

'Yes, of course, and now give me peace to read the letter.'

She was smiling as she read it. Laura wrote a good letter and some of it amusing. Connie put the pages back in the envelope. 'I would say that Laura has landed on her feet. There is a cook and someone to do the housework and all Laura has to do is look after the child and supervise the staff. For the first time that girl doesn't have financial worries and she seems to think the world of her employer. Indeed he must be a thoroughly nice man and he has made quite an impression on your son. Aren't you jealous?' She looked up.

'Mmmmm.'

'I must address the next letter to Ronnie and I'm glad Laura suggested it. How very thoughtful of her.' She paused. 'I know, I'll address every alternate one to the boy.'

'Do that if you want. I don't see the need myself since Laura gives the letters to Ronnie to read.'

'Not the same. The boy wants to feel that he matters as an individual and not just as Laura's young brother. I shall print it very clearly on the envelope: MASTER RONALD MORRISON.'

George grinned. 'Don't overdo it, MASTER RONNIE MORRISON will do.'

Connie noticed his greyness that was always worse when he was tired.

'You do look tired, are you?'

'No more than usual.'

'Oh, dear.'

'Sorry, didn't mean to sound sorry for myself. I'm not desperately tired and from now on I'm going to be very hard on myself. It's time I did more and I don't just mean about my disability.'

She looked up quickly. 'What do you mean?'

'I don't need you to tell me that I haven't been much of a father to my two. It's a bit late for Laura but I would like to feel that I could do something for Ronnie.'

'Such as?'

'He's a clever lad, hopeless at sport and that used to annoy me.'

'It shouldn't have. You should be proud to have a bright son.'

'Likely to get a university place.'

Connie heard the pride in his voice and smiled to herself. 'You would like to put him through university?'

'Yes, I would but I don't know how that can be managed.'

'Without too much difficulty I would say.'

'Where would the money come from? You keep me as it is,' he said bitterly.

'You make a contribution.'

'Don't patronise me.'

'I am not patronising, I would never do that. You under-estimate your worth. Hands are important, darling, but not all important. A brain is. My strength is in designing and in persuading wealthy women that I can make them look a million dollars. My weakness is in calculations and in knowing when it is safe to expand and when it would be foolhardy. Me, I would rush at it whereas you would think the whole thing through carefully before coming to a decision.'

He looked wistful. 'I'd like to think what you say is true.'

'Then believe me.' She could almost see him throwing back his shoulders and there was a new determination in his voice.

'That is exactly what I am going to do. From now on, Connie, I am going to study the books and check all the transactions.'

'Lovely! Just what I was waiting for you to say but we have rather strayed from the point, if you remember we were discussing Ronnie and university.'

'A few years before he is that length.'

'Enough time for us to have made a success of our venture. We are going to succeed, George, never fear. Apart from the confidence I have in my designs there is Harry. He can be kindly as we both know but first and foremost he is a hard-headed businessman. Harry Lambert doesn't throw away money, he makes it work for him. He will be expecting a good return on his wife's share of the business.'

'With due respect your sister doesn't do much.'

'Don't forget she was the means of me getting started. None of this would have been possible without her.'

'A sleeping partner?'

'Not quite. To begin with her friends came to me out of curiosity and were favourably impressed. They came back. Lottie goes to coffee mornings, bridge parties and afternoon teas and those are the ideal way of spreading the word. Lottie does her bit, never fear.'

'Selfish of me but you know what I was hoping?'

Connie shook her head. She crossed her silk-stockinged legs and sat back.

'In a year or two would we be able to buy Lottie out?'

'No, George, I could never bring myself to do that.' Connie was slightly shocked and not a little annoyed.

'Why not? She doesn't need to make money. Harry has plenty of it.'

'That isn't the point. Lottie needs an interest outside the home and she enjoys thinking of herself as a business woman.'

'Which she isn't.'

'She does her bit.'

'If you say so.'

'I do, and listen to me, George. As long as we have Lottie we have Harry and he is our insurance against disaster. He can smell trouble long before it happens and not even the most successful business can be one hundred per cent sure that they are protected against the unexpected.

He looked at her admiringly. 'I hadn't thought of that.'

'Let us get back to the family, your family. Much to my surprise I am beginning to see the advantages of having a family.'

'A stake in the future?'

'Yes. With no child of my own I find I want to share yours and I mean to become a model stepmother.'

He grinned. 'How are you going to become that?'

'By not interfering which shouldn't be difficult with the miles between us. I will try to be helpful but I will only give advice when it is asked.'

'Sounds admirable.'

'Do you know what I am looking at George?'

'The letter rack?'

'That's right, and whose letters are waiting to be answered?'

He groaned. 'Peggy's and Vera's.'

'Long overdue.'

'Oh, God! Couldn't we leave them for another day?'

'That is what we have been doing. The letters from them are mounting up. Three of Peggy's and two of Vera's.'

'They know that I can't write and you have enough to do. Laura keeps them informed and surely to goodness that should be enough.'

'Sadly it isn't and I can't help but feel sorry for them. They are very anxious about you.'

'Then write to one or the other.'

'That wouldn't do, one or the other would be peeved.'

'So what?'

'So again I feel guilty. It isn't so much getting down to the writing but what on earth do I find to say? Your progress will take one small paragraph and the weather here another few sentences.'

'Rubbish, you could tell them about your business.'

'No,' she said firmly.

'Why not? It would fill up the page.'

'Perhaps it would but I don't want to. I'm certain within myself that we are going to make a big success of this but until that time I shan't say anything about it. That said, I don't see your sisters all that interested in the latest fashions.'

'Now! Now! How can you be so sure?'

'Just a feeling.'

'Shame on you. Admittedly neither of my sisters were fashion plates but neither were they dowdy. You do Miltonsands an injustice, my love, it is not quite the back of beyond.'

'I never suggested it was but I imagine it to be rather a tweed and plus-fours small town,' she teased.

'That's the gentry for you and our golf courses are the envy of you Londoners.'

'That may well be, but to get back to your sisters—'

'I suggest we leave their letter for another week.'

'Again?' Connie smiled with relief. Writing to a stranger wasn't easy and she hoped the day would come soon when George could answer his own letters. To begin with it had been the same with her step-daughter. Each sentence had to be thought out. Now writing to Laura was a pleasure. Connie found that she could fill the pages effortlessly. On occasions she asked Laura's opinion of colour schemes. She also asked what was currently popular in the old country. Laura would reply telling her what was appearing in the magazines and what she would go for herself. Her letters were a delight and she could be funny too. She was genuinely interested in hearing about Connie's business.

Heaven knew the girl had plenty to complain about but she never did. Once she had explained in a letter her reasons for giving up the house there had been no more about it. Yet Connie sensed that she still had her worries and more than likely they would concern her brother. His welfare seemed to be her main concern.

She would see to it that George didn't forget his promise and that financial assistance would go to Laura as soon as it were possible. In doing that she would be helping to remove the burden of her own guilt. When she had persuaded George to accompany her to New York she had given no thought as to how it would affect his family. She had only considered her own happiness.

That George was deeply worried about being unemployed Connie was only too well aware. An even bigger worry for him was the dreadful thought that because of his accident, he had perhaps become unemployable. Even the doctors were less optimistic about his hand. Time was running out for George, his age was against him. New York was looking for young, ambitious men of good education and vacancies in his own age group were few and far between.

The well-paid job he had been promised turned out to be no more than Harry making a place for him. George had been shattered. Connie hadn't understood his bitterness. If he was unhappy with Harry as an employer it was a job until he found something more to his liking. To Connie a civil service appointment was no better or worse than any other employment. She wasn't to know that George, like so many in the provinces, had been brought up to believe that he was one of the privileged. No one, but no one, thought of throwing away a job that represented security, a decent living standard and good working conditions.

Only his love for Connie had made him sacrifice everything for an uncertain future. Connie knew that it was up to her now. It was important to give her husband back his pride and his independence. The only way she could do that and not be accused of being patronising, was to make him an equal partner. That would have to be done legally and she would have her solicitor draw up the necessary documents.

She, George and Lottie would all play their part. Hers was the leading role. The success of the business depended on her flair for fashion. No extremes but for all that always keeping one step ahead. Her clientele were in the main mature women who wanted to look fashionable but never to look ridiculous. The young could wear ridiculous outfits and get away with it. It was all part of growing up – the need to shock, the need to be different and eye-catching.

'You are happy, you really love this life, don't you?' George asked as they sat down to eat.

'I do, I feel fulfilled. All I need now is to see you well again. Together we can go forward. Fate takes a hand sometimes, George. Had you found employment for yourself I could only have expected limited support—'

'Whereas I am totally committed. Lottie didn't object to the three of us being equal partners?'

'She most certainly didn't. It was what she expected.'

Chapter Twenty-Three

'Laura, could you spare me a minute?'

'Of course, Mr Cunningham,' she said quickly.

Laura had been sitting at the bureau doing the accounts and segregating those requiring immediate payment. They went under the paperweight and those paid monthly were put into the front of the ledger. She had been working with the door open and at the sound of her employer's voice she had swivelled round then got to her feet.

'My study, I think, we'll get a bit more peace there.'

'I really am sorry.'

'For what?'

'I could have kept Sylvia quiet and sent Ronnie upstairs.'

'I wouldn't want that. I enjoy having them around and if it was peace and quiet I was after there are other rooms in the house,' he smiled.

They crossed into the hall and Fergus held open the study door. 'Do sit down, this won't take long.'

Laura sat straight-backed and looked at the man who now sat opposite her, the desk between them. Always at the back of her mind was the fear that this very pleasant life would come to an end and she felt a ripple of panic.

'That's what it is! I knew there was something different about you, you've cut your lovely hair.'

The remark was so unexpected that Laura almost laughed out loud. It was such a relief after what she had been half expecting. Then the sobering thought came that perhaps this was just an opening, a way of softening the blow to come.

She touched her hair a little self-consciously. 'I decided to have it cut short.'

'Such a pity. It isn't that you don't suit it that way,' he added hastily, 'but I have to confess that I prefer you with your hair longer, the way you had it at Christmas.'

'So does Ronnie but I thought it too long and short hair is more fashionable.'

'You aren't a slave to fashion, are you?'

Laura thought about it. 'No, I don't think so but that doesn't mean I don't like to be in fashion.'

His hand went to tidy some papers on his desk and for a few moments Fergus concentrated on just that. In those last moments he had been in danger of blurting out his feelings but it was too soon. The moment passed.

'I asked you in here to discuss what you suggested some time ago.'

She looked blank.

'I must now give some thought to returning the hospitality I have enjoyed.'

'Oh, you mean you would like me to arrange a dinner party?'

'Only if it would not involve too much work. The hotel proved to be perfectly satisfactory.'

'I would like to do it, Mr Cunningham, if you can trust me with the arrangements.'

'I have every confidence in you.'

Laura smiled. 'Do you think I could have a page of that writing pad?'

'By all means.' He placed it in front of her and a pencil.

Laura picked up the pencil, suddenly businesslike. 'Did you have a date in mind?'

'I thought the last Friday in March.'

'How many guests?'

'Let me see, we'll keep it small. Make it eight of us round the table.'

She jotted that down. 'That should do meantime.' She raised her eyes to him. 'I take it I'll be able to get further details nearer the time?'

'I can't think of anything else you need to know but why not ask me now?'

'I'm not sure about the invitations, do these need to be sent out and have I anything to do with that?'

'No. This is just an informal dinner party. The invitations will be by word of mouth. Mine.'

Laura nodded. 'The time?'

'Sherry served in the drawing-room at seven-thirty and dinner at eight.' It amused him to see her so businesslike and serious.

'The menu, you'll want to see that beforehand?'

'Not at all. I'll leave that to you and Mrs Barclay. Between you I'm sure you will come up with a dinner to please all.'

'Yes.' She nodded her head several times.

'Something worrying you?'

'Not exactly. I was thinking about Sylvia. Seven o'clock is her bedtime but then again I wouldn't be required to assist with the serving. My duty will be the preparations beforehand.'

'I'm glad you brought Sylvia and her bedtime to my attention. And, Laura, I would like you to be on hand to supervise the kitchen and the dining-room and that you most certainly cannot do with Sylvia to see to.' He smiled. 'My daughter would choose that evening to play up, children always do. Leave it, Laura, and I'll see if Betsy would take her for the night. That should take care of everything, and now tell me what the news is from America.'

'My stepmother has written to say that Dad's fingers haven't straightened properly and perhaps they never will but he is able to hold a pen and write a few words.'

'A beginning, and once he is making use of his fingers they should strengthen and in time even straighten. You'll be getting a letter in his own handwriting one of these days,' he said kindly.

'That's what I keep hoping. But I have to say I would miss Connie's letters if she stopped writing. She is one of those people who write as I imagine she talks. Everything is brought vividly to life.'

'A gift.'

'Yes, I think it is. Occasionally she admits to bouts of homesickness but not for England. What she misses is English food and so does Dad.'

'Good old English roast beef and Yorkshire pudding,' he smiled.

'Dad's favourite but the beef would be Aberdeen Angus.'

'Of course, I stand corrected. There is no equal to Aberdeen Angus beef.' He seemed in no hurry to let her go. 'This has turned out to be a good marriage,' Fergus surprised himself by saying.

'Yes, Mr Cunningham, a very good marriage. I was so wrong and so unfair to Connie. You see, I hated to think of Connie in my mother's place. Selfish and silly of me but perhaps you can understand—' She stopped, confused. She had been thinking he would understand because of losing his wife and unable or unwilling to replace her.

'Perhaps,' he said quietly.

'I haven't only gained a stepmother I've gained a friend. She is so good for Dad. Like my mother was, she is the managing type but in the nicest way. I do wish that we had been able to meet before they went off to America.'

'One day you and Ronnie may make a visit to the States.'

'Lovely thought but I don't see it happening.'

When Laura left the study it was as though she had taken the brightness with her, Fergus thought. He would stay where he was and do some serious thinking. For too long he had allowed this state of affairs with Davina to drift on. So many of his friends were now inviting them as a couple and to refuse their invitations or accept just for himself was impossible. In fact it was an impossible situation.

Davina was beginning to annoy him. She could be the limit. How could she fail to notice his lukewarm response to the invitations she gaily accepted on behalf of them both? Eventually he had brought himself to say, 'Davina, I do wish you wouldn't accept invitations on my behalf.'

'But, darling, I check first to find out that you are free and our friends would be so disappointed if you were not to be present and I couldn't possibly go on my own.'

'Perhaps we should be seeing less of each other,' he said desperately. And she had playfully patted his cheek.

'Does having our names coupled bother you? It doesn't me.'

'Too much is read into it, ours is just friendship.'

'If you say so. For myself I'm perfectly happy as things are.'

'I'm not.'

'You, Fergus, are too easily embarrassed and too sensitive. Others, naturally enough, want to know when we are going to name the day,' she said coyly. 'I like to keep them guessing.'

Fergus was coming out in a cold sweat. They were seated in the drawing-room of Davina's home, a tall, elegant building that had once been the family house. It was where Davina lived with a skeleton staff. The house had that slight air of neglect brought about by a need to cut expenses. The family solicitor – not Fergus Cunningham – had advised his client to sell up and buy a smaller house. Should she do that there was enough to keep her in moderate comfort but Davina chose not to. There was prestige living in the old house and when she left it it would be for something bigger not smaller.

She knew perfectly well what Fergus was trying to do. He was trying to slip away from her but he wouldn't find it so easy. Most certainly he wouldn't, she would put up a fight to the bitter end. She mustn't show her concern but Davina was becoming very alarmed.

'In future, Davina, please do not take my acceptance for granted. I need to be consulted.'

'Of course, dear, you are absolutely right and I was just a teeny bit naughty. Forgiven?'

'Yes.' What else could he say?

'Don't go just yet, I want to make a suggestion. It would give me a great deal of pleasure to do this for you and now that you have that smart little girl, Jinny, to serve at table —'

'I'm lost.'

'Dearest, I want you to give the hotel a miss and let me organise a dinner party at Braehead. You said not so long ago that you wanted to repay some of the hospitality—'

'I did and that has been taken care of.'

'I don't understand,' she faltered.

'Your offer comes too late.' For a moment he was sorry for her, she looked so taken aback. 'But do keep the last Friday in March free. Seven-thirty sherry, eight o'clock dinner,' he said almost flippantly.

Davina had recovered. 'Of course, dear, and I'll be happy to be your hostess for the evening.'

'No, Davina,' he said firmly, 'you will be a welcome guest.'

Davina drew herself up and looked at him haughtily. 'May I ask who is to be doing the arrangements?'

'Laura. As a matter of fact she offered.'

'I bet she did,' Davina said viciously.

'I am aware of your animosity towards Laura but this is my—'

She didn't let him finish. 'You are so blind, so hopelessly, stupidly blind,' she almost spat.

'Far from it, you have opened my eyes.' The cool mask had slipped from the woman's face and Fergus was seeing another Davina. A vicious, spiteful woman. Laura had done nothing to deserve her venom.

Davina made a determined effort to pull herself together and the smile she gave him held apology and regret.

'Forgive me, I let my feelings run away with me. I do not like Miss Morrison nor do I trust her. I think she is a scheming young woman who is out to get you and plays on your weakness.'

With difficulty he held on to his temper but his eyes were stormy. 'My weakness?' He raised his eyebrows.

'Your daughter. She falls over that child to keep in your good books and as a result she is ruining the child.'

'That is nonsense.'

'I am entitled to my opinion of your housekeeper which I accept you do not share. However, the day will come and hopefully soon when you will see her for what she is. There, I've got that off my chest and it won't be referred to again.'

They were both on their feet, two tall people facing up to each other. Davina's thoughts were frantic. She had gone too far, she saw that now, but to think of that chit of a girl organising a dinner party when she should have been doing it was almost more than she could bear. The cheek of her suggesting it in the first place. Why hadn't she thought of it sooner?

It wasn't easy to swallow her pride but if she didn't all would be lost. Her brain was working frantically. Eight people around the table, three married couples and Fergus and herself. The host at the head of the table and only she could occupy the chair at the other end. There was no other possible seating arrangement. She smiled. The others would see her as the hostess and a very gracious one. She would look her loveliest and Fergus couldn't but be captivated.

As for that Miss Morrison, she would be behind the scenes. With Jinny serving at table there would be no reason for her to appear. All was not yet lost.

Davina's smile was brilliant and Fergus marvelled at how quickly she could recover.

'Thank you for your invitation and of course I shall be delighted to accept.'

'I'm so glad,' he said insincerely. A refusal would have suited him better but no, perhaps this was the better way. This way they could remain friends but with no more misunderstandings.

* * *

LOST DREAMS

Fergus had a spring in his step as he left Davina's home and walked down the drive to his car. That had been a difficult hour but it was over and now he could turn his thoughts to Laura. What on earth would she think, he wondered, if she were ever to learn that he had checked through the mail each morning to see if there was one with a Manchester postmark? He hadn't seen one so surely no letters meant that Laura and this Michael were only friends?

There would be no more trouble from Davina, she had got the message. If he felt guilt it was only a very little and he quickly consoled himself with the thought that, beautiful woman that she was, she wouldn't be long without a partner. That unpleasantness disposed of he could plan for the future, a future with Laura if she would have him. What would her reaction be when he asked her to marry him? Would she be shocked, pleased or just very surprised? He didn't have to remind himself that she was a very lovely young girl and life with a widower and a small child might not appeal to her. Age wasn't a great problem, ten years not too much of a gap.

Laura was very mature for her years. How could she not be, left as she was? Sylvia loved her and the two of them got on very well. Ronnie fitted in and the four of them were like a family. More than anything he longed to free her of worry. She had such an expressive face and he knew that her main concern was for her brother's welfare. Marriage to him would give her all the security she could want. Ronnie would become his responsibility and he would willingly put the boy through university and give him the support he needed. It was something he wanted to do. So many boys with a good brain like Ronnie were denied the opportunity to make use of a superior intelligence. All to do with the accident of birth. There was no fairness in life, he thought, and anyone who thought otherwise was a fool.

Laura didn't go back to her accounts. Instead she went straight to the kitchen where Mrs Barclay was on her own. Laura found her standing in front of the cooker and leaning over a big black pot. After taking a spoonful of soup she supped it then raised her eyes to the ceiling. It was what she always did and it never ceased to amuse Laura. What was it up there that decided her whether or not the soup required more seasoning?

'A wee thing more salt, I'm thinking.' She added some, stirred the soup and had another taste. A few nods of her head showed her satisfaction, then the lid went back on. That done, she gave her attention to Laura.

'And what can I do for you, lass? It's very pensive you're looking as though you had the cares of the world on your young shoulders.'

'No, Mrs Barclay, I'm not worried, just thinking. I came to talk something over with you.'

'We'll talk better over a cup of tea. There's enough in the pot and it's fresh, just made this five minutes.'

Laura went to collect two blue and white cups and two plain white saucers from the cupboard. She set them out on the scrubbed table. The sugar bowl was already there and Mrs Barclay brought a jug of milk from the cold slab in the pantry.

'Bring over the biscuits for yourself,' she said, pouring out the tea.

'Not for me, thanks.'

'Nor me. That's the worst of this job, the food is too handy. Have you ever seen a skinny cook?'

'Can't say I have.' Laura sipped her tea then put down the cup. 'Mr Cunningham wants me to arrange a small dinner party for the last Friday of March.'

'Mercy me, what's come over the man? There's been precious little entertaining done in this house since—'

'His wife died,' Laura said clearly and firmly. She couldn't understand this reluctance to mention the late Mrs Cunningham.

'As you say, since his wife died. Mind you, I was none too pleased at him going along to that hotel.' She sniffed. 'Put me in a bad light and I was offended.'

'If you felt slighted it was unintentional, I can assure you. Mr Cunningham didn't want to make more work for you, and remember there was no one to serve at table.'

'That would be right enough but there is Jinny now. I'm weakening, I'll have a biscuit after all. Are you going to be tempted?'

'No, I'm not, but here you are,' Laura said, offering the tin.

'It wasn't me the master didn't want to bother, it was Mrs Mathewson. She ran the house and with her looking after the bairn she could do what she wanted.'

'Mrs Barclay, tell me about the accident, no one else seems to be prepared to talk about it.'

'There are things better left unsaid.'

'I get the distinct impression that there is a mystery.'

'No mystery, at least it wasn't a mystery to some. Lass, all I can tell you is that there was a car accident and the poor soul was killed outright. That could have been a blessing. To my mind death is better than being left a hopeless cripple or, even worse, if there was brain damage.' She pressed her lips firmly together and Laura knew to ask no more. 'To get back to this dinner, how many guests?'

'Eight around the table?'

'Is that all? It would be a bad show if we couldn't manage that between us.'

Laura smiled. The cook was pleased at the thought of a dinner party and a chance to show off her skills.

'You and Jinny will be seeing to the setting of the table?'

'Yes.'

'The master will be seeing to the wine.'

'I forgot about that, I didn't ask.'

'No need, that is the way it is done. You won't be knowing about these things?'

'No, but I'm a quick learner.'

'That you are. Just remember two glasses at each place and as to the coffee—'

'That is to be served in the drawing-room.'

The cook frowned. 'What I was going to say was don't rush it. Give the guests time to get their meal down. Fifteen minutes is about right with them going from dining-room to drawing-room. There'll be more drink consumed by the men.'

Laura nodded. She did have a lot to learn.

'Will you be serving the coffee or Jinny?'

'Jinny. I'll be behind the scenes.'

'And the bairn, is someone to be looking after her?'

'Sylvia is to be staying with Miss Yeaman overnight.'

'You are well organised, I'll say that for you.'

'The menu, Mrs Barclay?'

'Leave that to me. I'll get my thinking cap on and write out one or

293

two sample dinners and you can get Mr Cunningham to decide.'

'He is leaving it to us or rather to you.'

'Better and better,' she said with satisfaction.

'I can leave the food to you and I'll see to the house. I want it to look welcoming and I'm quite desperately hoping that there will be masses of daffodils out by then.'

'Sure to be, I had a wee look about the garden and there is quite a bit of yellow showing already.'

Laura looked pleased. 'I want vases of them in the hall to give a welcome splash of colour. Then some in the dining-room and the drawing-room unless Jack thinks I am being too greedy.'

'He won't think that and I bet with all those picked you would hardly notice the difference. You can get me some for the kitchen window. I like to see a touch of spring.'

Laura got up to go.

'Before you go satisfy my curiosity – is Mr Cunningham still seeing that besom, Dorward?'

'I wouldn't know. She was here on Christmas Day, evening actually, and they were going off somewhere together.'

'Men,' she said, her voice heavy with disgust, 'even the clever ones are such fools when it comes to a scheming woman. Is she to be one of the guests?'

'I haven't seen the guest list but I would expect so.'

Mrs Barclay put her hands on her ample waist. 'Acting like she was the mistress already, shameless hussy that she is. Mind you she could well be the next mistress and when that day comes I think I'll be looking elsewhere.'

'Surely not as bad as that.'

'This is just between us but I don't have to tell you that.'

'No.'

'My job is safe enough until I find myself another I would think but I wouldn't say so much for yours.'

'I know she doesn't like me.'

'I don't suppose she does but she'll want rid of you because you are too bonny, she'll see you as a threat.'

'I wouldn't be that but are you saying you see them getting married?'

'He'll have a job getting out of her clutches.'

Laura tried to make a joke of it. 'You would have me looking for a new job?'

'No, don't do anything hasty but keep your eyes and ears open.'

'Thanks for the warning,' Laura said dully.

Chapter Twenty-Four

The day before the dinner party everything was going according to plan. Mrs Barclay had taken a great deal of care over the menu and both Laura and she were confident that it would meet with everyone's approval. Nothing was left to chance, Laura saw to that, and if there were quiet smiles behind her back she chose not to notice. To the others this was just a small, not very important dinner party while for her it was so much more. She wanted to impress her employer. The evening's success would let her employer see that she could be trusted to organise his entertaining and hopefully that would help to make her job more secure.

She threw on a coat and let herself out of the back door and hurried along the tidy pathways. The day was bright and springlike with a little warmth in the sun that shone out of a blue sky. Across the blueness white puffy clouds drifted lazily by.

At Braehead the front garden was beautifully landscaped but not so the large area to the back. Jack was of the opinion that nature should be allowed its freedom provided it wasn't allowed to run riot. Only those knowledgeable about gardens knew the work that went into capturing the natural look. Laura thought it all delightful. High, mature trees gave complete privacy to the house, and shrubs showing pale green buds, divided the walks. The garden was on two levels with rockery plants and heathers on the slope between. To one side and partly hidden was the kitchen garden and Laura could see Tim working in it and hear his tuneless whistling. Away in the distance and on the lower level Jack was leaning on his spade and taking a breather.

'This you admiring your display, Jack?' Laura smiled as she drew near.

He turned at the sound of her voice. 'Ah, it's yourself, Miss

Morrison, didn't hear you. Not bad is it, supposing I say it myself?' His voice held the satisfaction of a man who knows he has done a good job.

'Simply wonderful, Jack. I don't think I have seen anything to equal it. It's like – she searched for a description – like a huge golden bedspread.'

'A fitting description I would say.' He paused to shift the weight to his other foot. 'I've always had a soft spot for the daffie. Mind you the roses make a fine show in the summer but to me there's nothing to compare with the bright yellow of the daffodil. Comes I suppose of being starved of colour in the winter.'

'I'm sure you're right.'

'This will be you wanting to rob my garden?'

'You won't miss a few,' she wheedled.

'Lass, take as many as you want. Armfuls if you like and I declare you'll see no difference.'

'When is the best time to pick them? I want them at their best for tomorrow evening.'

He nodded. 'I'll get Tim on the job in an hour or two. Keep the daffies indoors overnight and you should have a fine show the morn's night.'

'I'm grateful, Jack. Thank you.'

His weatherbeaten face creased into a smile. 'Never could resist a bonny face and that's a fact.' He gave a huge wink and she laughed.

'Shall I come for them?'

'No need. That's a job for the lad. There's plenty of work ahead of him.' He waved a hand. 'Once these have withered away it'll be a clearing-out.'

'You aren't digging them out? You wouldn't? You couldn't? Jack, it would be such a shame,' Laura said, horrified.

'Don't fret, lass, a good thinning-out and we'll get bigger heads by another year.'

'You have to know best,' she said in a voice that sounded unsure.

'Nothing too drastic I promise you and while I mind I've cuttings for your friend.'

'For Jane? She will be pleased.'

'Tell her I'm keeping the cuttings to bring them on. That'll give them a better chance.'

'I'll tell her, Jack, and many, many thanks,' she said, hurrying away.

The daffodils arrived. Tim had to make two journeys and Laura had looked out vases and containers. She would arrange the flowers first thing in the morning and leave the afternoon for setting the table in the dining-room.

Laura wanted to concentrate on the hall where the guests would be greeted. First impressions were important. The hall was spacious and she wanted it to be especially welcoming. There were healthy plants on the broad window-sill and plenty of greenery but it needed colour to bring it all to life. On her hunt for vases Laura removed two large crystal ones from the breakfast room. She had wondered what two such lovely vases were doing there.

Once they were filled and arranged, Laura placed one vase on the hall table and the other on a side table which held gleaming brass ornaments. Then she went to the door, turned round to take a critical look, moved the brass a fraction and smiled. Quite, quite perfect.

More daffodils went into the drawing-room and on the sideboard in the dining-room. Still some remained after Mrs Barclay had taken what she wanted and Laura took them up to her own room. Returning to the dining-room, she found Annie giving a final polish to the furniture.

'All this carry-on and folk could be forgiven for thinking royalty was expected.'

'Annie, am I overdoing it? Are there too many daffodils?'

'You couldn't have too many of those. No, this is just me having my wee bit of fun. If you ask me —'

'I am asking you,' Laura smiled.

'Then I'd say everything looks champion, real pretty and springlike. The master is going to be pleased with all the trouble you've taken.'

'If he notices.'

'He'll notice. Men do but they don't always say so.'

'When you finish that would you give me a hand with the tablecloth? Jinny is busy and I could make a start on the table.'

Annie got stiffly to her feet. 'Every picture tells a story,' she grimaced. 'Any more polishing and I declare I'll away the wood worn away.' She looked down at her hands. 'Clean enough I'd say but to be on the safe side I'll away and wash them.' She picked up her tin of polish and cleaning cloths and went to the kitchen to wash her hands at the sink.

Almost tenderly the dazzlingly white starched tablecloth was taken out of its folds and placed on the table. Great care was taken to have the same length of overlap at each end.

'A fraction this way, Laura, I'd say.' Annie tut-tutted. 'I should be remembering to call you Miss Morrison.'

'I don't mind, Annie, it isn't important. This is. Have we got it even?'

They both had a good look, Annie with half-closed eyes.

'I would say so.'

'So would I. Thanks, Annie.'

Jinny came in and was looking none too pleased. 'I was coming to help you with that, Miss Morrison.'

'You were busy, Jinny.'

'I was but I'm not now.' She walked around the table and shook her head. 'There should be slightly more at the window side,' she announced.

'Do you think so?'

'Yes, I do.'

Laura helped to make the adjustment, then Jinny moved it back to where it had been in the first place.

'There, that's it now?' she said in the voice of the expert.

On her way out Annie winked to Laura and Laura hid a smile.

'You do the cutlery, Jinny, and I'll see to the wine glasses.'

'If you don't mind me saying so, Miss Morrison, the glasses will be all the better of another polish with a soft cloth.' Jinny had been taking the silver cutlery out of the sideboard drawer and looked up to add, 'It gets them sparkling.'

'Yes, Jinny, thank you, I intended doing just that,' Laura said with a slight edge to her voice.

By early evening there was an appetising smell coming from the kitchen and Mrs Barclay was clattering pans and talking to herself. Jinny had changed into her tablemaid's uniform and looked fresh and efficient. In the last month the shy, plain tablemaid had blossomed. No longer did she keep her eyes downcast, now she held her head high and it seemed to have added two inches to her height. Mrs Barclay and Annie put it all down to her romance with Tim and told each other that it was a pity it hadn't had the same effect on the lad. He was as gormless as ever but a nice obliging lad for all that.

There was no need for Laura to take extra care over her appearance.

She was neat and tidy in her brown dress with the cream collar and cuffs. No one would see her and if they did it wouldn't matter. She was the housekeeper.

Jinny put down the laden tray on the kitchen table and rubbed her arms.

'Wouldn't have put so much on if I'd known it was to be so heavy.'

Mrs Barclay pushed a stray hair from her perspiring face and took a good look at the tray. 'That's what I like to see,' she said in a voice rich with satisfaction. 'They've done justice to my cooking.' The plates were clean and only a very little food remained in the serving dishes. Early on in Jinny's career she had been informed that dishes were never scraped out. Waste it might be but it just wasn't the done thing.

The remains in the fish dish would feed two hungry stray cats, one grey, one black. Each day they came sniffing around the back door to see what they could scrounge. They didn't try to sneak into the kitchen nor were they likely to. Once had been enough and on that occasion Annie, with blood-curdling threats, had chased them out with the broom handle. Now they waited out of sight until the cracked plate with food on it was put down at the side of the door together with a saucer of milk.

Jinny was rolling her eyes. 'I wish you folk could see her, Miss Dorward, I mean. She looks like a film star, all glamorous and everything.'

'That's a pleasure I'll happily deny myself,' Mrs Barclay sniffed, then, because she was curious, forced herself to ask, 'What's so special about what she's wearing?'

'You do want to know after all.' Jinny was pleased and proud. Only she got to see the guests and in between the serving of the meal she had the chance of a good look.

'Come on then, what is she wearing?'

'A bright red gown and I saw it properly before she sat down. Very, very fitting, like she would need a shoe horn to get into it.'

'What a blether you are, Jinny, I don't know where you hear such expressions.'

'I'm only trying to make it as plain as I can. You'll know what I mean when I say it shows all the places where she goes in and out.'

The cook rolled her eyes. 'My, but when it comes to describing fashion you're a genius. What you should say, my girl, is that the dress hugged her body.' Mrs Barclay beamed as though she had said something very clever. She remembered reading it somewhere.

'That's the expression I was trying to remember, Mrs Barclay, and I'm not finished. The dress, the gown I mean, has a plunging neckline that just about showed —' she giggled and covered her mouth with her hand. 'I would never have the nerve—'

'Never mind nerve, there isn't enough of you to hold anything up.'

Laura had come in quietly and heard the last part.

'That makes two of us, Jinny,' she said kindly. Jinny, as she knew was very sensitive about being flat-chested.

'Nothing of the kind, Laura, you've a nice, slim figure.' She turned to a glowering Jinny. 'Is there more?'

'No, only that the other two ladies looked quite nice.'

'But not sensational?' Laura smiled.

'No, one of them is wearing a black velvet dress and lots of jewellery. The other one has on mauve. I don't like it but then I don't fancy mauve.'

'Must say I do like black velvet,' the cook said, busying herself as she spoke, 'there's something rich about it.'

'Black is slimming,' Jinny said with a malicious gleam in her eye. 'Fat folk like you should wear black all the time.'

Mrs Barclay bristled. 'Stout women, I'll have you know, can look well in any colour. Not like scrawny women who always manage to look half dead.'

'If you say so,' Jinny smirked.

'I do say so. I'd rather be jolly and fat than skinny and miserable.'

'You'll be happy then,' Jinny said cheekily.

Mrs Barclay pursed her lips. 'I do not like impudence, Jinny, and that is no way to speak to your elders and your betters.' She took a deep breath. 'You would do well to remember that it was me that got you this job and I wouldn't like to be in your shoes if I was to have a word with your grandma.'

Jinny looked frightened. 'I'm sorry, Mrs Barclay,' she muttered.

Laura thought the exchange had gone on long enough and surely it was time for Jinny to serve the coffee.

'Jinny, the coffee.'

'It's here ready and has been for the last five minutes,' cook said.

'You told me not to hurry, to wait fifteen minutes,' Jinny shot back.

'Take it through, Jinny,' Laura said firmly. They were all tired and tempers were getting frayed, she thought, as she went along to the dining-room. On the way she heard the sound of laughter coming from the drawing-room and smiled to herself. The evening appeared to be going well.

Laura was gathering up the tablecloth in readiness for the laundry when Jinny burst in. She looked close to tears and was holding her right hand and sucking her fingers.

'Jinny, what is it? What's the matter? What have you done to yourself?' Laura felt panicky.

'My hand, I've burnt it. I went to get the coffee pot and I didn't notice and I went too near the kettle and it was boiling and I got some on my hand and its stinging and Mrs Barclay said I was making a fuss over nothing and it was my own fault for not looking what I was doing,' she babbled without pausing for breath.

Laura let out a sigh of relief and just managed to hold back the 'is that all?' that she was on the point of saying. Poor Jinny, a burn was very painful and obviously she hadn't been getting much sympathy.

'You go and see to your hand, Jinny. I can't remember whether it is cold water or soap for a burn but Mrs Barclay will know.'

'What about the coffee? It's still in the kitchen.'

'I'll see to the coffee.'

'I really am sorry, Miss Morrison. Maybe I could manage to pour, it isn't stinging so much now. Only I'm scared in case my hand shakes and I spill some in the saucer.'

'We can't risk it, Jinny.' Laura hurried ahead and into the kitchen where a rather subdued cook had the silver coffee pot on a cork mat.

'What a carry on about a wee burn. Is she serving the coffee or not?'

'I'm seeing to it.' Laura lifted the pot and hurried away when she all but bumped into Fergus Cunningham.

'Whoops! A near thing,' he said, steadying her, 'that could have been nasty for one of us.'

'I'm sorry.'

He smiled. 'Would you happen to know if there is a bottle of brandy in the dining-room?'

'Yes, on the sideboard.' She remembered seeing it.

303

'Good. That was a lovely meal and enjoyed by all,' he said as he moved away.

Laura continued on her way with slightly flushed cheeks. After knocking she entered the drawing-room and for a moment all eyes were turned to her.

'Excuse me,' she said quietly as she put down the coffee pot on the silver stand. The cups were set out on the Queen Anne table.

'Leave that, Miss Morrison,' Davina Dorward said imperiously. 'I'll see to the coffee when Mr Cunningham returns.'

'Thank you.' Laura went out, glad to make her escape. Had she but known it, Davina Dorward had done her a good turn because she did feel nervous.

One week had gone by since the dinner party and Fergus was feeling happier than he had been in a long time. The final break had been made with Davina and whether she accepted it or not it no longer concerned him. As for the social scene he would give that a miss for the time being. A discreet word to his friends was all that had been necessary. They said they fully understood the situation and sympathised. The ladies were secretly pleased and one or two very relieved. They were not fond of Davina, she was too sharp and there was a cruel edge to some of her remarks. When she used her charm on their husbands they were extremely uneasy and as a result Fergus found that he had their whole-hearted support.

After Fergus had gone they gossiped among themselves and there was a good deal of speculation as to the possibility of Fergus having a lady love tucked away somewhere.

With all that behind him Fergus began to think about the evening ahead. He wouldn't plan, just play it by ear. Very likely the evening would follow the pattern of those others he spent at home. About seven o'clock Laura would put a sleepy Sylvia to bed and read her a story. Or perhaps she would make up one. She had a fund of them. Laura, he was discovering, was a young lady of many talents.

He smiled, thinking how good she was with her young brother. The boy was looking for more freedom and Laura, very sensibly he thought, was letting him have it. Not too much though, there were rules and Ronnie had to obey them. The boy must say where he was going and be back in Braehead by a certain hour. On Fridays and Saturdays this was extended by half an hour. According to Ronnie everybody, but everybody, was allowed to stay out longer but Laura was adamant. Fergus had laughed when she told him, it brought his own boyhood back.

Too much petticoat rule was bad for a growing boy and Fergus sought to have the occasional man-to-man talk. On one such occasion the rules set by Laura had come up in the conversation.

'Your sister is being fair, I would say, Ronnie. At your age my brother and I had to obey the rules.'

'Did you always – obey them I mean?'

'We found it more comfortable to do so,' he said drily.

'Suppose you have to with parents but you don't have to when it's only your sister.'

'In your case you should. Laura has taken on the responsibility for you. Sometimes, Ronnie, I wonder if you fully appreciate all your sister has given up for you.'

Ronnie was thoughtful. He liked Mr Cunningham and had a lot of respect for him.

'You mean like getting married?'

'Like that, yes.'

'Michael was going to marry her but then he went to live in Manchester and she didn't want to go there.'

'Perhaps she only said that,' Fergus said carefully.

'You mean because of me?'

'It's a possibility.'

'I liked Michael and I missed him when he didn't come to the house. He liked me too, Mr Cunningham, I could have gone with them. I think I could. Anyway it doesn't matter now. She still likes him but she doesn't want to marry him. Laura likes living here and that goes for me too.'

'I'm very glad to hear you are both happy at Braehead.'

'Is the little imp asleep?'

'Sound asleep, Mr Cunningham, I had read only a few lines before her eyes were closing.'

'I was sure a cup of coffee would be welcome and I had Jinny bring another cup.'

'Thank you, it would be very welcome,' she smiled. It wasn't the first time they had taken coffee together but it was usually when there was something to discuss.

The coffee pot was beside him and he poured coffee into the other cup. She took it from him and put it down on the circular table between them.

The silence lengthened as they both drank a little. She wondered if she should break it or wait for him to do so. For his part Fergus was admiring the attractive picture she made. How young and fresh the girl was and so natural. He was fascinated by the way the gold in her hair shone through and he had an urge to feel its softness between his fingers. When she looked across at him he thought there was a veiled worry in those lovely eyes. She was plainly dressed yet the most ordinary clothes looked well on her. She didn't have an extensive wardrobe, she had worn that tweed skirt many times before.

Fergus Cunningham was never nervous but at this moment he was. Was this a good time to propose marriage? Was it too soon? On the other hand this was probably as good a time as any. There was little fear of them being interrupted. He cleared his throat.

'Laura, there is something I want to say to you and I don't quite know how to begin.' He stopped and watched in fascinated horror as every vestige of colour left her face. She had been holding her cup and when she put it down it rattled on her saucer.

Fergus had half risen. 'Laura, my dear girl, what is the matter? Are you unwell?'

She shook her head and made an attempt to pull herself together. She even managed a small smile. 'I'm sorry, it was just the shock.'

'The shock?' he repeated.

'Stupid of me, Mr Cunningham, I saw it coming and I should have been prepared.'

'You saw it coming?'

Laura frowned. Why was he repeating everything she said?

'Yes.'

'How could you possibly know what I was going to say?'

'I just did.'

'You just did?'

There he was again, 'I knew it had to come sometime.'

'And you found that upsetting?'

'Of course it was upsetting.'

Fergus was dismayed and shattered. Had he made his feelings so very obvious? He must have done and the poor girl had found it embarrassing. He was beginning to feel all kinds of a fool.

'I'm sorry about that,' he said stiffly.

'You don't have to be, it wasn't your fault.'

'It wasn't?'

'No, you wouldn't have found it easy, I know that. And I just want to say,' her voice was wobbling and she stopped to compose herself, 'that I'll always remember your kindness to me and to Ronnie.'

'Does this mean that you want to leave Braehead?'

She looked at him curiously. 'You know I don't but I accept that I must.'

Fergus pushed his hands through his hair. 'Laura, I am becoming more bewildered by the minute and I am beginning to think that we are talking at cross-purposes.'

'It seems clear enough to me.'

'Not to me it doesn't. Just tell me in the simplest of words why you are going to leave Braehead when you don't want to?'

'It is not my place—'

'It is your duty to explain this muddle to me.'

Laura pursed her lips. 'Since you insist I have no alternative – Miss Dorward doesn't like me,' she said abruptly.

'I know that.'

She stared. 'That's what all this is about.'

'Laura, will you kindly stop talking in riddles? What has Davina to do with this?'

'Everything, I would have thought, since you are going to marry her and she most certainly won't want me here when she becomes mistress.'

'What may I ask has given you that impression?' There was a hint of grimness in Fergus's pleasant voice.

It was Laura's turn to be mystified. 'N-nothing, I just thought—'

'Then you thought wrong.' His expression relaxed into a smile and Laura felt dizzy with relief. 'Let me explain,' he continued, 'Davina is a very old friend and she was extremely kind to accompany me to those functions where one is required to bring a partner. I see now that it was unwise.'

'You don't owe me an explanation but thank you. You must have thought me mad?'

'For a time I must confess I was concerned about my own sanity and as for you all of a sudden you have lost that strained look.'

'It was the relief, you see. I thought you wanted me to go so that you could engage another housekeeper.'

'I may well be doing that,' he said wickedly. Then, seeing the light leave her face, he hastened to add, 'I wondered if you would be interested in another position?'

'In your household?' She looked puzzled.

'Very much so. No, enough of this. There are to be no more misunderstandings.' He paused and looked into her face. 'Would you consider marriage to me, Laura? I am asking you to be my wife.'

She stared at him incredulously. 'You are asking me to marry you?'

'I had hoped the suggestion would appeal to you.'

'I think it does but are you really sure?'

'Very sure.'

'I can't take this in.'

'I'm sorry, I don't seem to have done this very well.'

'It isn't that, I mean a proposal is a proposal, isn't it?'

This wasn't going according to plan but then there hadn't been a plan. The girl was in shock and was it any wonder?

'You will give the matter some thought?'

'Of course I will. I'm very flattered, Mr Cunningham.'

'That had better be Fergus, don't you think?'

'All right,' she said shyly.

The initial shock was beginning to wear off and Laura was thinking of all that marriage to Fergus would mean. No more worries and a secure future for herself and Ronnie. She would be mistress of this lovely house. What more could she ask? The trouble was she did want more. One little word that would have made all the difference. Fergus hadn't said he loved her. That he liked and respected her, she knew that, but was it enough for marriage? Perhaps it was. Fergus was honest and he would only say what was true. There would be only one love for him, his first wife, and all she could expect was second best. Then her own feelings, she was confused about those. Hadn't she thought that she had loved Michael but it had turned out not to be the case? Now she believed herself to be in love with her employer but he didn't love her. His reason for this proposal was because she got on so well with his child. Could she settle for that?

'Laura,' he said gently, 'let us leave it there for the present. I don't want to rush you.'

'Thank you,' she said tremulously and reached for her cup.

'Leave that, it will be stone cold. I think after the shocks and misunderstandings we both need something a little stronger.' He got up to fill two glasses, one with sherry and one with whisky topped up with water.

She took the glass from him.

'There is more I should have said, Laura. Should you decide to honour me with an acceptance I shall do all in my power to make you happy and it will be my privilege to put Ronnie through university. We could be a happy family,' he said wistfully, 'the four of us.'

She nodded, too full for words. He was such a kind man but he still couldn't say the one word she wanted to hear.

Chapter Twenty-Five

They had come a long way, she and George, and in a remarkably short time. Harry's money, his backing, his business expertise and his contacts had paved the way. Premises, as he had been quick to point out, could be improved but not a district. The importance of being in the right place to attract the kind of customer they were seeking couldn't be emphasised enough, he explained. Also important was the room for expansion. Start small, think big. When Harry chose the premises he had all that in mind.

Connie was well pleased, more than well pleased, she was over the moon. This was her world of dreams and creativity and she was seeing it all happen. Finding a name had not been easy. It had to be something eye-catching, something memorable, but none of the suggestions put forward had met with enthusiasm. In the end it became Connie's Fashion House and then it was just Connie's.

The entrance to Connie's was in a prestigious corner some distance from the bustle of the main shopping area. It was on Eighth Avenue, a thoroughfare of exclusive shops patronised by a rich clientele. There were expensive jewellers, an antique shop, shoe shops, a hair stylist and a rather quaint establishment with a long narrow window that advertised hand-made chocolates boxed and packed to requirements.

For months Connie had studied displays and learned from their mistakes. Simplicity was the keynote and that was the look she was after. One carefully selected gown would grace the window with nothing to detract the eye: only one arrangement of flowers in a tall vase in the far corner to soften the effect. With the window to her satisfaction Connie could indulge in the luxury of a dream well on the way to being fulfilled.

The Fashion House occupied two floors in beautifully appointed premises. There was a sewing room and two excellent machinists worked in it. She had chosen young married women who had left their previous employment to start a family and were anxious, in one case frantic, to return to the world of fashion and away from nappies and feeding bottles. The tiny, gorgeous baby gurgling in the pram had suddenly turned into a demanding, noisy and exhausting toddler. It was sheer bliss to hand over the responsibility to an obliging grandmother who was blessed with an abundance of time and patience.

Connie's own room had two large windows that gave plenty of light so that she could judge the true colour of a fabric. Always her mind was busy working on new designs and she liked to shut herself away to do her thinking. Her rough sketches would be pinned to the wall to be pored over and then later they would either be discarded or improved upon.

Another room had been made into an office and had a very large desk in it which had been picked up at a sale. This was George's sanctuary and the difference George had brought to the office was quite amazing. Into the chaotic mess of unfiled statements, bills, invoices and second demands that were due to an oversight, George brought order. He had the floor quickly cleared of papers for which Connie had found no home. Old advertisements were thrown into the wastepaper basket and a miscellaneous file opened for the others. No longer were there frantic searches for an invoice or a receipt. They were produced on demand and George revelled in the sense of power it gave him. New York had captivated George Morrison and he marvelled to think that he and Connie were a part of this huge, exciting, pulsating world.

For a time his crooked fingers had both distressed and embarrassed him and he mourned the loss of his long, straight fingers. Now he hardly noticed as his pen flew across the pages. He was essential to the smooth running of the business as Connie was quick to tell him but as he himself already knew. George was happy.

Connie was amused. She hadn't realised what an asset it would be to have a good-looking man on the premises, particularly in an all-women business.

George was a natural with his pleasant manner and his quiet, well-modulated voice. Walking through the store in his dark, tailormade suit he would smile and when asked, which was quite often, would stop to give his considered opinion. In other words George told the customer what she wanted to hear but in such a way that it could not be mistaken for sales talk.

'George,' Connie smiled into his face, 'that lady was hard to convince until you told her how well she looked in that dress.'

'She did, I told her the truth.'

'I know, but she kept swithering and looking at another which was totally unsuitable for her figure.'

George smiled knowingly. 'She believed me because she knew that I wouldn't sin my soul by saying one thing and thinking another.'

'Tell me, dear, if someone looked a mess would you tell them to their face?'

'Hardly, I'm not stupid. I would suggest that they tried on something else before making up their mind.'

'Just as I would do. It is important to me to have my customers feeling happy about their purchase before they leave these premises. I would rather forgo a sale.' She smiled. 'We make a good team, darling.'

By evening they were usually exhausted. Connie quite often brought work home with her and on these occasions George would prepare the meal. He had become deft domestically and discovered that he actually liked to cook. The kitchen of the apartment was bright and cheerful with floral curtains in pinks and blues. The woodwork was light brown and a large calendar on the wall showed gardens with the flowers blooming for that month. The kitchen was small and compact and had been well planned. There was little walking to be done since everything was within easy reach.

George was in shirt-sleeves and had a blue and white apron, like a butcher's, tied round his middle. He was slicing onions.

'Darling, I'm keeping my distance, if I go too near an onion I weep oceans.'

'An original excuse anyway,' he said drily.

'Lots of people suffer this way. What are we having?'

'Steak and onions.'

'Oh, good! Just what I'm in the mood for,' she said, kicking off her shoes in the doorway. She dabbed at her eyes with a handkerchief. 'Even at this distance would you believe and I'm weeping? I'll come back once you have them in the pan.' She lifted her shoes and padded away.

It wasn't all work and no play and once a week they went to a show or had a meal at a good restaurant. Most nights they were in bed by ten-thirty. One or other of them might fall asleep at once but often they would talk well into the night.

'George, are you asleep?'

'Yes.'

'You're not.'

'I was very nearly over. Can't you sleep?'

'I wasn't trying to.'

'You'll be a wash-out in the morning.'

'Very probably. I got thinking about Laura.'

'She's all right.'

'So she says. Have you done any more about arranging to send money?'

'Not yet but I will.'

'You're off-putting and it isn't fair on your daughter.'

'She appears to be managing all right.'

'You can't know that for sure.'

He sighed and turned on to his back. The curtains hadn't been properly closed and a chink of light was getting through. Was it worth getting up to adjust it, he wondered? The shaft of light was beginning to annoy him but not sufficiently to have him make the effort to get up.

'You closed the curtains, didn't you?'

'I always do,' Connie said.

'You didn't make a very good job of it.'

'So I see. Does it bother you?'

'Yes.'

'You are nearer, I would have to go all the way round the bed.'

George groaned, got up, arranged the curtain and managed to stub his big toe on the way back. He muttered a number of oaths.

'Naughty! Naughty! I heard that.'

'I'm beyond sleep,' he said in an aggrieved voice.

'So am I. We were talking about Laura.'

'No need to worry about her. She is doing well enough. Free food and free lodgings for both of them. That can't be bad and what she gets will be found money.'

'Perhaps not so very much in her hand. Remember the girl has

314

clothes to buy for them both plus all the extras one forgets about until needed. Are you listening?'

'I'm listening.' George gave a deep sigh which she ignored.

'Admittedly I have no experience but I imagine that Ronnie is of an age when he is quickly outgrowing his clothes. Laura did say in one of her letters that her brother was stretching. You have to remember, George, that it all costs money.' She put her arms above the bedclothes and gazed into the darkness.

'Connie, I would like to send money to Laura, not just an allowance. I didn't tell you and only recently have I thought about it myself—' He stopped.

'Go on, dear, we must share our problems.'

'Ellen was left money which was to be used for Laura's education. She was to go on to college but then her mother died and she had to look after the house.'

'And where is that money now if I am permitted to ask?'

'Gone, but I'll make it up to her sometime.'

'Sometime is now, George,' Connie said firmly.

'No, Connie, it'll have to wait. We have a huge debt to pay off which you seem to forget.'

'Don't be silly, I know exactly how much we are in debt but it can wait. Your debt to your family is on my conscience, George. Had it not been for me the three of you might well be together today.'

George was becoming exasperated. 'None of this bothered you before. In fact you were quite happy to ignore my family.'

'And don't you think I'm ashamed?' she snapped. 'I was totally selfish and completely mistaken in thinking that your family could threaten our happiness.'

'We need to get our priorities right, Connie. It worries me to be so heavily in debt to Harry and I want to start reducing it as soon as possible.'

'Harry doesn't want that. You are supposed to be the one to know about finance.'

'I was a civil servant not a businessman.'

'I know, dear, and you are doing marvellously but this is one area of business you don't understand. Harry neither expects nor wants the debt reduced at this early stage. As far as he is concerned it is an investment and a good one. With his wife involved he'll keep a close watch on the way things are going.'

'Take years then?' he said gloomily.

'Of course it will. What happens is that we take out enough for our personal needs and some extra. Already we are doing far better than we dared hope and as the business improves so does our standard of living.'

'You have it all worked out.'

'I've had a lot longer to study the situation than you have, so stop worrying and get that money to Laura.'

An ocean away in the Cunningham residence the evening meal was over and Laura had tidied the sitting-room of toys. Sylvia was asleep and Ronnie was upstairs reading or perhaps doing his homework. Laura was alone when Fergus entered. She felt shy and her cheeks grew hot but he appeared exactly as normal. They smiled to each other and Fergus, deciding the fire could do with a log, picked a large one from the brass bucket and placed it carefully on the coal before pressing it down with his foot.

'I'm sorry, you should have let me do that.'

'My dear Laura, I am not completely useless in the house.' She's nervous, he thought, as she crossed to the window and examined one of the plants on the sill. With her fingers she removed one brown leaf and another that was beginning to curl. After appearing to be examining them she dropped the leaves into the fire.

'Do stop wandering around, Laura, and come and sit down. I do hope you are not trying to avoid me?'

'Of course not. Why would I do that?'

'If you were embarrassed you might.'

'Perhaps I am a little.'

'Don't be. My dear girl, I know that this is a very big step for you and for both our sakes you have to be sure.' He gave a short laugh that showed he wasn't as relaxed as he made out. 'Believe me, the last thing I want is a reluctant bride.'

Laura smiled at that. 'I do need a little more time. You did take me completely by surprise, you know.'

'You should be getting used to it by now.'

'I should, but I was so sure that you were going to ask me to leave and even yet—'

His hand covered hers. 'Whatever the outcome you need have no fears there. In any event where would you and your brother have gone?'

'I don't know but that would have been my worry.'

He got up to hide his expression. What had he hoped? That she would have had her answer for him. The words he wanted to hear. That she could be in love with him was only wishful thinking but in time it might turn to that. She might accept him because she was desperate to stay at Braehead. They had nowhere else to go. Fergus made a face. It wasn't a good foundation for marriage but he knew he would settle for it because he loved her and he couldn't bear the thought of her not being at Braehead. Going over to the decanter he put whisky in his glass and looked enquiringly at Laura.

'Just a very small sherry, please.' She didn't want it but it was something to hold in her hand.

How kind and considerate he was, Laura thought, and hated herself for keeping him guessing. If she said yes there would be no drawing back and she would have committed herself to a loveless marriage. What she felt for her employer could be love but she would never have his. On the other hand could she afford to say no? Would she ever forgive herself if her brother was forced to leave school and find a job?

She took the sherry and he sat down with his long legs stretched towards the fire. 'I have news for you, we are to have a visitor staying at Braehead. I shouldn't call him that since the visitor in question is my brother, Roger.' He smiled. 'I only heard this morning.' He paused. 'I seem to recall telling you that my brother was home from India.'

'Yes, you did. He was to be staying with your parents, you said.'

'I believed that to be the case but life with the parents is too quiet for Roger. He uses it as his base and spends much of his time in London with friends.'

'Is this a holiday or is your brother home for good?'

'Your guess is as good as mine.' He shrugged. 'I'm not sure that Roger knows himself.' He laughed. 'When he is out there he complains about the heat and just about everything else and when he is home—'

'He complains about the cold.'

'Exactly.' He was playing with his glass and gazing mournfully into the amber-coloured liquid.

Laura hoped he would say more. She was curious about Fergus's brother and wondered why his name was so seldom mentioned.

'Since we are to have Roger here it might be better if I put you in the picture. Roger is one of those people who cannot stick one job for any length of time.'

'Perhaps he hasn't found one to suit him.'

He chose to ignore that. 'Laura, Roger was given every chance but he wasn't prepared to study, all he wanted was a good time. There was – I won't go into that – but it ended with him going out to India. We have an aunt and uncle out there. My mother's brother has a jute mill in Bengal and a managerial position was arranged for Roger. He appeared to take to the life and we all breathed a sigh of relief then as I feared he became bored and dissatisfied.'

'He wanted back to this country?'

Fergus nodded. 'The usual stint is for four years but Roger can't have done more than three, perhaps not quite three. Mother has always doted on Roger and she managed to persuade her brother to bend the rules for his nephew.'

'Did your father agree with it?'

'No, he thought as I did that he should stick it out but mother won the day as we all knew she would.'

'Your brother doesn't sound a bit like you?'

'No, he is much better-looking,' he smiled, 'and has a brand of charm that appeals to women of all ages.'

'When is he expected?'

'The end of the week, Friday he suggests. Could you see to that, Laura, getting a room prepared for him?'

'Of course. Which of the guest rooms?'

'It doesn't matter, I'll leave it to you. As you know, this was once the family home and Roger will still think of it as that.'

'Annie, don't bother about the drawing-room. Leave it for another day.'

Annie took her hand off the door knob. 'That'll save me looking for dust that isn't there. It's folk that makes dust and there has been no one over that door for well over a week.'

'That is all to change, Annie. We are expecting Mr Cunningham's brother on Friday. He's home from India and wants to spend some time here.'

'And which room is this I have to prepare?'

'I thought the one with the window overlooking the rose garden. Too early in the year for roses but he'll see beyond it to the flower-beds.'

'If he ever takes the trouble to look out. Men don't as a rule and when they do it is to see what kind of day it is and whether he needs to take a brolly with him or not.'

'I never knew that,' Laura said, poker-faced.

'Always learning, aren't we? If that room is to be made ready I'd better move myself.'

'Were you here before Mr Cunningham married, Annie?'

'No. The young mistress engaged me and Mrs Barclay. Mrs Mathewson would have known all the family.'

'I see. Once I've had a word with Mrs Barclay I'll bring the linen.'

The drawing-room was far too hot but Fergus had requested a fire as, according to his mother, Roger was still taking bad with the cold. If he was feeling cold in Devon, Laura thought, he would feel it a lot worse up here. She opened the window which she would close before Mr Roger Cunningham was due to arrive. Some time late afternoon he was expected. Sylvia was excited and only after the threat of not seeing her uncle at all was she persuaded to rest for half an hour. When Laura went up to waken her she had been asleep for a good hour.

Now she was dressed in her frilly pink dress. It hadn't been Laura's choice but she had given in to avoid tears. The child wanted to look her best for the uncle she had never seen and best meant her party dress. Laura had brushed her fair hair and coaxed it into a curl at the ends.

'A ribbon. I want a ribbon.'

'Your hair looks nicer without a ribbon.'

'Please, I want one.'

Laura found a pink ribbon and tied her hair back with it.

'Will Uncle Roger bring me something?'

'I don't know, but nice little girls don't look for presents.'

'Why not?'

'Because it is greedy to ask and bad manners too.'

'Is Daddy home?'

'I don't know, we'll go along and see.'

Fergus Cunningham was home and coming out of his study. Sylvia ran to him and caught him round the leg.

'Are you going to a party?'

'No, I've got on my bestest dress for Uncle Roger.'

'I felt it easier to give in,' Laura laughed. She left father and daughter.

A half-hour later she heard voices in the hall and heard the brothers greeting each other.

'How are you, Roger?'

'Very well, Fergus, apart from being chilled to the bone. You haven't changed,' he added.

'Did you expect me to? Were you looking for grey hairs and a bald patch?'

'Heaven forbid! There is only a couple of years between us.' His eyes moved to the child. 'And this very pretty little girl must be Sylvia,' he said, bending down. 'Does your Uncle Roger get a kiss?' All of a sudden the child became bashful and clung to her daddy.

'Just an act, I can assure you. Go on, Sylvia, say hello to your Uncle Roger.' He gave her a little push.

Roger scooped her up, lifted her above his head then set her down.

'Hello, Uncle Roger,' she dimpled prettily.

'Like a princess.'

'Am I?'

'We'll leave your cases at the foot of the stairs and someone will take them up.' The cab driver had brought in two large cases and left them in the vestibule and Fergus had moved them to the foot of the stairs. Two large suitcases could only mean he was contemplating a lengthy stay. Fergus felt depressed then ashamed. Three years was a long time and perhaps it was time to forgive and forget.

'Thank God for heat,' the visitor said, going over to the fire then looking about him. 'No changes here, at least I don't see any.'

'There aren't, the drawing-room is just as it was. It's not a room that is much in use.'

'You don't do much entertaining then?'

'Very little.' They were both seated. 'Parents well when you left them?'

'Dad's legs are giving him some trouble. Too much sitting around I told him but he wasn't having that.'

'No wonder. Rheumatism is very painful and he is the type that suffers in silence.' He got up to pour Roger a drink. 'Runs in families they say so we may know something about it one day.'

'Cheerful soul, aren't you? Mother tells me that old Ma Mathewson got her walking ticket.'

'I'm quite sure she said nothing of the sort. Mrs Mathewson retired,' Fergus said coldly. 'She served this family well and she was due a rest.'

'Managed to get someone else?'

'Yes.'

'Any good?'

'Very efficient.'

'One of those,' he said dismissively. 'India does have its advantages. A snap of the fingers or a shout brings immediate attention.'

'I deplore that. The poor wretches are human beings,' he said with distaste.

'There to serve. It is what they are paid to do.'

'Don't make me laugh, all they get is a pittance. One day it may all be different.'

'Never.'

'Give it a few more years and the unrest will begin.'

'I won't be there.'

'Aren't you going back?'

'Haven't decided but one thing is for sure I'm taking a long holiday.'

'Perhaps your job will be filled?'

He grinned. 'No danger. The job was made for me.'

'Meaning you won't be missed?'

'I wouldn't say that.'

Sylvia had grown tired of adult conversation and gone in search of Laura.

She left the door open and Fergus got up to close it when he saw Sylvia with Laura. 'Laura, come and meet my brother.'

Roger had been lounging but got up when Laura entered the room. Laura's first thought was that he was the most handsome man she had ever met. He was as tall as Fergus but his shoulders were broader. His face was lightly tanned and his features regular. His thick black hair had a suggestion of a wave in it and the eyes, admiring eyes, were a startling blue with long thick eyelashes that were the envy of many a woman. Laura felt a queer little thrill go through her and for some reason felt unnerved.

'Roger, this is Miss Morrison, my very efficient housekeeper.'

'Delighted to meet you, Miss Morrison,' Roger said in a deep, pleasant voice while he held on to her hand rather too long. He turned to his brother with raised eyebrows. 'You are a dark horse. Here was I expecting a dear old soul a few years younger than Mrs Mathewson and instead—' He shook his head and grinned boyishly. 'Just let me say it is a very pleasant surprise.'

Sylvia came in. 'I've been looking all over for you, Laura.'

'And I was looking for you.'

'Uncle Roger,' she said, sidling up to him.

'What is it, princess?'

'I haven't got to ask you,' she said, looking down at her shoe and going over the side of it.

Laura frowned. She had a good idea of what was coming but apart from a warning look there was nothing she could do.

'You can ask me anything, whisper it if you want.'

'Whispering is rude.'

'Who told you that?'

'Daddy,' she said swiftly.

'Did I? I don't recall.'

'Come on, you can ask me.'

'Did you bring me something?' she said in a rush then looked fearful.

Fergus was frowning and he looked angry. 'You are behaving very badly, Sylvia,' he said sternly. 'Little girls who ask for gifts don't get any, instead they are sent to bed early.'

'Steady on, old chap, she's only a baby.'

It was the worst thing he could have said. 'I'm not! I'm not!' Sylvia screamed, then burst into tears and flew to Laura.

'It's all right,' she said soothingly.

'I'm not a baby,' she said, looking up at Laura with swimming eyes.

'Of course you aren't a baby.'

'Uncle Roger said I was.'

'He didn't mean it.'

'No, I didn't mean it, princess, and if you don't give me a big smile I might burst into tears myself.'

'Big men don't cry.'

'Don't you believe it.' Roger had no gift for his little niece. It had never occurred to him to buy one. Fortunately for him his mother had put in a package for her grand-daughter. He was saved.

'There is something for you, of course there is. How could I forget something important like that? You'll have to wait until I open my cases.'

'What is it?'

'That would be telling and spoil the surprise,' he said. He hadn't a clue as to what was in the package.

'Come along, dear,' Laura said, taking the child firmly by the hand.

She felt his eyes on her and willed herself not to turn when she got to the door but she couldn't stop herself. The look in his eyes had her blushing in confusion and a kind of breathlessness seized her.

Fergus watched it all and his eyes were bleak.

Chapter Twenty-Six

For the first few days Laura saw little of Roger Cunningham and wasn't sure if what she felt was relief or disappointment. She knew from Fergus that Roger was looking up old friends.

Below stairs the guest was not making himself popular. Mrs Barclay was tight-lipped with disapproval. In her book there was no excuse for a healthy young man to remain in bed long after everyone else was up and about. When he did manage to drag himself to the breakfast table he was bleary-eyed and in need of a shave. Not dressed either, would you believe, cook had announced with indignation, just that gaudy silk dressing-gown over his pyjamas. Probably bought the thing in India for little or nothing. Well known it was that those poor natives got precious little payment and had to work damn hard to get that.

Annie clucked in sympathy. As for herself she could see the man far enough, preferably back in India.

'A sight easier for you if he had breakfast in bed,' she said.

'Just what I was saying to Jean. It would get it over and let me get on.'

'Jinny could take the tray up,' Annie said, 'though God knows she might drop it if he as much as raised his head and gave her a smile.'

'Some lassies are that silly,' Mrs Barclay said as her fat fingers worked the pastry ready for rolling out. She sprinkled flour on the table and took a rest. 'Mind you, I thought her gran had instilled some sense into her.'

'The lass is going through a daft phase.'

'She is that. I made the mistake of thinking Jinny had more sense but she's as bad as the rest of her generation.'

'Comes from getting too much freedom, not like it was in our day.'

'As you say, Annie. I despair at times wondering what the world is coming to. Still, we'll no' be here so we'll be spared the finding out.'

It was all very upsetting and affecting the smooth running of the house. Tempers were frayed and Mrs Barclay had taken to banging the pots about as a way of expressing her anger. Annie fretted because she couldn't get in to tidy the bedroom and with the drawing-room being in daily use there was a lot more work to get through. It meant cleaning out the fire every morning and setting it ready to put a match to. As for the bedroom that was a perfect disgrace and it had to be seen to be believed. Clothes were left lying on the floor where they had been dropped. Drawers were half open with the contents spilled over. Jackets and trousers – he changed during the day and again in the evening – were draped over chairs. The master smoked a pipe but his brother favoured cigarettes and ash was everywhere. Added to that was the disgusting smell of stale smoke lingering in the room since he didn't believe in opening the window.

Annie had flounced out of the bedroom to complain to Laura.

'It is just not good enough,' she said, two spots of angry colour on her cheeks.

'You have to make allowances, Annie, Mr Cunningham's brother has been used to having everything done for him in India.'

'This isn't India and don't you be making excuses for him.' She looked at Laura through narrowed eyes. 'Surely a sensible lass like you isn't taken in by a handsome face. I gave you credit for more sense.'

Laura was used to Annie's outspokenness and was usually amused by it. Although she was the housekeeper she never used her position of authority. She hadn't done so until now that is. Laura was angry. Roger might leave his bedroom in a mess, no question about it he did. That wasn't the point. He was a guest, more than that he was family and with a perfect right to make himself at home. She accepted that she wouldn't like the cleaning of his bedroom but they were all paid hands and expected to fulfil their various duties.

'Annie,' Laura said sternly, 'you will refrain from making derogatory remarks about a guest in this house. You will remember that he is your employer's brother.'

Annie gave Laura a look of surprised disbelief then sniffed.

'Is my nose still on?' she said and marched away.

There had been no major upsets since she'd come to Braehead but in this case she had been forced to take a firm stand, Laura told herself. Annie would no doubt see it as throwing her weight around and that was a pity. She consoled herself with the thought that the incident would soon be forgotten and harmony restored.

Sylvia was asleep and Ronnie was doing his homework. Fergus was in his study where he had taken to spending a lot of his time since his brother's arrival. Before his daughter was taken upstairs to bed Fergus did spend time with her but when Laura returned to the sitting-room he had gone and the newspapers with him. Laura wondered if it were deliberate and that he was avoiding her. An awkwardness had developed between them and this, she knew, was because Roger was paying her too much attention. Laura didn't feel it was her fault, she hadn't encouraged Roger Cunningham. But then neither had she discouraged him.

Feeling restless and vaguely discontented, Laura put on her coat and let herself out by the back door. The lovely golden show was no more, the daffodils had withered and died, but there was still colour where clumps of primroses grew beneath the hedges. The sky was sinking in a golden-red glow and Laura breathed in the evening air. It was a mild, pleasant night and she was enjoying the peace and tranquility as she strolled along the path. Since it was so pleasant and there was nothing hurrying her she decided to go further afield and opened the door into the lane. She would walk the length of it and back. That would help her to get to sleep because of late she had tossed and turned before sleep claimed her.

Behind her she heard the sound of a car stopping and voices then the car starting up again. In a few moments the vehicle had passed her. Laura paid little attention apart from keeping well into the side until she heard hurrying feet, then she looked back feeling alarmed.

'It is you, Laura, I couldn't be sure. Did I startle you? That was me getting a lift back.'

'Only a little,' she smiled.

'Not safe for a lovely young woman to be out on her own.'

'I wasn't venturing far, just to the end of the lane and back.'

'May I walk with you?'

'If you wish, Mr Cunningham.'

'Roger, please.' They smiled to each other as they fell into step. 'Since you now have a companion we could do a round tour and save retracing our steps.'

Laura had no objections and said so.

'Mind if I smoke?'

'Not at all.'

He stopped to light a cigarette, then apologised for not offering her one first.

'I don't smoke, thank you.'

He put his cigarette case back in his pocket, then inhaled deeply before speaking again. 'How do you like living at Braehead?'

'Very much.'

'Not too quiet for you?'

'No.'

'I'm curious as to why a girl like you should be working as a house-keeper or childminder or is it a bit of both?

'It is a bit of both,' she smiled.

'And you actually like the work?' he persisted.

'I do as a matter of fact but it is far from what I had hoped to do.'

'What was that?'

'I had hoped to teach.'

'Then why aren't you?'

'Circumstances,' she said shortly.

'I've been in that position myself,' he said grimly.

He sounded sincere and sympathetic and Laura told him a little about her life and her father going off to America.

'Fergus agreed to let the boy live at Braehead?'

'Yes. I couldn't have come otherwise and it was very, very kind of your brother.'

'Kind-hearted, would you say?'

'He is and to Ronnie he is a kind of hero.'

'Don't run away with the idea that Fergus is a soft mark.'

'I wasn't.' Laura wished now that she hadn't said so much.

'He can be as hard as nails.'

'That I don't believe. Mr Cunningham would always be fair.'

Roger was thoughtful. 'Is there something between you and Fergus?'

'No,' she said a little too quickly.

'Stupid of me to ask.' He was silent, then decided to say more on the subject. 'My brother won't remarry. Had he been so inclined the gorgeous Davina would by now be the second Mrs Cunningham.

There again he isn't totally blind and he can't but fail to see how lovely you are.'

She blushed and Roger was intrigued. He was almost sure now that there was an attraction and come to think of it Fergus's eyes had followed his housekeeper and when he spoke her name there was almost a caress in his voice. Roger prided himself on being observant. He grinned maliciously. It might be rather fun to woo this girl and it would be one in the eye for Fergus.

'You won't object if I ask you a personal question?'

'I won't know until I hear it.'

'Not that personal,' he grinned. 'I wondered what was to hinder your brother making his home with your father and stepmother.'

'It was never considered.'

'Why not? He is your father's responsibility not yours.'

'They were never close.'

'But the boy and you are?'

'Yes.'

'Spoilt your own chances, it must have?'

'Perhaps.'

'Could be a millstone round your neck for years to come.'

'Then so be it,' she said lightly.

They were nearing Braehead. 'Tell me, Laura, does a hardworking girl like you get time off?'

'Of course, and I also have a full day off.'

'Which day?'

'Thursday.'

'How do you usually spend it?'

She shrugged. 'Visiting my aunts or friends and occasionally going into Dundee to shop.'

'Hardly riotous living,' he grinned.

'I'm not that kind of person.'

'Perhaps you are but chance hasn't come your way.'

Laura laughed. 'I'm still trying to work that one out.'

'I bet you could be a lot of fun. By the way, who looks after the little 'un when you aren't available?'

'Betsy. Miss—'

'I know old Betsy.' He made a face. 'Never had much to do with her.

329

Disapproves of me but adores Fergus as you must have noticed. He's the good boy and I'm the black sheep.'

'You do talk a lot of nonsense.'

'You've been spared my escapades?' he said lightly but when she turned her head he was looking at her intently.

'Apart from you hating the heat in India and moaning about the cold here your sins have been hidden from me.'

She didn't hear Roger's sigh of relief.

'Laura, I do have arrangements made for Thursday and it would be deuced awkward to get out of them but how about the evening? We could have dinner somewhere?' He smiled engagingly.

The invitation had taken Laura completely by surprise. She wanted to accept but how could she? True, there was no understanding between her and Fergus but he had proposed marriage and she had not as yet given him answer.

'It is very kind of you, Roger, to invite me but I'm afraid I must decline.'

Roger Cunningham was taken aback. The look on his face showed that it hadn't been the answer he expected. Laura could understand that. Not many would refuse and she hadn't wanted to.

'Why must you decline?' He was frowning heavily. Was this just her trying to play hard to get? 'Do you happen to have a previous engagement for that evening?'

'No,' she said truthfully.

'Then I am at a loss to understand your refusal.'

'Nevertheless that is what it is. I don't have to give you a reason.'

'Ah, I think I've got it. You think big brother wouldn't approve?'

'You are being ridiculous.'

'Am I? I don't think so.' He had opened the back door into the garden and Laura followed him in. He shut the door. A light breeze had sprung up and blown her hair into attractive disorder. What a wonderful colour it was, he thought, like spun gold. Unlike the women of his acquaintance Laura wore very little make-up but then she didn't need it with her clear, peach-coloured skin.

She turned to find him close behind her and when he gently touched her face and traced the finely arched eyebrows she made no objection. There was no pretence, no coyness about this girl. When she gave her love it would be wholly and completely. Roger felt a surge of excitement and knew that he wanted this girl and not just to spite his brother. Going about her duties he had thought her attractive but too quiet for his liking. In fact she wasn't his type, not by a mile.

His lips brushed her cheek, a butterfly touch, and she drew in her breath.

'You are a very sweet girl. Now go and get your beauty sleep, Laura, and —' He paused and looked deep into her eyes. 'Goodnight,' he whispered.

'Goodnight, Roger,' she said breathlessly and almost ran indoors.

Once in her bedroom Laura sat down at the dressing-table and in the mirror looked at her flushed cheeks and shining eyes. She put her fingers to her face where his lips had touched and then she found herself saying his name aloud. Roger. She said it a few times, then got up to take off her coat and prepare for bed.

When she turned out the light and lay down in bed she wondered what had happened to make her feel like this.

For once Roger had made the effort and was up and dressed before Fergus left home for the office. Roger found him in his study.

'Good heavens! This is early for you, isn't it?'

'Wanted a word with you before you left.'

'Make it smart then. I do have an appointment.' Secretly he was hoping that this was Roger deciding to return down south.

'Shan't keep you. Just wanted to mention that I have asked your charming housekeeper to have dinner with me on her day off which I've discovered is Thursday.'

'Why are you telling me?' Fergus didn't raise his eyes but concentrated on his briefcase. He gave an unnecessary check to the contents, then the lock clicked. When he looked up his face was controlled.

'I told Laura it wasn't necessary but for some unknown reason she appeared to think it was.'

'What nonsense.'

'Thanks, old boy. Wondered if perhaps you were interested yourself but I see I was wrong. I take it that I can tell Laura it is all right with you?'

'For God's sake, I am her employer not her keeper. Now if you will excuse me.'

Roger watched him go and there was a satisfied smile on his face.

The poor fellow had tried to hide his feelings but it was plain enough to him that his brother was in love with Laura. Humming, he went along to the breakfast room and as luck would have it Laura was coming out.

'Don't reach for the smelling salts, it really is me,' he grinned. 'Don't you go.'

'I have to.'

'No, you don't. I am a guest and —'

'And what?' But she was smiling and making no attempt to leave him.

'Presumably you've had breakfast?'

'An hour ago.'

'Then you can drink a cup of tea to keep me company.'

'A quick cup, then I must see to Sylvia.'

'You take your duties seriously.'

'Of course I do, that is what I'm paid for.'

Roger had gone to the hot plate to help himself to scrambled eggs and bacon and Laura poured tea into two cups.

'Getting up at this unearthly hour was for you, my dearest Laura.'

'Am I supposed to believe that?'

'It's true, I assure you. I wanted to see Fergus before he left for the office.'

'That has nothing to do with me.'

'Oh, but it has. Everything to do with you. You see, I wanted his permission to take you out.'

'You had no business to do that,' Laura said angrily. 'For your information I make my own decisions.'

'Fergus said much the same.'

'Did he?' She wondered what Fergus had said.

Roger was looking at her carefully from across the table. He forked a piece of lean bacon, put it into his mouth and swallowed it before speaking.

'Yes, he did. In fact he went as far as to say that an evening out would do you good, that you don't go out a lot.'

'Did he say that?' she said faintly.

'More or less word for word.'

Laura nodded. There was no reason for Roger not to tell the truth.

Perhaps Fergus was having second thoughts and this was an easy way out for him. It had been no more than an impulse of the moment to propose marriage and now he was embarrassed about it. Well, if that was how he wanted it then it suited her too. She drank some tea and put down her cup. If the invitation for Thursday evening still stood she would accept. Why shouldn't she?

'Roger, you would agree that it is a woman's privilege to change her mind,' she smiled.

'I would indeed.'

'Then if the invitation for Thursday evening still stands—' she hesitated.

'It does and I couldn't be more pleased.'

She blushed and got up quickly. 'You must excuse me.'

He stood up. 'Be ready at seven-thirty. I thought The Oasis, it has just opened and according to friends of mine is well worth a visit.'

'Where is it?'

'A few miles outside Perth. Meet you in the drawing-room.'

Laura dressed carefully, lingering before the mirror. It was important that she looked her very best. She had brushed her hair until it shone and fell into its natural soft waves. The blue dress bought for Christmas would be very suitable and she was glad that she had been persuaded to splash out. She was smiling to herself as she gave a light dusting of powder to her face and put on more lipstick than she usually did. Her expensive perfume she dabbed behind her ears and on her wrists. A glance at her clock told her it was seven twenty-five and time to go. Ronnie had already been informed that she was going out but he hadn't asked where or with whom.

Showers had fallen during the day but it was warm. May was an unpredictable month and it wasn't unknown to get a flurry of snow. Scotland, it was said, and with a lot of truth, could experience all the seasons in one day. Laura wished that she possessed a cape or a silk shawl to drape over her shoulders but since she didn't her short jacket would have to do. Fortunately it was a safe colour, an oatmeal shade that went with everything. Laura was carrying it over her arm when she went along to the drawing-room, hoping against hope that she wouldn't meet Fergus. She didn't and breathed a sigh of relief. It could have been embarrassing.

Roger, glass in hand, was stubbing out a cigarette when she knocked and entered.

'Punctual,' he smiled, 'and unusual in my experience but welcome since we have a journey ahead of us.' Laura felt a little uncomfortable at his lengthy appraisal but she remained standing where she was.

Roger's eyes had travelled over the blue dress noting how well it showed off her slim, shapely figure. She wore no jewellery apart from a silver bracelet.

'Will I do? Have I passed the test?'

'With flying colours, and forgive my rudeness in staring but you do look delightful.' He had expected confusion after his lengthy gaze but he had seen none and that both surprised and pleased him.

'If I am permitted to pay you a compliment you look very well yourself.'

He cocked an eyebrow and grinned. 'Thank you, fair lady, your car awaits you at the front of the house. Up to you we can leave now or there is plenty of time for a drink.'

Laura didn't want a drink and neither did she want Roger to have another. He did seem to drink rather a lot. 'If you don't mind I would prefer to leave now.'

He downed the rest of his drink, put down the glass and lifted his car keys. Then, going ahead, he opened the door and frowned at the coat she was carrying. It was cheap and certainly not the kind of garment one would take into a first-class restaurant. He would make sure that it was left in the car.

Before switching on the ignition he enquired if she was comfortable.

'Yes, thank you.' He had thrown her coat on to the back seat.

'This is just a hire. No point in buying a car if I should decide to return to India.'

'You haven't made up your mind?'

'No, whether I return or not depends on a number of things.' He didn't enlarge on that.

'Would you like to live down south?'

'Where do you mean by down south?' He took his eyes off the road to smile to her.

'Your parents are in Devon aren't they?'

'Yes, but good Lord, I wouldn't want to live there. Too quiet for me. London is a possibility but as I say I haven't made up my mind. This was meant to be a short stay in Braehead but it has suddenly become very attractive to me.'

Laura couldn't mistake his meaning and felt a rush of pure happiness.

'After all this time it must be nice to meet up with your old friends?'

'It has its attractions,' he smiled.

Laura wanted to sparkle but she didn't know what else to say. Maybe if she asked him to tell her about India she would just have to put in a word here and there. It was awful to be tongue-tied and so unlike her.

Happily for the remainder of the journey Roger spoke about India and had some amusing tales.

'You must have enjoyed it then?'

'Indeed I did for some of the time but it was boring too. Dead boring.'

The restaurant was secluded and only those with transport would patronise The Oasis, Laura thought. Roger parked behind the building and on the grass. Six or more cars were already there and from the restaurant came men's laughter, loud and cheerful.

'Don't be alarmed. The village isn't so very far away and the locals will be drinking in the public bar,' he explained. 'Where we are to be dining is quite separate and none of that noise will reach there.' He pulled her hand through his arm and she shivered in the cold of the evening.

'My coat, Roger, I meant to bring it.'

'You don't need it. There won't be time for you to get cold. We only have to walk round to the front of the restaurant.'

Laura said no more but two couples going in ahead of them hurried to get out of the cold and the ladies wore fur capes. Laura wasn't stupid and she remembered the way he had looked at her jacket. Was he ashamed to be seen with someone who wore such an unworthy garment or was he protecting her? She hoped it was the latter but she didn't need protecting. Clothes didn't make the person. Her head went a little higher.

'Heaven help my friends if we have come all this way for a mediocre meal.'

'I'm sure it's going to be lovely,' she said as they went in.

The entrance hall was brightly lit and tastefully decorated. They were barely inside when a middle-aged man in evening dress came over to greet them.

'Welcome to The Oasis,' he smiled. 'Do you have a reservation?'

'Yes, Cunningham.'

'Ah, yes,' he said, checking the names and ticking one off. He looked at Laura. 'Madam does not feel the cold,' he said as he waved away a young man who had clearly arrived to take her coat, cape or whatever.

Madam did, Laura thought but madam couldn't say so. 'Hardly ever,' she lied.

'This way, please.' They followed him along a broad passageway to the dining-room. The subdued lighting made it look romantic and inviting. The tables were well spaced and covered with a brilliantly white starched cloth. In the centre was a candle in a holder. Once they were seated the candle was lit and they were each handed a leather-bound menu. The wine list, also leather-bound, was placed on the table beside Roger.

A very thin, narrow-hipped young waiter arrived to see if they would like a drink.

'Laura?' Roger looked at her questioningly.

'I don't—' she said hesitantly.

He frowned. 'Is it sherry or gin or—?'

'A small sherry, please.'

'And whisky.'

The waiter bowed and departed.

'This is a minus point with most restaurants. I much prefer to have a drink in the cocktail bar and study the menu there. Never mind,' he smiled, 'we'll go to an hotel next time.'

Next time! There was to be a next time! Laura's hands were shaking as she began to study the menu.

Roger was nodding his head and looking impressed. 'Full marks for an excellent choice and from all accounts they enticed one of the best chefs by giving into his every request. A chef is all-powerful these days, Laura.'

'I imagine he would be. After all, the food is the main attraction.'

'Exactly, and speaking of food Mrs Barclay is good, but hardly imaginative.'

Laura looked up swiftly. 'I can't agree with that.'

'You may after tonight.'

336

'Don't be too sure. You may be disappointed in me, Roger, I'm afraid I don't have sophisticated tastes. Mine are simple.'

'Then I must take you in hand, my dear Laura, and introduce you to the finer things in life.'

The words sent a frisson of excitement down her spine.

The meal was delicious and Laura thoroughly enjoyed it. There had been, she had to admit, something extra special about it. Roger, who seemed to know all about food, congratulated the chef when he came round each table to hear the comments on the dinner.

'Is that usual?' Laura whispered.

'Fairly common in this type of restaurant. The customers like it and nothing pleases a chef more than to be showered with compliments.'

'His moment of glory,' Laura smiled.

They were outside and if it was cold Laura didn't feel it. The stars twinkled out of a dark sky and only their feet on the gravel broke the silence. Then as they reached the grass the silence was complete. It was a night for lovers and when Roger put his arms around her Laura leaned into him.

'Did you enjoy that?'

'It was wonderful,' Laura whispered and turned her face to him.

'I'm so glad,' he said and smiled down at her but made no attempt to kiss her. Instead he just gave her a tight hug.

Laura felt acutely disappointed and embarrassed. Would he think that she had thrown herself at him? Her face burned and she drew away.

It had been quite an effort on Roger's part not to crush her to him, feel the softness of her yielding body, but not yet. She was like a fluttering bird, poised to take flight if scared, and he didn't want to risk that. Roger liked to think that he understood women. Those in his own set were hardened and experienced and he knew how to handle them. Laura was different. There was no pretence with her. When she loved it would be completely. Roger smiled to himself thinking of the pleasure ahead. He held the car door open and she got in, then leaned over to stretch for her jacket. She put it on and hugged the warmth to her.

Roger was concentrating on his driving and Laura was alone with her thoughts. How wrong everybody was about Roger. He was a thorough gentleman like his brother. Much as she had wanted his kisses wasn't it better this way? A first date when they were just beginning to know one another was too soon to show one's feelings. There would be other times, he had said so.

In the days that followed Laura tried to keep Roger from her mind. She did her work and whenever she thought of him, which was most of the time, she tried to calm herself by working all the harder.

Fergus saw what was happening and was afraid for Laura. His brother was unscrupulous and would dazzle the girl until he had grown tired of her. How would Laura cope with being dropped when he left Braehead? Would she be broken-hearted? On the other hand there was just the possibility that this time his brother could be serious. What then? Would he take her away, perhaps to India? How could anyone fail to love Laura?

And Laura so honest, so straightforward. The flushed cheeks and sparkling eyes told their own tale. She was in love and didn't mind who knew it.

If he could believe that Laura would be happy with Roger then he would try to hide his own heartbreak and be glad for her. But he couldn't, knowing Roger as he did, he couldn't believe he was the one to bring her happiness.

Was he mistaken, seeing something that wasn't there? The trouble was he didn't trust that self-satisfied, triumphant smirk that he saw on his brother's face. He couldn't understand it either.

They were all watching, Betsy, Ronnie and the kitchen staff. Betsy was deeply concerned but it was none of her business. What distressed her most was to see Fergus looking so wretched. His face looked grim and grey and there were dark hollows under his eyes which could be due to work or worry. Betsy had long suspected that Fergus was in love with Laura and if so this must bring it all back. Poor Fergus hadn't had all his sorrows to seek. The pity of it was that Roger had ever come to Braehead. No two brothers could be more unalike.

Ronnie was noticing and he was becoming increasingly anxious and angry. Just of late both Betsy and Mrs Barclay had thought he looked peaky but Laura didn't seem to notice. No one could find fault with her work. She performed her tasks with her usual efficiency and Sylvia wasn't neglected. It was just that for most of the day she had her head in the clouds.

Laura had come into their sitting-room where Ronnie was writing in an exercise book. He looked up and that could have been a scowl on his face.

'You going out again?' he growled.

'Yes, as a matter of fact I am.'

'With him, I suppose?'

Laura didn't answer.

'You never stay in.'

'That's an exaggeration, Ronnie, and is there any reason why I shouldn't go out? You don't need me, do you?'

'No,' he said shortly. 'What would I need you for?'

'Nothing that I know of and I am entitled to some enjoyment you know.' In spite of her words Laura was feeling some guilt. Of late she had been out a great deal.

'I know that and I wouldn't mind if it wasn't with that smoothie.'

Laura gasped. 'Smoothie! How dare you describe Roger like that. It is the height of impudence and where may I ask did you get hold of that word?'

'It doesn't matter where I got it,' he shouted, 'that's what he is and it isn't only me that thinks so.'

'Listening to gossip in the kitchen I suppose? Gossip won't bother me, Ronnie, and it certainly won't bother Roger.'

Ronnie looked miserable. 'He isn't like our Mr Cunningham.'

'I know that, Ronnie,' Laura said gently, 'they are quite different but both nice in their own way.'

'Our Mr Cunningham likes you and I bet he doesn't like you going around with his brother.'

Laura thought there was more to this than she was getting.

'Ronnie, I have to go in a few minutes but tell me what is really bothering you.'

'If you want to know I like living here and I thought you did too.'

'I do, when have I ever said otherwise?'

'It stands to reason we cannot go on living at Braehead if you go and get married to *him.*'

339

'What you are talking is absolute nonsense, no one has mentioned marriage.'

He had cheered up slightly. 'Why haven't Dad or Connie written?'

'Ferg – Mr Cunningham noticed something in the paper about a hold-up in the mail, not here, in America. Something should arrive any day now.'

Chapter Twenty-Seven

Laura was thinking of Ronnie's outburst when she went along to the drawing-room. It had been so unlike him, and describing Roger as a smoothie – where had he heard that? It could only have been someone at Braehead and the thought angered her. Poor Roger to be so misunderstood and if he had been spoilt it hadn't been his fault. He was such a handsome darling and he had opened up a whole new world for her. An exciting world and dare she say exhausting too. Roger could sleep on in the morning but he seemed to forget that she couldn't. She had work to do

A warm June had given way to an even warmer July and still Roger showed no signs of leaving Braehead. As he couldn't fail to know he had long outstayed his welcome but as he laughingly said to Laura, poor old Fergus did wish him gone but couldn't bring himself to say so.

'I'm quite sure Fergus doesn't wish that at all,' Laura had replied though she thought it was probably true.

'He does, my sweet,' Roger said, drawing her close to him on the settee. 'I would have gone long before now had it not been for you.'

'For me?'

'Don't sound so surprised, you must know.'

She smiled and snuggled closer. She did know but she had wanted him to say the words.

'Alas, this can't go on forever,' he said softly.

Laura's heart plummeted. He was going away. 'I can't bear the thought of never seeing you again,' she said unsteadily.

'That's life, my darling, but we must make the most of what is left of our time together.'

She knew it would have to end. This idyllic life couldn't go on and she had to face it.

'Don't think about it, my darling, until it happens. Be like me, live for the moment and enjoy what is on offer. The future is best left to take care of itself.'

'We can't all live that way, Roger.'

'You worry too much.'

'I know.'

'You worry about that brother of yours and would always put him first. That in my book is just plain stupid.'

'What would you I did?' Laura was playing for time and wondering how she would answer if – when he proposed marriage. He loved her, had told her so often, and she loved him. Why then did she keep refusing? If she truly loved him she would give herself completely was what he said and lately he had shown irritation with her continued refusal to give herself to him.

'What would you I did was how you phrased it. Easy, my dear Laura, your father would have to stump up for the fare and then take charge of him until he was of an age to look after himself.'

'I couldn't do that to Ronnie.'

'You've made that clear.' Roger was secretly relieved. This whole affair was getting out of hand because he was becoming too fond of Laura. Heavens! Maybe he was in love with her and as for Laura she was head over heels in love with him. Roger didn't find that surprising, he had that effect on women. All that he had intended was taking her away from Fergus and that had been very easy. Perhaps it was time he took his leave from Braehead.

Roger would be waiting for her, very likely with a glass in his hand, and she just wished he wouldn't drink so much. She kept quiet, but in the car she was sometimes scared, particularly when he put his foot down and drove at a reckless speed. Fergus only drank in moderation. She frowned at her own thoughts. Just of late she had taken to comparing the brothers and Roger was suffering in the comparison. Was she growing tired of this life, the endless pursuit of pleasure, all this wining and dining and dressing up? If she was honest she was and it was expensive. Laura was spending more on clothes than she wanted but felt she had to.

Connie had come to her rescue and had given her some tips on how to look a million dollars without bursting the bank. Forget evening gowns, she had written to Laura, unless you can afford to throw them away after a few wearings. Too easily remembered, my dear. Go for long skirts, one of them should be black and team them with different tops and blouses. I can see from your photographs that you are blessed with a lovely, long neck. Wear jewellery on some occasions then on others be unadorned. It is unusual and for that reason eye-catching. Laura had followed Connie's advice and was glad when Roger paid her the compliment of remarking on her good dress sense. She was learning and learning fast, he said.

Why did Fergus come so often into her thoughts these days? She felt the tears sting her eyes when she remembered how understanding he had been.

'You must know, my dear Laura, that I would never hold you to a promise. In any case you gave me none. If I recall I was to allow you more time.'

'You are very kind,' she said awkwardly, 'but what about – does it make any difference – but it must —' she stumbled over the words.

'To your position in this house?'

She nodded.

'None at all.'

'Are you sure?' Her lovely eyes searched his face for an answer. Anxious, pleading eyes.

'I see no reason to dispense with your services,' he said gently.

'Thank you.'

'By the way, is young Ronnie all right?'

'Yes. Why do you ask?' she said quickly.

'Just that I thought him quiet and withdrawn, not like his usual self. Perhaps he has problems at school?'

'If he has he hasn't mentioned them.' But then would he? she wondered. Once he would have confided in her but they had been growing apart.

'Probably just down in the dumps,' he smiled, 'we all have spells of that.' He glanced at his watch. 'I must go.' She saw that he was dressed for an evening out and wondered if it were all on again with Davina Dorward. She found the thought strangely depressing. Not only that, she had felt a stab of something very like jealousy. What was wrong with her? She couldn't be in love with both brothers, could she?

She thought without enthusiasm of the evening ahead. It was to be a foursome and she didn't like Roger's friends. They were so loud and always trying to attract attention to themselves. How pleasant instead to spend an evening as she once had: companionable and enjoyable as she and Fergus sat listening to gramophone records or reading a book or just talking. He was so easy to talk to. They had lively discussions about just everything and didn't always agree but that didn't matter. Ronnie was always welcome and very protective of Sylvia who adored him. Such happy times and she had thrown them away. Almost reluctantly Laura went along to the drawing-room and went in.

Roger finished his drink and got to his feet. 'There you are, darling, and looking gorgeous.'

She wore a coffee-coloured dress with cream trimming. It was in the fashionable long-waisted style that suited her figure. Roger wore a lightweight suit. He was immaculate as always when he was going out and insisted that his suits were sponged and pressed regularly.

Laura accepted the compliment with a smile and when he held out his arms she went to him and for a few blissful moments she forgot everything but the joy of being held close and the feel of his lips on hers.

He drew away. 'I did tell you that we were meeting up with Derek and Kathryn?'

'Yes, you did,' she replied with a marked lack of enthusiasm.

'Try to be a bit more sociable, will you?'

Laura was stung, but before she could say anything he had spoken again.

'Take a drink for God's sake when you are offered one.'

'Why should I when I don't want it?'

'Might help you to unwind, you don't exactly—'

'Shine in their company? Is that what you were going to say? Well, it's true I don't, for the simple reason I do not like them. I cannot abide people who take such pleasure in ridiculing others behind their back. No doubt I come in for some of it myself.'

'All harmless fun. You are too sensitive, my darling, and if you aren't careful you will be in danger of being called Miss Prim.'

She shrugged. 'As if I care.'

'That's better.' He was smiling again. 'You are available Friday evening?'

'Once Sylvia is in bed, yes.'

'We have an invitation to a party at Hillend, and Hillend for your information is the home of Wilma and Howard Menzies.'

'Where is Hillend?'

'In Pebblesands. Know it?'

'Yes, I do, a lovely little place. Our Sunday School picnic used to go there.'

Roger gave a loud guffaw and threw his head back. 'This is a very long way from being a Sunday School picnic.' He began laughing again and Laura wondered how it should be so funny. It made her uncomfortable but she tried to shrug it off.

'It was very kind of Mr and Mrs Menzies to invite me but you have to remember, Roger, that I am a working girl and I can't have too many late nights.'

'You're not exactly overworked are you?'

'No, I'm not.'

'For a moment I thought this was you making excuses not to go. You do want to accompany me, don't you?'

'Of course I do.' Laura could see that he was getting annoyed and tried to make amends. 'Think how awful it would be if I fell asleep during the evening.'

'Not much likelihood of that but even if you did no one would bat an eye.' Roger lit another cigarette. 'Incidentally it isn't Mr and Mrs. Wilma and Howard are sister and brother. They lost their parents but still live in the family house. Howard is a lot older than his sister and likes to feel he is keeping an eye on her. Wilma is a super girl, lots of fun, but you'll see that for yourself when you meet her.'

Laura knew that she could be fun to be with, others had said so, but somehow she was never at ease with Roger's friends and it made her appear stiff and staid. She must make a bigger effort.

'Laura, two letters from America, one for you and one for me,' Ronnie said happily. He was in school uniform and had picked up the letters from the hall table.

Laura took hers and glanced at it. It was in her father's writing.

'I'll read mine later and it is time you were away, Ronnie.'

'I know. I'll take mine with me and read it in the playground.'

Laura waited until Sylvia had finished her breakfast and was occupied with her colouring book before opening her letter.

Sylvia looked up. 'Who is your letter from, Laura?'

'My daddy.'

'Why doesn't he come here and see you?'

'Because he lives far away in America.'

'With your mummy?'

'No, my mummy is dead, Sylvia, but I have a stepmother.'

'Is she wicked like in fairy stories?'

'No, she is a very nice lady. And now, Sylvia, please let me read my letter and you finish colouring in that picture without going over the lines.'

'That's hard.'

'No, it isn't, you just have to be careful.'

Laura started to read her letter and as she did her eyes widened in amazement. She couldn't believe the change in him. This was a very different person to the one she had known. Laura began it again.

My dear Laura,

Life is pretty hectic but even more so for Connie. Fortunately she seems to thrive on it. I have my very strict instructions to have this letter written to you before she returns. Connie is a woman who gets things done and I, according to her, am a ditherer.

The fashion business has really taken off and Connie's creations are becoming more and more popular. Her clientele, her expression I may add, is mainly with the middle-aged woman of means who is anxious to dress attractively and fashionably without earning the label 'mutton dressed as lamb'. Enough of that. Just let me say that we are taking on extra staff and the future looks very promising indeed. As a canny Scot I thought we should be concentrating on reducing our debt to Harry but that is not the way business is done. We pay ourselves a salary which gives us a good living allowance plus a bit over. The bit over is for you.

I am well aware that I left you with an unfair burden and now I am anxious to make your life easier. The bank will be sending you a regular allowance.

To be honest I do not like the thought of my daughter being employed as a housekeeper even though you appear to be happy in such an occupation. You are too young to be a paid housekeeper, that is a job for a middle-aged woman. I accept that your employer must be a very understanding man when he agreed to have Ronnie in his home. Even so, Laura, I want you as soon as it is possible to give in your notice and look for something more suitable.

The money which your mother intended for your education belongs to you and this together with a further sum which Connie and I have agreed on, will allow you to rent and furnish a two-roomed house. Contact our old landlord and since it is unlikely he would rent you a property the house can go in my name. This I shall put in writing when necessary. Are you reeling from shock? I wouldn't blame you if you were.

Probably you read each others letters and if so you'll know that I very much want to put him through university. Him being Ronnie. Excuse the untidy writing. My hand still gets tired when I write for long periods.

One day in the not too distant future we both hope to give you and Ronnie a holiday in New York.

With love,

Dad.

Laura felt light-headed with relief. It was quite a heady feeling, this unexpected independence. She wouldn't rush into anything, it needed a great deal of careful thought. Leaving Braehead would be a wrench but in the circumstances it would be a sensible move. She would, of course, make as sure as she could that Fergus found a suitable replacement and someone who would be kindly and take good care of Sylvia.

'Why aren't you answering me, Laura?' the child said petulantly.

'Sorry, dear, I was dreaming.'

'But you didn't have your eyes shut, you weren't sleeping.'

'Day-dreaming,' Laura smiled, 'but I'm wide awake now and we are going out to the park to play.'

'Do I have to put on a coat?'

'No you don't. Look, the sun is streaming in the window.'

'I'll go and get my new ball,' the child said, rushing out of the room.

Laura had never felt less like a party, at least one with Roger's friends, but she must make the effort. She was seldom short of energy but even for her the late nights and early rising were taking their toll. A few early nights was what she both needed and wanted. Roger would have to understand that but since she had promised to go to the party she couldn't back out now. Roger would be furious.

Roger was looking very smart and summery in his flannels and blazer and an open-necked white shirt. His face registered surprise when she came in.

'Well, well, sweetheart, you look as though you could be going to a Sunday School picnic.'

'You don't approve?'

'Make you the odd one out, I told you a long skirt.'

'No, you didn't.'

'Then I must have just thought you would know.'

Perhaps Roger was right and she should have but it had been so hot all day and indoors would be stifling. Wanting to be cool and comfortable, she had decided on a sleeveless yellow dress with a wide collar and full skirt. Her feet were in white sandals and her long legs were bare. Those hours in the park with Sylvia had given her a nice tan.

'I'm not going up to change,' she said stubbornly.

'No one is asking you to do that and there isn't time in any case.'

'You are in summer clothes,' she said accusingly.

'Leave it, Laura,' Roger said irritably.

It wasn't a good start to the evening and neither of them had much to say on the journey. When they arrived several cars were already parked on open ground behind the house. Together they walked round to the front and Laura got her first good look at the house. She liked it. It was a solid stone-built structure that was quietly pleasing to the eye and not in the least pretentious. Whatever she had been expecting it wasn't this.

'Roger, I love it, I adore these old houses.'

'Not too austere?'

'No, not at all. The position is excellent too. What a wonderful view your friends must have.'

Roger was amused. 'You have a thing about old houses, don't you? You profess to love Braehead.'

'I do.'

Taking her arm they went up to the heavy oak door and rang the bell.

Roger rang it again and again but the shrieks of laughter and the music must have drowned out the sound. Just as they were about to move away to try the back, the door opened and a young girl, slim and pretty and about Laura's own age, grinned at them both before flinging her arms round Roger and kissing him.

'Lovely to see you, Roger, darling, and I'm just so glad you could come.' Laura, for the moment ignored, saw that the girl was wearing an evening skirt and a wide-sleeved blouse in a very fine material. 'Someone thought that must be the bell and I thought I'd better check. Have you been waiting long?' she asked as she invited them both in.

'Hours, Wilma, we were just about giving up. What a reception,' he teased.

'So sorry, darlings, I do apologise, and Roger, sweet, you haven't introduced me to your friend.'

'Give me time. Laura, meet the irrepressible Wilma and our hostess for the evening. Wilma, meet Laura.'

'Hello, Laura, you look delightfully cool, I wish I'd had the sense to dress like that.' She gave a friendly smile. 'We don't stand on ceremony as Roger would tell you. You just do whatever you want, within reason of course,' she giggled. 'Our dragon of a housekeeper has been given the night off and Maggie, who is as deaf as a door post, is the only servant on the premises.'

'You have a lovely home—' Laura began.

'You've only seen it from the outside but how kind of you to say so. Howard, my brother, will love you for it. He's an architect by the way. There were suggestions that we should sell this barn of a house and look for something smaller.' She chattered on. 'I wasn't bothered one way or another but Howard would never move from this house.'

'Speaking of Howard, where is he?'

'Keeping himself as far away as possible.' She turned to Laura. 'Much as I love my brother he is an old fusspot.'

Laura found herself warming to this vivacious girl but rather sorry for her brother who had to keep an eye on her.

They were being led through a spacious hall then along a wide passage to a room where the door stood open. They went in. It was a particularly large room and Laura was of the opinion that it had once been two rooms and the wall knocked down to make it one. An untidy pile of records was on the floor in one corner and a

gramophone ground out a dance tune. Three couples were swaying to
the music in the space where the carpet had been lifted. Sofas and
chairs were against the wall and a few couples were locked in an
embrace.

Wilma took Laura's hand with Roger following and led her over to
meet a group of people standing together. All the women were wearing
evening gowns or long skirts and Laura wished quite desperately that
she had gone up to change.

'Do shut up everybody and pay attention. I want to introduce you
to Laura, Roger's friend.' For Laura's benefit she rattled off
the Christian names of those nearest and Laura smiled brightly.
Apart from one other girl and Wilma, Laura thought they all
looked jaded. They had the look of too many parties and too much
to drink. In that moment she could almost hear her Aunt Peggy using
one of her favourite expressions that you can't burn the candle at
both ends.

A glass was put in her hands, Roger disappeared and Laura felt ill-
at-ease. Her dress was wrong and she felt uncomfortable but it was
much more than that.

She was completely out of place in this gathering.

One heavily made-up blonde girl looked her up and down, then
drawled, 'New to these parts are you?'

'No, I was brought up not so very far from here.'

'Really! Where would home be then?'

'At the moment Braehead,' Laura said quietly.

'You must be a guest of Fergus Cunningham then?'

'No, an employee.'

Roger had returned. 'Laura looks after my little niece, Ena.'

She raised her pencilled eyebrows. 'A nanny, how quaint.'

'Heaven help any infant left in your care, Ena,' Wilma said sharply.

Another voice and this one with eyes only for Roger. 'How
absolutely divine to have you back in our midst, Roger darling.'

Roger smiled and gave a small bow. 'How kind of you to say so,
Ursula.'

Ursula's eyes fixed on Laura. 'You must be careful our Roger has
quite a reputation.'

'I wouldn't know,' Laura smiled and put her arm through Roger's.

Wilma gave a shriek as a young man twirled her into a dance and at the same time a voice yelled, 'Wilma, honey, someone at the door.'

'Then go and let them in,' Wilma's partner shouted as he tightened his hold. 'She's busy.'

Roger felt a tap on his shoulder. 'Is this you finished with India, old boy?'

'Can't say, Jack, haven't made up my mind.'

'Good life they tell me?'

'Some of the time.'

'Did you know,' he said, turning his attention to Laura and giving her a broad wink, 'our Roger, here, was packed off to India because he had been a bad boy?'

'Cut that out.' Roger looked nettled but at that moment Ursula sailed over.

'I don't care if this is ladies' choice or not, I want this dance with you, Roger darling. Come along.' She took his arm.

'Do you mind, Laura?'

'Not at all.' She smiled weakly and as they moved away so did Jack. Laura was alone when the latecomers arrived. She half turned at the sound, then froze.

Wilma managed to disengage herself and hurried over.

'Hello, Davina. Hello, Kenneth, we had all but given you up.' They pecked at each other's cheek.

'Don't blame me,' Kenneth Patterson smiled. 'I was bright and early but Davina took an age to get ready.' Kenneth was tall and thin with swarthy skin and springy black hair. When Davina had asked him to partner her he couldn't believe his luck. Previously the gorgeous Davina had scarcely given him a glance but then it was changed days now that Fergus Cunningham had deserted her.

Davina, bored with life, wondered if she had any chance with the elusive Howard Menzies. Usually when he put in an appearance it was to hasten the departure of the partygoers. Not that she could altogether blame him, one or two did go over the score. Fergus, like Howard, had no time for such parties. She sighed. The truth was she was tired of them herself but she had to keep in circulation.

'Help yourselves to drinks,' Wilma was saying. 'You know everyone – oh, no, sorry,' she corrected herself as she caught sight of Laura and at the same moment Davina did too. She gave a start of shocked surprise. Wilma saw it.

'You know Laura?'

'Hardly,' Davina said at her haughtiest. 'Miss Morrison is the house-keeper at Braehead.' She made sure her voice carried. Her eyes looked Laura up and down, making Laura even more conscious that she was unsuitably dressed.

'Wilma,' Kenneth said quietly, 'I haven't had the pleasure of meeting Miss Morrison.'

'Sorry.' She made the introductions. Wilma was uncomfortable and not quite sure how to handle the awkwardness. 'Laura came with Roger,' she said lamely, 'but heaven knows where he is.'

'That someone taking my name in vain? Davina, you look wonderful as always,' Roger beamed. Davina looked cool and elegant in the pale apple-green long dress with its attractive halter neckline.

'Thank you, Roger.' They kissed and Davina managed to get a smile back on her face though inwardly she was seething. How did that girl, that nobody, manage it? Fergus, now Roger.

The buffet was set in the dining-room and guests could come and go as they wished. There was masses of food and a table of drinks.

Roger was in great demand by the ladies and Laura was never without a partner. As the evening wore on Laura was becoming concerned by the amount Roger was drinking. Didn't he remember that he had to drive home? Perhaps she should remind him. He could hold his drink and only the very bright eyes showed him to be under the influence. Driving was a different story. Drink made him aggressive and reckless and though she knew that it wouldn't be well received she must have a quiet word with him.

Laura hated her partner's clammy hands and longed to be rid of him. When the record came to an end she tried to move away but he held on to her.

'The next one, sweetie pie, I must have the next one and the next—' His speech was slurred.

'Excuse me, I'm going over to Roger.'

'Roger, my pet, is otherwise engaged.'

'I want to talk to him so would you please—' She removed his hand from her waist.

He was otherwise engaged, very much so. Ena was sitting on his knee and planting little feathery kisses on his face and Roger seemed perfectly happy to let her.

'Roger?'

He looked up. 'Laura, honey, enjoying yourself?'

'Yes,' she lied and watched him reach for his glass.

'Darling,' she said, keeping her voice deliberately light, 'do remember you have to drive home and I would hate it if we ended up in the ditch.'

'No danger of that with me driving.' And as though to emphasise the point he drank some more and held up his glass to be filled. 'I know that road blindfolded.'

'Perhaps you do,' she said desperately, 'but I have to work tomorrow.'

'So what? Am I supposed to jump to it whenever you decide it is time to go?'

'Of course not but—'

'But nothing, I wish I hadn't brought you. You're nothing but a wet blanket.'

Laura saw Ena's glittering, spiteful eyes, the triumphant look, and without another word turned on her heel. She had to get out of this room before she made a fool of herself. Angry tears stung the back of her eyes at the way Roger had spoken to her. Certainly it was the drink that had spoken but she didn't let that be an excuse. How was she to get back to Braehead? Seven miles was too far to walk. There was no chance of anyone leaving and she wondered if they just slept it off and left in the morning when they had sobered up. Laura was out of the room and unaware of where she was going. There was a light under one door and as she looked it opened.

'Cloakroom the other way,' said a pleasant voice. 'This is out of bounds.'

'I'm so sorry,' she whispered and he thought he heard tears in her voice.

'You are upset, I can see that. Look, come in, this is my den,' and when she made no move he apologised. 'Sorry, you are a stranger and I haven't introduced myself. I'm Howard Menzies and Wilma is my young sister. Is that party of hers getting out of hand?'

She shook her head. 'I feel all sorts of a fool.'

'Don't we all at times? Perhaps you could begin by telling me to whom I have the pleasure of speaking.'

'I'm Laura Morrison and I came with Roger Cunningham.'

353

'Well, Laura, come in and have a seat. Before that lot got at it I collected sandwiches and I have the necessary to make myself a cup of tea. You'll join me, of course you will?'

'Thank you.'

He had been working at his desk and moved the books to make a space for her cup and saucer. Laura knew he was giving her time to compose herself.

'I did hear that Roger was back in the country and staying with Fergus at Braehead.'

'I'm a friend of Roger's, Mr Menzies, but I'm also an employee of Fergus Cunningham. I look after his small daughter.'

'The name is Howard and now tell me what was distressing you.'

'Getting back to Braehead. Roger is in no state to drive.'

'You would like to leave now?'

'I would but I don't see how.'

'No problem. I'll drive you.'

'But I couldn't ask you to do that—'

'You didn't. I offered,' he smiled, such a nice smile.

'I can't tell you how grateful I would be.'

'Have you a coat or something?'

'A cardigan but I don't mind leaving it.'

'Nonsense, Wilma would have put it in the cloakroom.'

'I'm worried about Roger. He thinks he is sober enough to drive.'

'I'll relieve him of his car keys and he'll find them returned when he *is* sober enough to drive.'

In a remarkably short time she had her cardigan and purse and Howard was dangling Roger's car keys.

'I'm wasted as an architect, I should have been a pickpocket.' Laura laughed her first genuine laugh of the evening,

Howard didn't talk much while he was driving and she thought him a comfortable person to be with. He must be well over ten years older than Wilma. His wasn't a handsome face, it was too long, but there was kindness and good humour. Laura found herself taking stock of her life and feeling an unexpected freedom. What a foolish girl she had been to be taken in by a handsome face and a lot of charm. Roger was weak and she had been just a distraction, someone to amuse him. He had never been serious about her and Fergus, how shabbily she had treated him. What must he think of her? When it was too late she had discovered that it wasn't Roger she loved but Fergus. Quiet, thoughtful Fergus, so different from his brother in every way.

Howard broke into her thoughts. 'Thought you had nodded off there.'

'No. Just thinking.'

'Have you a key to get in?'

'Yes, in my purse.'

She saw his smile. 'At least you won't have to disturb the household to get in.'

Laura shuddered. 'That would have been the last straw.'

He shook his head. 'Fergus is a good lad and if you would forgive me saying so a better man than his brother.'

'I'm inclined to agree.' The car stopped. 'Howard, I can't even begin to thank you.'

'My pleasure and I hope we meet again. I wish Wilma could see beyond that mob she goes around with,' he sighed.

'I like Wilma, to be honest she was the only one I did.'

'Nice if you two became friends, nice for me too. Off you go then and I'll wait here until I know you are safely indoors.'

'Thank you. Goodnight, Howard.'

Laura hurried along the path with the key in her hand. She wished now that it had been the back door key, then she could have gone up to her room without going through the main house. Her fingers were clumsy but eventually she was inside and through the hall. There was enough light to see by as she tiptoed to the stairs. A noise made her look up.

'Sorry if I startled you,' Fergus said. He was in his dressing-gown.

'I–I'm sorry I disturbed you.'

'You didn't.'

'Where is Roger? Putting the car away?'

'No. No, he isn't here.'

'Where is he then?'

'Hillend.'

'How did you get back? No, tell me in the sitting-room, we cannot stand about here.'

Laura wanted to escape to her own room, she had had just as much as she could take but there was no way out. A command was a command. She went ahead and sat down, her legs suddenly weak.

He sat down, but a good distance from her.

'Howard Menzies brought me back.'

'From that I gather Roger was incapable,' he said with a show of distaste.

'Yes.'

'I hope the fool doesn't attempt the journey.'

'He won't. Howard relieved him of his car keys.'

A glimmer of a smile crossed Fergus's face. 'Well done, Howard.' He paused. 'Howard is a decent sort and since his parents' death has been responsible for that empty-headed sister of his.'

'I liked Wilma,' Laura said, looking across at him. 'As Howard said she is just in with the wrong crowd but he thinks his sister is getting rather tired of them.'

'I hope so for Howard's sake.'

'Would you excuse me, I'm really very tired.'

'Hardly surprising considering the hours you keep.'

She flushed.

'Not that it is any concern of mine. It would be if your work suffered.'

'It won't.' Laura felt an overwhelming sadness. Fergus had only spoken to her once before in that cold voice. She got up. 'Goodnight, Mr Cunningham,' she said unsteadily and fled from the room.

In bed sleep wouldn't come but then she hadn't expected it would. Too many thoughts going through her head. Of one thing she was certain, her days at Braehead were numbered. At the first opportunity she would do as her father wished and see the landlord about a small house to rent. Ronnie would be upset but that couldn't be helped. He had been upset about leaving Fairfield Street and got over it. It would be the same leaving Braehead and the future was much more secure. There was money where before there had been none. That settled in her mind, Laura drifted off to sleep and awoke unrefreshed.

Roger appeared at midday and set off in search of Laura. Sylvia had a small friend from nearby and the two were playing happily. Laura had taken the chance to pen a letter to America. At his approach she looked up to find him smiling broadly but behind the smile was some unease.

'What made you disappear like that?'

'I'm surprised you noticed,' Laura said sarcastically.

'Meaning I neglected you?'

'You did.'

'One is supposed to circulate at a party, my dear Laura, and you were never short of a partner. Some people there I hadn't seen for a very long time.'

'So I gathered.'

'Howard ran you back, I believe.'

'Yes, he very kindly offered to do so.'

'Just as well you went with him.'

'I know that.'

'No, I meant the wretched car keys, I couldn't find them anywhere.' Laura hid a smile. 'But you did eventually?'

'Thought it was some joker but no one admitted to it.'

'Is this just you back?'

'Yes, slept it out like some others. Good bunch they are, great for a laugh. Must say they all found you a bit standoffish.'

'I found them insufferable, all but Wilma, and I quite liked her.'

'Never mind, we can forget it and I'll make it up to you. How about the theatre and dinner? Don't know what they are doing but I'll find out.'

'No, thank you, Roger, I won't be going out with you again.'

'Just because of last night?' he said disbelievingly.

'No, not just because of last night.' She looked at him and smiled.

'Thank you for all the good times and those I shall remember but this is the end as far as I am concerned.'

'Maybe it is for the best, Laura. Time I was leaving here but truthfully I'll miss you.'

'Will you go back to India?'

'I have a feeling I just might. Who knows, we may meet again one day, we may even be related through marriage.'

'You are hopeless.'

'I know. Do I get a goodbye kiss to say all is forgiven?'

'Of course,' she said, holding up her face, and it was at that moment that Fergus came in, saw them and went out.

'Poor devil,' Roger grinned. 'Never mind, I'll put the smile back on his face when I tell him I'm leaving Braehead.'

Laura felt miserable and depressed when she left Braehead to see the factor and what accommodation he had to offer. The sky was overcast and a thin drizzle of rain was falling. For the moment summer had deserted Miltonsands but if nothing else it matched her mood. She carried no umbrella, uncaring if she got soaked.

It was a very shabby office she was shown into, much shabbier than she remembered.

'Take a seat, Miss Morrison, and tell me what I can do for you.' What a lovely girl, he thought, but so sad-looking.

'I'm looking for a small house to rent.'

He smiled. 'You are to be married? Well, I can't say I'm surprised and I envy the very fortunate young man.' He did too. Looking at her fresh beauty he thought resentfully of his nagging wife at home. Never pleased, never satisfied with her life, but wanting and wanting. All right for her to tell him to put up the rents but she wasn't at the receiving end of the mutterings and the black looks.

'No, Mr Atkinson, I'm not getting married,' Laura said quietly.

'Difficult, Miss Morrison.' He shook his head and put his fingers together.

'You mean there is nothing meantime?'

'My dear young lady, you are not of an age to be renting property.'

'Oh, I see,' she said quickly. 'I'm sorry, I should have explained. The house will be in my father's name—'

'I seem to recall hearing that Mr Morrison had remarried and was abroad.'

'That's true.'

'Miss Morrison,' I accept that your mother, a lovely lady, paid the rent regular as clockwork.' He gave a little laugh. 'I mean, of course, that she was never behind with payment and much as I would like to oblige—'

She cut him off. 'There would be no problem with money, Mr Atkinson,' Laura said with a slight toss of her head, 'the bank will give you all the references you need.'

'In that case I may be of assistance as a very special favour to you.'

'You do have something on your books?'

'Not immediately, but there is a chance that a two-bedroomed house quite near to your old house in Fairfield Street may shortly become vacant.'

She smiled. 'Will you let me have it, Mr Atkinson? I would be very much obliged to you if you would.'

'May I ask if you would be living on your own?'

'No. My brother will share the house.' She got up, anxious to be gone, and shook his sweaty hand. 'Goodbye, Mr Atkinson.'

'Goodbye, my dear.'

Once outside Laura used her handkerchief to wipe her hand. Henry Atkinson was quite harmless and a little pathetic but even so she was glad to be out of his office.

Henry Atkinson had sighed and gone back to his ledger.

Chapter Twenty-Eight

Laura was nervous and on edge but doing her best not to show it. The day's work was over and Sylvia sound asleep. She knew that Fergus Cunningham was in the sitting-room and she forced herself to go there and not put it off any longer. The sooner it was over the better. Better for whom? Better for Fergus most certainly.

'May I have a word with you, Mr Cunningham, if it is convenient?'

'Quite convenient. Please be seated.' He put aside his book and waited.

She sat down, twisted her hands together and moistened her lips.

'I want to give in my notice.'

'I see.'

'Not right away, of course, I'll wait until you have a suitable replacement.'

'That won't be easy and this is going to be very upsetting for Sylvia.'

Not for him though, she thought. He was too polite to say it but he must be greatly relieved.

'Perhaps for a little while.'

'It is none of my business, I know, but have you and Ronnie some place to go?'

'Our old factor has promised me a house and,' she smiled, 'my father, rather belatedly, is accepting his responsibilities and a regular allowance will be coming.'

'That must be a big relief to you?'

'Yes, I don't know what I would have done otherwise.'

'Stayed on at Braehead, I imagine.'

'You wouldn't want that any more than I would.' Unable to stop them the tears coursed down her cheeks.

Fergus longed to comfort her but forced himself to remain where he was. A murderous anger against his brother took hold of him and he said harshly, 'He isn't worth one tear.'

'Who isn't?'

'Roger.'

'I know that.'

'He's gone.'

'I know that too.'

Fergus was at a loss to understand her. Was she in love with Roger or was it over between them?

'What is Ronnie saying about it all?'

'He doesn't know. I'll tell him this evening.'

'I have a feeling he won't be too happy about it and I must confess I'll miss him, as will Sylvia.'

No word about missing her but what could she expect? 'Ronnie was upset when we had to leave Fairfield Street and he got over it. He'll do the same again. He'll have to.'

'Won't you miss us even a little?' he said gently.

Laura swallowed hard. 'Yes, Mr Cunningham, more than a little. You have been more than kind to both of us and I'm sorry, truly, truly sorry —' She couldn't go on, her eyes were swimming. With a strangled sob she got up and made for the door but he was there before her. His back was to the door and when he opened his arms she went into them as naturally as a bird to its nesting place.

'Darling, I can't bear to see you unhappy. I love you, Laura—'

She moved back in his arms. 'What did you say?' she said wonderingly.

'I love you but then you knew that?'

'I didn't. You never said you loved me.'

'But I asked you to marry me,' he said as he drew her over to the sofa.

'I know, but I thought that was because you wanted – wanted someone to look after Braehead and Sylvia.'

'You couldn't possibly have thought that.'

'I did though. You see, Fergus, I do understand that no one will ever take the place of your first wife.'

'That's what you thought? Why have there been so many misunderstandings between us?' he said almost despairingly.

'I don't know.'

'Before you leave this room we are to promise each other to be completely honest. Can you promise that, Laura?'

'Yes.'

'Then tell me about Roger.'

She took a deep breath. She owed him the truth. 'I thought at first that he was the most handsome and charming man I had ever met and I was more than flattered when he seemed to – to want me.'

'You wouldn't be the first,' he said drily, 'Roger has that effect on a lot of women.'

'Thinking back, I was never in love with him but I did enjoy being with him. He showed me a whole new life but after a very short time I grew very tired of the wining and dining and when he began to want foursomes I found that I didn't care for his friends and they thought I was the original country mouse.'

Fergus laughed, a lovely carefree laugh. 'Some mouse.'

She laughed too. 'I didn't fit in and I told Roger I didn't want to go to that party at Wilma's home but he persuaded me and you know how that ended up?'

'I am indebted to Howard for his part and Roger was left in no doubt as to my opinion of him.'

'Don't blame Roger for everything, Fergus, I was very foolish and I don't deserve your forgiveness.'

'There is nothing to forgive, my dearest, we all make mistakes, I've made plenty in my time.' He paused. 'You have been honest but there is more I need to know. Are you still in love with Roger?'

She turned to look him straight in the face. 'I never was. What I felt for Roger wasn't love, I told you that. I was fascinated for a time and now I feel nothing except perhaps some sadness. He isn't happy and occasionally I got the impression that there had been a personal tragedy in his life.'

He nodded. 'Thank you and now let me be equally frank with you. I loved you from the first moment I saw you and I admired your devotion to your brother. Being a widower with a small child, how could I expect a lovely young girl to love me? There was, however, a chance that she might have enough affection for me to consider marriage in return for security and a home for her brother.' He waited.

'It's true that went through my mind but I knew I couldn't go

363

through with it. I wasn't sure if I loved you then, but I thought it very possible that I would grow to love you. When that happened I couldn't bear the thought of loving you and only getting second best in return.'

'If only you knew.'

'That was why I had to get away: I loved you and I couldn't bear to go about each day knowing that I'd hurt you.'

'About my first wife, you have a right to know about Mavis.'

'You loved her very much, didn't you?' Laura said softly.

'When I married her I did love Mavis but it was an unsuitable match. As you know I am a dry old stick — '

'You are nothing of the kind.'

'Thank you, dear, but Mavis thought I was and I have to confess that I did neglect her. Mavis was a vivacious, fun-loving girl and heaven knows what she saw in me in the first place. At the time of our marriage my father was in poor health and mother persuaded him to give up the practice and retire to their home in Devon. Mother's family home, actually, and being the one and only it was left to her. It was a good move for them both but it meant a tremendous amount of work for me. Apart from the new responsibility there were one or two very difficult and complicated cases outstanding.' He sighed. 'I neglected Mavis and she grew resentful which was natural enough. She liked to entertain and there were times when the meal had to be started because I was to be very late.'

'She should have understood.'

'You would have, my darling, but to get back to my story. Sylvia was born and for a while she delighted in showing off her beautiful baby. Then she grew tired of that and bored with her life. She had engaged a very efficient nursemaid who took charge of Sylvia and about that time Roger came on the scene. He had been down south and had a flat in London which he let out for spells when he wasn't to be using it. I'm rather straying but it is just to put you in the picture. Mavis and Roger had always hit it off and I was happy to see Mavis content. It shows how aloof I was from it all not to see where it was leading.' He sighed and took her hand in his.

'You mean they were—'

'Having an affair. Yes, under my nose and I didn't suspect anything.'

'Did others suspect, do you think?' Laura found herself asking.

'Must have, but perhaps out of consideration for me no one thought to tell me.'

'Would you have believed them?'

'My wife and my brother? Possibly not but then again with the seed of suspicion sown I would have been looking for possible signs. And now we come to the accident and that is a day I shall never forgot.'

'If it upsets you, Fergus, you don't have to tell me.'

'I must and I want to.' He paused. 'The police came to the office to tell me there had been a bad accident and that my wife had been killed and my brother injured. Roger had means of identification on him and, of course, Mavis had enough in her handbag to say who she was. That was when they got in touch with me.'

'How dreadful for you—' Laura gripped his hand tighter.

'Yes, I suppose I was in deep shock myself. Anyway, to get on with the story, Roger had been taken to hospital with cuts and bruises and suffering from shock. Later I was informed that Roger had not been speeding but the car must have gone out of control and careered into a tree. No other vehicle was involved.' He paused and gave a sad smile. 'As you can imagine I was unable to think properly but the fact that they were both in Roger's car didn't trouble me. Why should it? He could have been driving Mavis to see her mother in Montrose. My mother-in-law was in poor health and Mavis did visit her fairly regularly.' Fergus got himself up to pour a drink. 'Would you?' His hand went towards the sherry bottle.

'No, thank you, Fergus.'

He joined her on the sofa and began again.

'It would all have happened so quickly that Mavis would have known nothing of it. And for that I am thankful. The passenger side got the full force of the impact and if Mavis had not been killed she would have been terribly injured. I hadn't been home at all and I was with the police when they forced the boot open. Two suitcases were in the boot, Laura. One his, one hers. Even then, would you believe, I didn't give a great deal of thought to it. There could be a perfectly simple explanation.' Fergus looked into Laura's concerned face. 'As you have probably guessed, Mavis and Roger were going away together. This was confirmed when I got home and found a note from Mavis.'

'Oh, Fergus, it must have been awful for you.'

He nodded. 'She left a note to say that she and Roger were in love and they were going away together. That she couldn't take any more and that our marriage had been a mistake.'

'What about the baby? What about Sylvia?'

'I'm sure that leaving her baby did upset Mavis.'

'But she was going to do it just the same?'

'Yes.' He paused. 'You have to remember, Laura, that Mavis didn't have a lot to do with her child. All that was left to our very efficient nurse maid who adored Mavis and Mavis I understood was very good to her.' He smiled. 'She got a lot of my wife's cast-offs and after two or three months of Mrs Mathewson who was in charge, she gave in her notice. That is all by the way. Mavis knew that Sylvia would be all right, that I wouldn't let my daughter go without a struggle.'

'Fergus, may I say something?'

'Of course.'

'My impression is that Mavis was probably in love with Roger or thought she was, but she didn't trust him. She was leaving the door open to come back.'

'You could be right. Mavis was anything but stupid. She wanted Roger but she didn't altogether trust him. She must, however, have found him—' He stopped.

'Irresistible.'

'Just as you did,' Fergus said gently.

'I can't deny that and I feel so very ashamed.'

'Don't be, but since I've started this long, unhappy story let me finish. Roger might well have denied everything and given a plausible excuse for the two suitcases had it not been for the note. Indeed, I'm sure he would have. As a lawyer I am not proud of what followed but I accept that it saved a lot of heartbreak. Mavis's mother, very naturally, was desperate that her daughter's name wouldn't be dragged through the mud and my parents were equally anxious to protect Roger.'

'You weren't?'

'Of course I was, but I also knew it was wrong and could well make matters worse. As it was it would have been a nine days wonder, then forgotten, whereas even to this day rumours persist.'

'No one could blame you for feeling bitter.'

'Perhaps not. I didn't blame Mavis so much but I did blame Roger

366

and went so far as tell him that he would never be welcome at Braehead. My parents have always had a soft spot for their younger son and it was they who decided Roger should be out of sight for a bit.'

'That was when he went to India?'

'Yes.'

'Probably the best thing that could have happened.'

He nodded. 'We were all together when I destroyed the note, and you, and only you, apart from immediate family, know about it.'

'It will remain a secret.'

'I know that.'

'Perhaps Roger will go back to India. He did say there was a possibility.'

'I hope he does,' Fergus said grimly.

'Can't you forgive him?'

He was thoughtful. 'Perhaps I can find it in my heart to do so now. I must have when I allowed him to stay here. There is one more thing that needs to be said, then the subject will be dropped for ever. In many ways Mavis and Roger were alike. Both liked a good time and if I may be forgiven both were shallow. Maybe if Mavis had been spared they would have been happy together.' He got up and brought Laura to her feet. 'We have some unfinished business, my darling.'

'Have we?'

'Yes, we have. Since you have not yet agreed to marry me I am going to propose again, this being the last time.'

'Then do it properly,' Laura said impishly.

'On my knees?'

'No, that won't be necessary.'

'Darling, Laura, I love you more than I can ever say and if you will agree to marry me you'll make me the happiest man in the world.'

Laura looked back at him, and she was flushed and radiant with happiness.

'I love you too with all my heart.'

'Do I take that as an acceptance?'

'Yes, yes and yes again,' she laughed. Then she was in his arms and their lips met in a kiss that left them both shaken.

'How soon?' he whispered.

'Very soon.'

'This landlord, this house—'

'I'll go along and tell him I no longer wish it.'

'No, you won't. You'll give me his name and address and I'll deal with it.'

'Make it a nice letter, he was really very kind.'

'Very well,' he laughed. 'And as for Ronnie, aren't you glad you didn't say anything to him about leaving Braehead?'

'Very glad.' She paused as they sat down with his arm around her. 'Fergus, Dad wants to put Ronnie through university.'

'I'm delighted to hear it. Much as I would have liked to do that it is better this way. In Ronnie's place I would have preferred it to be my father rather than my future brother-in-law.'

'Fergus, you are the kindest man and I love you dearly. I think myself very, very lucky to be getting —'

'I'm the lucky one to be getting such a lovely wife. My friends are going to love you and you'll like them.'

'Sure to when they are your friends.'

'Davina won't be—' he said gently.

'It doesn't matter, truly it doesn't.' And it was true, Laura thought, Fergus loved her and nothing else mattered. In fact she could feel sorry for Davina and she said so.

'Davina will be all right. She'll find her happiness with someone else.'

'I hope so.' There was something about happiness that made one want everyone else to be happy too.

'I have a feeling that your clever stepmother is going to make a name for herself in the fashion world and be famous the length and breadth of New York.'

'I do hope so, she deserves it. How I wish we could all meet,' Laura said wistfully.

'I'm sure that could be arranged. In a year or two the four of us will spend a holiday in New York. How does that appeal to you?'

Her eyes were shining. 'You really mean it is possible?'

'Would I raise your hopes otherwise? Of course I mean it.'

'Isn't life exciting?' she said.

'It is now,' he smiled.